HEALTH CARE
IN MULTIRACIAL BRITA

Penny Mares / *Alix Henley* / *Carol Baxter*

'*It may be that blacks are in the same boat as poor whites; but we are on different decks.*'

Tony Ottey

'*. . . the availability of good medical care tends to vary inversely with the need of the population served.*'

Julian Hart

'*Washing one's hands of the conflict between the powerful and the powerless means to side with powerful, not to be neutral.*'

Paolo Freire

HEALTH EDUCATION COUNCIL / NATIONAL EXTENSION COLLEGE

ACKNOWLEDGEMENTS

It would be impossible to mention all the people who have given their time to talk to us and help us work through the issues we have covered in this handbook. We would especially like to thank all those people who gave us permission to quote them but who asked to remain anonymous.

We would like to thank the following people who contributed material:
Liz Anionwu, Brent Sickle Cell Centre, who contributed background material for Chapters 9 and 10;
Ann Brownlee, who is co-author of Chapter 14;
Kit Sampson, who contributed background material for Chapter 10;
Antoinette Satow and Hilary Homans who contributed material to Chapter 7;
Professor Peter Sever and Dr Bernadette Modell, who contributed background material for Chapter 9.

We would also like to thank:
Clara Arokiasamy, Mavis Clarke, Jenny Douglas, Jo Larbie and Shaama Saggar-Malik of Training in Health and Race;
Cathy Ballard, West Yorkshire Language Link;
Alistair Cameron, General Practitioner;
Pauline Goodbourne, Barrack House Community Health Education Co-ordinator;
Sue Kilroe, Senior Lecturer in Nursing;
Selina Leung, Cantonese interpreter;
Mark McCarthy, Specialist in Community Medicine;
Sherea Miah, Bengali interpreter;
Maggie Pearson, Centre for Ethnic Minority Health Studies, Bradford;
John Roberts and Staff of Leeds Community Relations Council;
Pammi Sahota, Asian Family Caseworker;
Lan Trinh and other field workers of the Refugee Action Northern Team;
And all the people who attended the Leeds seminar in 1981 to discuss HEC/NEC project materials.
Finally, special thanks to:
Fred Adelmann, Jo Bradley, Phil Coyne, Jean Harmer, Celia Hall, Margaret Levin, Ros Morpeth and Ian Sutherland.

With very grateful thanks to the following for permission to use extracts from their publications: Susan C. Walsh, *Overseas Nurses – Training for a Caring Profession*, reproduced with permission from the author. CRE Employment Report, April 1981, p. 9 reproduced with permission of the Commission for Racial Equality. A. Henley, *Asian Patients in Hospital or at Home*, King's Fund Centre, 1979, reproduced with permission of the King's Fund Centre. Sherham and Quick, *The Rickets Report*, Haringey Community Health Council, 1981, reproduced with permission of Haringey Community Health Council. Berger and Mohr, *A Seventh Man*, Writers and Readers Publishing Cooperative Ltd., 144 Camden High Street, London NW1 0NE, pp. 68–78, 1975 (reprinted 1982), Copyright © John Berger, text; Jean Mohr, pictures; reproduced with permission of the authors. David J. Smith, *Racial Disadvantages in Britain*, Pelican Books, 1977, pp. 75–77, Copyright © PEP 1977, reprinted by permission of Penguin Books Ltd. The Open University, *Racism in the Workplace and Community*, Unit 10, Copyright © The Open University Press, reproduced with permission of The Open University.

ISBN 0 86082 613 9
Published by the Health Education Council and the National Extension College,
18 Brooklands Avenue, Cambridge CB2 2HN
Printed by NEC Print
Design and illustration: Vicky Squires
Typesetting: Cambridge Photosetting Services
Photographs: Phil Coyne

Contents

Foreword

This handbook sets out to explore some of the key issues involved in developing health services to meet the needs of a multiracial population.

Discussion about the delivery of health care to ethnic minority communities has tended, so far, to happen in a disjointed and piecemeal way. This book is a first attempt to bring together a number of issues that have so far been considered separately, but which are really different aspects of the same debate. The difficulties in trying to do this for the first time are enormous. We are aware that, to people already familiar with the issues, some sections of the book may seem to be stating the obvious; we are also aware that there are other important issues we have had to leave out due to lack of space.

It must be emphasised that the handbook is intended only as a starting point, a tentative first step on which we hope other people will be able to build. The issues involved in any discussion of race and health are complex and highly sensitive. It is likely that some readers will disagree with part or all of the analysis presented. There are no simple answers to some of the questions we are discussing here, and professionals and black* and ethnic minority community members may disagree with our analysis for very different reasons. If nothing else we hope this handbook will prompt others to attempt something better. There is an urgent need for more detailed research into the effectiveness of health care delivery to Britain's black population and for practical action on these issues. If future initiatives are to be successful, it is also essential that steps are taken to involve more black health professionals in this field and more members of the community in the consultation process.

Penny Mares
Alix Henley
Carol Baxter

---

* See Notes on Terminology on p. 3

1

About this handbook

Who is it for?

This handbook is designed for health professionals and especially trainers, tutors and students. We expect it will be of most use in the following ways:

- to **students and learners** who are unfamiliar with the subject, as an introduction to the issues involved in providing health care in a multiracial society;
- to **practising professionals**, as a means of clarifying some of the issues they are already familiar with, and as a source of ideas for practical action;
- to **tutors and trainers** who are increasingly concerned to address the issues discussed here in their training programmes, but who are often prevented by a lack of resources: this handbook is intended as a useful reference and guide to other resources and sources of more detailed information.

How is it organised?

This book is divided into four parts:

Part One: Explanations of health inequalities
Part Two: Health needs and expectations
Part Three: The health services
Part Four: Resources

The material in the first three parts is presented as a series of essays, each of which focuses on a particular issue and examines it in detail. Many of the issues are, of course, interlinked, and there is inevitably some overlap in the topics explored in each chapter.

The book is not intended to be read from cover to cover. We have tried to design it so that it can be used in a range of situations. Each chapter begins with a short introduction summarising the contents, and includes material at several different levels.

- discussion of issues and principles;
- factual information;
- illustrations and examples (interview extracts, quotations, case studies, etc.);
- suggestions for practical action;
- questions and propositions for further discussion.

How to work through the material

The handbook can be used in several ways. We hope you will select and adapt it to suit your own needs. For example:

Skimming

By working through the **bold typeface** and picking out the quotes and illustrations that interest you, you should get a good sense of the main issues and ideas covered in the book.

Working through one chapter

Some chapters are likely to be more relevant than others, depending on your particular field of interest. It may be useful to work slowly through one or two of the most relevant chapters, taking time to think about the questions, the suggestions for practical action, and perhaps following up some of the suggested further reading.

For reference

If you want to find all the references to one particular issue or topic, there is a detailed list of contents at the beginning and cross references throughout the text and at the end of each chapter.

For group work

Most chapters include questions and exercises that can be used as a basis for group work. Tutors or study groups may find it useful to use some of the questions and exercises as a starting point for discussion *before* working through the arguments presented in the text.

Conventions and symbols

Finally, here is an explanation of the conventions and symbols used in the text, indicating the kind of material included in the section you are working through.

Bold typeface is used to emphasise the key points in each section.

Material which has come from another source is shown in italics. The source may be people's personal views, or quotations from books, articles, etc.

Some of the longer quotations, examples and case studies are shown in boxes. Material in boxes is referred to in the main text, but is not part of it, and the boxes can be read on their own.

Questions to think about, questions for discussion, and exercises are indicated by this symbol in the margin. Some of the activities are more appropriate for group discussion, while others can be done just as well by students working on their own.

Where there are suggestions for **practical action** this symbol appears in the margin. Often practical action is divided into two sections: 'Policy' and 'Individual practice'. Many health workers feel they are not in a position to influence policy, but we hope that including these issues will at least provoke discussion about how such influence might be achieved!

This symbol indicates a cross-reference to relevant information in another part of the book.

Notes on terminology

The definitions in this section are taken from:
Race, Children and Cities, E361, Open University, 1978, pp. 11–13
Racism in the Workplace and Community, Open University, 1983, Unit 1
Ouseley, Herman *et al.*, *The System*, Runnymede Trust/South London Equal Rights Consultancy, 1982, p. 26

One controversial aspect of writing about race and health issues is the terminology used. There is a great deal of confusion in this area: words such as 'multiracial', 'multicultural' and 'multiethnic' are used in different contexts by different writers as though they had the same or crucially different meanings. Should minority ethnic groups be described in terms of their ethnic origin and cultural, religious and language differences, or is skin colour the most important factor? It is clear that there is no one answer completely acceptable to everyone, and that the most appropriate criterion will vary according to the issues under discussion. There is, however, an extensive body of factual information, based on authoritative research, which shows that skin colour is the most vital factor determining unequal treatment.

It may be helpful therefore if some of the terms used in this handbook are clearly defined at the start.

Race

The definition of this term has never been very clear. Sometimes the word is used for convenience to define *social* groups, such as people from different parts of the world or with some special characteristic (for example skin or hair colour, but not height or eye colour). Sometimes the term is used to define *biological* groups, as if people were varieties of cabbages or cows. But most scientists argue that the biological differences between humans are so superficial and so spread out and intermingled that the term is meaningless.

Racial inequality

So 'race' in itself is of no social importance, since it is a biological fact that has as little influence on essential human nature as differences in height or eye colour. But when 'race' is used as a means of *classifying* people socially it *does* become important. In other words race is important because people *think* it is important, and because it has come to be used as an arbitrary criterion for giving and denying rights, choices and opportunities to groups of people on the basis of their skin colour.

'Black'

There is no word in general use that embraces all members of minority racial groups in this country. The word increasingly used by people of Afro-Caribbean and Asian origin is '*black*'. For the black people who have adopted it, it underlines a unity of experience of discrimination and exploitation among peoples whose skin colour is not white, both in Britain and abroad.

For the purposes of this handbook, therefore, we have used the term 'black', particularly when discussing questions of racial discrimination and inequality.

'Migrant' and 'settler'

We have tried to avoid the term 'immigrant' because the way it has come to be used popularly has moved it a long way from its original definition. It is a term that is now rarely used to denote the *majority* of recent immigrants to Britain, namely white immigrants from the EEC and the white Commonwealth. Instead popular usage of the word is generally restricted to black immigrants, and extended to include British-born people who are black or of mixed race. Thus the word has come to have a racial connotation.

This popular usage tends to divert attention away from the fact that it is also British-born black people, the children and grandchildren of settlers, who are being treated differently from other British citizens in some respects. Defining British-born black citizens as 'immigrants' negates the necessity for action by suggesting that the problems they face will go away once the 'immigrants' have become established. Certainly members of the black community in Britain see the term 'immigrant' as a kind of diversionary label, and as a discriminatory one.

In this handbook we have therefore preferred to use the terms 'migrant' and 'settler' when discussing issues related to the process and effects of migration.

'New Commonwealth'

'New Commonwealth' and 'Old Commonwealth' are official terms used to distinguish between Commonwealth countries whose populations are predominantly black (for example India and the West Indies), and countries whose populations are predominantly white (Australia, Canada, New Zealand). In official terminology, the majority of black settlers in Britain are described as 'New Commonwealth immigrants'.

'Ethnic group'

An ethnic group is a group of people who have certain cultural characteristics such as language or religion in common, which provide the group with a distinct identity, as seen both by themselves and by others. The word 'ethnic' is often used inaccurately to describe black or ethnic minority groups, as in phrases such as 'the ethnics' or 'ethnic families'. Such terms are fairly meaningless as, of course, white people also belong to an ethnic group.

Prejudice

Prejudice is literally 'pre-judging'. A prejudiced person is someone who holds views about an individual, or group of people, which are not based on knowledge. People are often unwilling to change these views even when presented with clear evidence that they are factually wrong.

Discrimination

Discrimination occurs when a person is treated differently from others, in an unfair way, simply because of his or her membership of a particular group. Discrimination does not only occur on the basis of race – people may be discriminated against because of their class, sex, age, physical disability, etc.

Racism

In the past few years the term 'racism' has come to be used in Britain in the way it has been widely used in the US for some time. In other words, 'racism' refers to beliefs based on racial prejudice, and to acts of racial discrimination, whether deliberate or unintentional. This is how we have used it in this handbook. 'Racialism' is often used synonymously with 'racism', and may be preferred by some people. But to avoid confusion we have used only one term throughout.

Disadvantage and inequality

A larger proportion of black people than white people suffer from social and economic disadvantages, such as poor housing, badly paid jobs, unemployment, and restricted educational opportunities.

Black people may experience additional disadvantages because of attempts by the majority society to suppress or dismiss the culture of minority communities. Uninformed social policy which ignores minority cultures can lead to discrimination and disadvantage in the form of inappropriate or wrong decisions in policy and practice.

Many people prefer to talk about 'inequality' rather than 'disadvantage' because the term disadvantage has sometimes been wrongly used to imply that people who suffer the effects of social inequality are themselves to blame for their own situation because they are in some way inadequate or inferior. It is more acccurate to say that social and economic disadvantages are the result of *unequal opportunities* and *unequal treatment*, not individual characteristics or behaviour, and that such inequalities are *structural*, built into and perpetuated by the structure and organisation of British society.

'Multiracial' and 'multicultural'

These terms are not, of course, mutually exclusive, but it is useful in this context to define the *multiracial* viewpoint as one which acknowledges the fact that 'race' is one of the most significant factors contributing to unfair treatment and social inequalities in British society. The *multicultural* viewpoint, on the other hand, tends to attribute such inequalities to the cultural differences that exist between different communities in Britain, and sees the solution in promoting greater understanding between cultures. The multicultural viewpoint has been criticised by many people because it avoids the issue of race, and does not provide an adequate explanation of how racial discrimination arises or how it can be eradicated.

The difference in emphasis has important implications for the training of health professionals. For example, a *multicultural* approach to training would see as its purpose the focusing of attention on all groups represented in society – Irish, Greek, Cypriot, Welsh, West Indian, Jewish, Scottish, Bengali, etc. – for the purpose of understanding their cultures. A *multiracial* approach to training, on the other hand, would focus in particular on the specific issues that arise from the area of black/white race relations, and racial inequality. Such a programme would of course look at ethnic minority cultures, but from the point of view of understanding how *white perceptions* of minority cultures may contribute to inequality and disadvantage among those minorities. We have therefore called this handbook *Health Care in Multiracial Britain*, because it is not just a book about ethnic minority cultures, but about the broader issues of racial inequality.

'Health workers' and 'patients'

In the text the health worker is referred to as 'she' and the patient or client as 'he'. This is to avoid confusion and awkward repetition of 'he/she' and 'himself/herself'. It is not, of course, meant to imply that all health workers are female nor that all patients are male.

Users of the health service are sometimes referred to as patients and sometimes as clients, to avoid clumsy repetition of the term 'client/patient'.

Health worker is used to indicate anyone who may be involved directly or indirectly in health care or health education.

1: Why is a multiracial approach necessary?

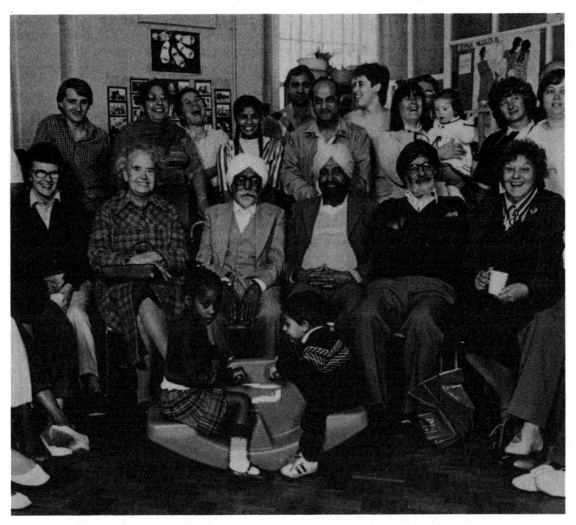

Introduction

The National Health Service (NHS) was set up in 1948 to cater for the needs of people from a fairly homogeneous British culture and background. Today health service provision and staff training programmes are still geared to the way of life, the family patterns, the dietary norms, the religious beliefs and the attitudes, priorities and expectations of the majority population. But over the last thirty years the composition of the population in many areas of Britain has changed significantly, and so too have health needs. This chapter looks at the implications of these changes for the health services.

1.1 Britain's black* population

Sizeable but isolated minority communities have been established in different parts of Britain for generations, and in some cases for centuries. The Liverpool-born black community, the Chinese in Cardiff and the Cypriots in Haringey are just three examples among many long-settled communities. But it was a booming economy in the 1950s and 60s which saw the brief but most intense period of migration, when **because of acute labour shortages in this country workers from the 'New Commonwealth'* countries were actively encouraged by British employers to come and work here.** It was this period of intense migration which brought about the settlement and growth of ethnic minority communities in most major towns and cities throughout the country. This process continued on a smaller scale with the refugee migration to Britain of Ugandan Asians, Chileans and Vietnamese in the 1970s and early 80s. **In 1983, almost half the black* people in the population (about 43 per cent) were born in Britain.**[1]

Most of the ethnic minority population is concentrated in the inner city areas. This means that, today, the 'ethnic minorities' in some areas make up 30, 50 or 70 per cent of the total population served by a particular hospital, clinic or health centre. Health workers in inner city areas may have a caseload of which three-quarters are patients of Chinese, Asian or Afro-Caribbean origin. What are the implications for health care of this population change, and how far are the health services meeting the new health needs that these changes bring?

1.2 The organisation of the health services

It has been argued that, like many institutions, the NHS has tended to develop an inflexible life and structure of its own.[2] There is a growing feeling among health professionals and community organisations that the policies and structure of the NHS have helped to prevent an adequate response to the health needs of many sections of the population, and in particular those of ethnic minorities. Health service provision and training do not yet fully take the various ethnic minority groups in British society into account. As a result they often fail to meet their needs. For example:

- Individuals from ethnic minority communites may have **life styles, family patterns, religious beliefs, dietary norms, expectations and priorities that differ significantly from those of the majority population.** Health care which is appropriate for an English Christian patient may be inappropriate and unacceptable to a Bengali Muslim; this means that valuable time and resources can be wasted on ineffective care.

Lack of knowledge and awareness among health staff in certain crucial areas can increase the danger of underdiagnosis and misdiagnosis in ethnic minority patients. For example:

- Health workers' awareness of illnesses such as sickle cell disease and thalassaemia, which particularly affect minority ethnic groups, may be less good than their knowledge of illnesses that affect the majority population.

* See Notes on Terminology, p. 3

- Psychiatric health staff may be unfamiliar with important cultural factors relating to mental health and illness.
- Medical and nursing staff may be less able to recognise symptoms of, for example, inflammation, jaundice and cyanosis in patients with black skin.
- Health workers may be unable to communicate with patients, making effective care impossible.

There is a growing concern among health professionals at all levels that the delivery of health care in multiracial areas is not as effective as it should be.

1.3 Poverty and racial inequality

Standards of health are not, of course, determined by medical services alone. **The effects of medical services on the state of health of a population are secondary to social and economic factors, such as income, housing, working conditions, education, unemployment, nutrition, and the quality of the environment and local amenities.** With economic recession, social inequalities have deepened, particularly among communities living in the inner city areas.

Poor housing, high unemployment and poverty are problems of class disadvantage that black people share with white people living in the same area. But ethnic minority communities face additional disadvantages that are not shared by the white population.

Census statistics, and a growing body of research evidence, show that far more black people are likely to live in poor housing, and to work in low-paid jobs or have no job at all, and that their children are more likely to attend poorly equipped under-staffed schools.[3]

Various explanations have been suggested for these cumulative disadvantages: language and communication difficulties, migration and 'newness' or 'foreign-ness', cultural differences, and racism (racial discrimination and prejudice).* But, although language, culture and migration may explain some of the disadvantages that affect the older generation (who migrated to Britain), they do not explain the continuing and cumulative disadvantages suffered by long-settled minority communities, and by black people who were born in this country (almost half the total black population). A growing number of research studies confirm that the position of black people in British society is largely due to the racial discrimination they experience in many areas of life.[4]

1.4 Poverty and access to health care

The Black Report on inequalities in health stated that it was not possible to point to any single and simple explanation of inequalities in health, but at the same time stressed the importance of **differences in the material conditions of life:**

In our view much of the evidence on social inequalities in health can be adequately understood in terms of specific features of the socio-economic environment: features (such as work accidents, overcrowding, cigarette smoking) which are strongly class-related in Britain and also have clear causal significance.[5]

The report, first published in 1980, confirmed the view put forward more than ten years ago by Julian Tudor Hart, that **inequalities in access to health care are also clearly class-related**, producing the phenomenon now known as the 'inverse care law':

In areas with most sickness and death, general practitioners have more work, larger lists, less hospital support and inherit more clinically ineffective traditions of consultation, than in the healthiest areas; and hospital doctors shoulder heavier case loads with less staff and equipment, more obsolete buildings and suffer recurrent crises in the availability of beds and replacement staff. These trends can be summed up as the inverse care law: that the availability of good medical care tends to vary inversely with the need of the population served. [our emphasis][6]

* See Notes on Terminology, p. 3

Because a high proportion of black people are affected by multiple social and economic disadvantage, ethnic minority communities are likely to be particularly affected by the inverse care law.

Difficulties of access to health care, shared with the white population in inner city areas, may be compounded for black people by direct or indirect discrimination, and by a lack of knowledge and awareness among health service staff of their way of life and economic circumstances. In addition, some sections of the black population face language and communication difficulties with health staff, and are unfamiliar with, and unable to get adequate information about, how the health service works. All these factors are clearly interlinked, but the net results, confirmed by various studies, is that black people tend to benefit less from health service provision than the population as a whole.[7]

1.5 Current health care policy

The National Health Service was set up to provide a comprehensive range of health services to the whole population on the basis of individual need, a service free at the point of delivery and equal for all. **Providing the same service in the face of differing need is not providing an equitable service.** It is *not* discriminatory to recognise that an ethnic minority patient may have different needs and face different problems from a white patient. It *is* discriminatory to treat black patients as though they were just like white patients in every respect but their skin colour. **There are significant variations among ethnic groups which are of crucial practical importance in the delivery of health care and which should not be ignored.** For example:

- Different ethnic groups are susceptible to different **illnesses**: the incidence of cystic fibrosis is high in the white population compared with other ethnic groups; thalassaemia particularly affects people of Mediterranean and Asian origin; people of Afro-Caribbean origin are more susceptible to hypertension than any other ethnic group;[8] babies with dark skin may be more susceptible to jaundice than babies with pale skin.[9] Health workers may fail to pick up important signs and symptoms if they are not familiar with these differences.

- The main sources of nutrients in the **diet** vary from one ethnic group to another. It is pointless to urge a pregnant Chinese or Vietnamese woman to drink plenty of milk if she has lactose-intolerance.[10]

- Research suggests there are important ethnic differences in **reactions to certain drugs**, producing more serious side effects in some ethnic groups than in others.[11]

- Aspects of existing care may be **unacceptable** for religious or cultural reasons, **making compliance difficult** or impossible for some patients. If Muslim women are reluctant to attend the local ante-natal clinic because they fear internal examination by a male doctor, it will be more cost-effective in the long term to arrange appointments on a day when patients can be examined by a woman doctor.

- Previous **experience of racial prejudice and discrimination** is likely to influence, consciously or unconsciously, ethnic minority patients' expectations of the health services and health staff. Some patients may withhold relevant information, for example, about family circumstances, or about other treatment being applied, because they think health staff will not understand, will not be sympathetic, or will make fun of them. Occasionally, ethnic minority patients may appear awkward or uncooperative to health staff because they are under stress and have difficulty in communicating, or because they expect, from past experience, to be treated with antagonism by many white people. This dimension has to be recognised in building up a caring relationship with black patients.

A health service which maintains a 'colour-blind' or 'culture-blind' approach in the face of these facts is likely to be less effective, and may even prove negligent of the health care needs of ethnic minority patients.

CASE STUDY

Mr and Mrs A

Mr and Mrs A were a Bangladeshi couple living in London. They had two small children and all four of them lived in one cramped room in a Victorian tenement building. They shared washing and lavatory facilities with two other families on the same floor. They did not know any other Bangladeshi families in the area. Mr A worked from early morning till late at night in an Indian restaurant. He spoke little English; Mrs A spoke none. She was very shy and rather nervous and hardly ever went out of their room. She had periods of depression.

Mrs A gave birth to her third child, a boy, in a London teaching hospital. The child was small and weak, and it was thought that he was probably developmentally delayed and possibly deaf. Mrs A became severely depressed after the child's birth and seemed to hospital staff to find it difficult to cope. It was decided that she should go home to her other children and leave the baby in hospital for the time being.

The baby was very lovable and the nurses were extremely fond of him. They gave him as much attention as they could, though they were pressed for time. Mr A came to visit him as often as he was able in his hours off from the restaurant, but Mrs A did not visit him at all. Mr A was keen to take the baby home once he was strong enough, but the hospital staff felt that this was not a good idea; the baby needed all the stimulation he could get and in their view Mrs A was clearly not interested in her child since she never visited him.

The staff at the hospital were not sure that Mr A knew that his son was in any way handicapped. Whenever they tried to explain he said the baby was all right, he was a lovely baby and so on. Whenever Mr A mentioned taking the baby home the hospital staff dissuaded him, saying that the child needed good care and lots of stimulation and play, and was better off in hospital.

By the time her little boy was nine months old Mrs A had only been to see him twice. Each time she had seemed very distressed. The hospital staff loved the baby, and felt very protective towards him. Mr A then came in and said he wanted to take the baby home. He was going to take him back to Bangladesh and leave him there. The hospital staff were appalled at this apparent total rejection and at the prospects the child would face back in Bangladesh with little or no medical care and no chance of speech therapy or other remedial work. They began to apply for a court order to take the child into care.

At this stage the hospital brought in an interpreter to discuss the position with Mr A and to make sure that he understood about the court order and what it would mean. The interpreter explained that because the boy was slightly mentally retarded and deaf he would need the best medical and social care and that this was what the authorities wanted to provide. If the parents didn't feel they could look after him it was in the boy's own interests that he should be taken into care in England.

During the discussion that followed the father said that he knew very well that his son was both mentally retarded and deaf.

He felt that such a child needed as much love and attention as possible. He didn't see, although the nurses were extremely kind and very hardworking, how they could give his son enough attention or stimulus. In fact he usually found him sitting silent and alone in the corner of his cot when he came to visit him and he felt that this was not right.

He knew that life was very difficult for his wife alone with the other two children for most of every day in a small room and he realised that she was probably too depressed and unhappy to cope properly with their third child. The one thing their baby really needed more than anything was love and lots of companionship and playmates. He felt that the baby could get those better than anywhere else at home with his family in Bangladesh. His family were farmers, they lived in a small *village, there were lots of other children and adults to look after him and love him. It was warm and sunny, there was lots of space, and children like his son were always loved and protected and looked after. He didn't understand why the hospital wanted to keep his son. He felt that they were trying to be kind but that in fact what they were doing was harming him.*

The hospital staff decided not to make any immediate decisions but discuss the whole matter further with Social Services and with Mr A.

1.6 Developing a multiracial approach

This handbook argues the need for health workers to challenge some of the conventional wisdom on which the NHS's current approach to ethnic minority patients is based. Much of this conventional wisdom is based on three false propositions: ethnic minority communities are immigrants who don't really belong here; they should conform to British ways if they want to live here; the health services are doing enough already for minority patients, and it is discriminatory to make 'special' or 'extra' provision for one particular patient group.

The aim of this handbook is to put the case for a multiracial approach in the delivery of health care, based on realistic principles which reflect the true position of Britain's ethnic minority population:

- **Almost half the black people in the population were born in this country.** Denying that black people belong here is to deny them their legal rights. Members of ethnic minorities are taxpayers like everyone else and entitled to a fair share of the services they pay for.

- **Arguing that ethnic minority patients should conform to British ways is a failure to understand the *nature* of cultural variation and the degree of adaptation to another culture that anyone, white or black, can reasonably make.** People who have migrated to Britain have already made major adaptations in their lifestyle and outlook. It is neither desirable nor possible for people to cast aside one set of cultural influences and adopt another just because they change their country of residence.

- **It is a mistake to suggest that 'British ways' are necessarily more desirable than those of ethnic minority communities**; many aspects of British culture (high-fat, low-fibre diets; smoking; inner-city deprivation; the breakdown of family support) are clearly harmful to health. An individual's level of confidence and self-esteem affects his or her ability to communicate effectively with health staff and to seek appropriate health care. If we accept this, it is essential to recognise and respect those aspects of his or her cultural identity on which that confidence is based.

- **Finally, making the service more appropriate to the needs of ethnic minority patients is not discriminatory, nor giving 'extra privilege'.** It is part of the wider argument, clearly set out in the Black Report, for a more effective allocation of resources on the basis of need. The health care needs of multiply-disadvantaged families, for whom racial inequality is a major contributing factor, are likely to be far greater than those of middle-class families with higher incomes.

There are immediate and practical ways of making services and individual practice more effective. **Many of the measures discussed in this handbook do not call for extra money. Rather they need the political will to re-examine existing practices and procedures and to alter those which are not as effective or as appropriate as they could be.** For example, scheduling appointments to take account of shift work, so that relatives can accompany a non-English-speaking patient; arranging for women to see a female doctor whenever possible if specifically requested; allowing post-natal patients to shower if it is possible and they express a strong preference, rather than insisting that they bath; organising the records of patients with different naming systems more efficiently to reduce confusion and delay; increasing the emphasis in professional training on knowledge and awareness of ethnic minority health needs and lifestyles; actively encouraging the recruitment and promotion of ethnic minority staff at all grades in all disciplines (not just at junior grades and in unpopular disciplines).

Certain measures, such as the provision of trained interpreters, would of course require additional allocation of resources. But it is clear from the evidence available in other countries that in the long term such measures are highly cost-effective, in that they reduce the amount of time and money wasted on unnecessary or ineffective care.

If resources are not matched to need, inequalities can only deepen. The ethnic minority population is an extreme case; **changes which improve the delivery of care to a particularly disadvantaged group will improve the quality of the service to the population as a whole.** The consequences of ignoring such needs are clear:

Notes

1. This estimate is based on data from the 1981 Census and from the OPCS Labourforce Survey, HMSO, 1981. Exact figures are not available but this percentage is likely to be an *underestimate* of the total number of British-born black people.
2. Townsend, Peter, 'Inequality and the Health Service', *Lancet*, 15 June 1974, p. 1179.
3. See for example:
   Rampton, A. (ed.), *West Indian Children in our Schools: Interim report of the Committee of Inquiry into the education of children from ethnic minority communities*, HMSO, 1981.
   Runnymede Trust and the Radical Statistics Race Group, *Britain's Black Population*, Heinemann, 1980.
   Smith, David J., *Racial Disadvantage in Britain: The PEP Report*, Penguin, 1977.
   Smith, David J., *Unemployment and Racial Minorities*, Policy Studies Institute, No. 594, February 1981.
4. See, for example, the publications listed above and also:
   Ouseley, Herman *et al.*, *The System*, Runnymede Trust and South London Equal Rights Consultancy, 1982.
   Scarman, Leslie George, *The Brixton Disorders: Report of an Inquiry*, HMSO, 1981, also available as *The Scarman Report*, Penguin, 1982.
   Simpson, Alan, *Stacking the Decks: A Study of Race, Inequality and Council Housing in Nottingham*, Nottingham and District Community Relations Council, 1981.
   Young, Ken and Connelly, Naomi, *Policy and Practice in the Multi-Racial City*, Policy Studies Institute, 1981.
5. Townsend, Peter and Davidson, Nick, (eds), *Inequalities in Health: The Black Report*, Penguin, 1982, p. 207.
6. Hart, Julian Tudor, 'The Inverse Care Law', *The Lancet*, 27 February 1971, p. 412.
7. For examples see:
   Ethnic Minorities and the Health Service, Wandsworth and East Merton Health District, September 1979.
   Second Report from the Social Services Committee *Perinatal and Neonatal Mortality*, HMSO, 1980. Chapter 17: Ethnic Minorities.
   Chinese Workers' Use of the NHS GP Services in the W.1 Postal Area, Kensington, Chelsea and Westminster North East District Community Health Council, 1977.
   Radio London/Merton, Sutton and Wandsworth Area Health Education Service Project, 'Health Problems of London's Asians and Afro-Caribbeans', *Health Visitor*, April 1981, pp. 144–147.
   North Kensington Moroccan Project Report, Kensington, Chelsea and Westminster Area Health Authority Health Education Department, 1979.
8. Langford, Herbert G., 'Is Blood Pressure Different in Black People?' in 'Ethnic Differences in Common Diseases', *Postgraduate Medical Journal*, Vol. 57, No. 674, December 1981.
9. Roach, Lora B., 'Colour Changes in Dark Skin', in Henderson, G., and Primeaux, M., *Transcultural Health Care*, Addison-Wesley, 1981, pp. 287–292.
   Tarnow-Mordi, W. O. and Pickering, D., 'Missed Jaundice in Black Infants: a Hazard', *British Medical Journal*, Vol. 286, 5 February 1983, pp. 463–4.
10. Mares, Penny, *The Vietnamese in Britain: A Handbook for Health Workers*, National Extension College, 1982, pp. 117–118.
11. Overfield, Teresa, 'Biological Variations: Concepts from Physical Anthropology', in Henderson, G., and Primeaux, M., *Transcultural Health Care*, Addison-Wesley, 1981, pp. 279–286.
12. Hart, Julian Tudor, 'The Inverse Care Law', *The Lancet*, 27 February 1971, p. 409.

Further reading

See reading list in Chapter 16:
16.1 **Why is a multiracial approach necessary?**
See also relevant publications in
16.2 **Racial inequality and health**

Part 1: Explanations of health inequalities

Part 1: Explanations of health inequalities

Social and economic disadvantages have a major impact on health and health care, but little has been written about the effects of racial inequality on the health of Britain's black population. In fact, it is an issue which is by and large avoided. We have seen that almost half the black people in the population today are British-born. **At best, migration, language and culture may provide partial explanations for some but not all inequalities in health among the black population; at worst, they may be marginal or irrelevant.**

Part 1 looks at each of these issues in turn.

Chapter 2: the nature of **racial inequality** and its possible effects on health.

The three following chapters outline and discuss other factors that may be linked with racial inequality, and where appropriate, make **suggestions for practical action:**

Chapter 3: the effects of **migration** on the generation who came to settle in Britain.

Chapter 4: the implications of **cultural variation**, and lack of cultural awareness in the majority population; ways in which health workers can improve their understanding of ethnic minority cultures and practical implications for health care.

Chapter 5: the effects of **language and communication** difficulties; ways in which English-speaking health workers can improve their communication skills.

2 Racial inequality and health

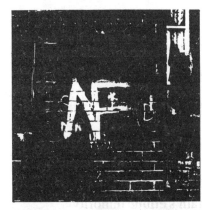
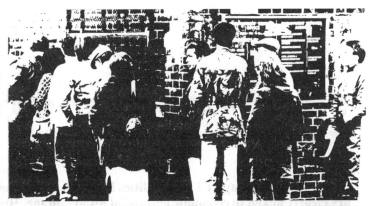
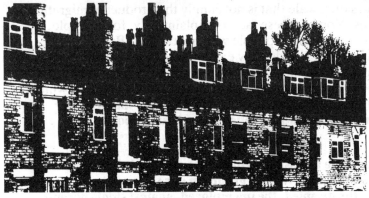
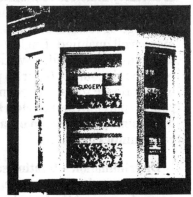

2.1 Discrimination, disadvantage and inequalities in health

2.2 Kinds of racial discrimination

2.3 A misleading 'explanation' of racial inequality

2.4 Discrimination, health needs and health care

2.5 Health service policies

2.6 Professional practice

2.7 Health workers' attitudes and expectations

2.8 Practical action

Introduction

This chapter discusses the relationship between racial discrimination, disadvantage and inequalities in health. It looks at definitions and examples of discrimination and examines some existing health care policies and practices that can work to the disadvantage of ethnic minority patients.

2.1 Discrimination, disadvantage and inequalities in health

As we saw in Chapter 1, **inequalities in health and in the availability of health care are clearly linked to economic and social disadvantage.** Britain's ethnic minority communities face disadvantages on a scale that is not simply the product of migration, language or cultural differences. None of these factors explains why, for example, many well qualified, English-speaking black people who migrated to Britain have ended up in low-paid, low-status jobs. Nor do they explain why black people born and bred in this country (over 46 per cent of the total ethnic minority population) continue to experience social and economic disadvantage on a scale far wider than their white counterparts. **Research clearly shows that racial discrimination is a major factor determining the position of, and opportunities available to, ethnic minority communities in Britain.**[1]

Discrimination – treating someone as less than equal because they belong to a particular social group – operates against various groups in our society. It operates, for example, against the homeless, the disabled, the unemployed, against single parents and women, but black people probably face more extensive discrimination than any other group in British society.

A government white paper in 1975 described how the interaction between material conditions and racial discrimination can create a cycle of disadvantage in which black people become trapped.

The possibility has to be faced that there is at work in this country, as elsewhere in the world, the familiar cycle of cumulative disadvantage by which relatively low-paid or low-status jobs for the first generation of immigrants go hand in hand with poor over-crowded living conditions and a depressed environment. If, for example, job opportunities, educational facilities, housing and environmental conditions are all poor, the next generation will grow up less well equipped to deal with the difficulties facing them. The wheel then comes full circle, as the second generation find themselves trapped in poor jobs and poor housing. If, at each stage of this process an element of racial discrimination enters in, then an entire group of people are launched on a vicious downward spiral of deprivation. They may share each of the disadvantages with some other deprived group in society; but few other groups in society display all their accumulated disadvantages. [our emphasis][2]

Discrimination, coupled with economic and social disadvantage, affects health in two ways:

• it influences the **state of health** of the black population;

• it influences the **quality and availability of health care** to ethnic minority patients.

We shall return to these issues later in this chapter, but at this point it may be helpful to define exactly what is meant by racial discrimination.

2.2 *Kinds of racial discrimination*

Discrimination can occur in various ways: it can be direct or indirect, it may be on an institutional or a personal level. The 1976 Race Relations Act draws an important distinction between 'direct' and 'indirect' discrimination.

Direct discrimination occurs when a person receives less favourable treatment 'on racial grounds' than someone else. Racial grounds refer to colour, race, nationality, citizenship or ethnic or national origins.

Indirect discrimination arises when policies or practices are discriminatory in effect, even though they are not intended to be so. There may be no deliberate desire to discriminate on the part of an individual or institution, but a policy or action can effectively work to the disadvantage of a particular ethnic group without being specifically directed at them. The fact that certain policies and practices *unintentionally* or *unconsciously* result in a particular group receiving unfavourable treatment does not diminish their discriminatory effect. **The possibility of indirect discrimination must be recognised in any discussion about the delivery of health care to ethnic minority patients.**

In many ways indirect discrimination is more difficult to perceive and to prevent. Because nobody has explicitly stated that black people will be treated worse than whites, it cannot be pinpointed as anybody's 'fault' or conscious decision. It is usually built in to the system and is part and parcel of the everyday running of things. Any attempt to do something about it may meet with hostility at two levels: firstly, because it is trying to change the way things have always been done, which most people dislike; and secondly, because it is 'bringing race in' where people feel it wasn't an issue before, which makes most white people very uncomfortable. And since indirect discrimination is often difficult to recognise, many people feel that things were fine as they were, and that bringing in race as an issue is crude, distasteful and 'political'.

There is, however, a growing body of well documented research from authoritative sources which shows that certain policies and practices in many organisations unintentionally work to the disadvantage of ethnic minority communities, and result in black people receiving less favourable treatment in many areas of life.[1]

Because indirect discrimination is inherent in the existing structure of things, any organisation which has not subjected its policies and procedures to review is more likely to be discriminating than not. The intention may not be discriminatory, but the effect is.

In the following pages we have set out a few examples of discrimination which have been identified by various investigations into housing, employment and education. Often direct and indirect discrimination are interlinked. Alongside the factual evidence we have included comments from black people talking about their own experiences and views of discrimination.

Employment

Asians and West Indians with academic qualifications lag far behind whites with equivalent qualifications in getting white collar, professional or management jobs; but Asians and West Indians with formal or informal qualifications for skilled manual jobs are in a position of near equality with similarly qualified whites, except that substantially more of the whites have progressed to white-collar or management positions. Thus, Asians and West Indians face their greatest difficulties in trying to penetrate to the better non-manual jobs.

It might be suggested that inadequate English is the explanation of the low job levels of Asian men, even after their qualification level has been taken into account, but this is not so. We have seen that there is a very strong relationship between fluency in English and academic qualifications – so strong, in fact, that nearly all Asian men with degree-equivalent qualifications speak English fluently. Nevertheless, a substantial proportion of them are doing manual jobs. [3]

Job levels of men with degree-standard qualifications in 1974 – white and minority men compared.[3]

Job level:	White men %	Minority men %
Professional/management	79	31
White-collar	22	48
Skilled manual	—	14
Semi-skilled manual	—	4
Unskilled	—	3

The table above compares the 1974 job levels of white and black men *with degree standard qualifications*. (This comparison is based on a system of equivalence which if anything undervalued non-British qualifications. For example, Asian first degrees were counted as equivalent to 'A' level.) The table shows that a substantial proportion of black people with the same qualifications and abilities as white people were doing manual jobs at the time of study. If this pattern was due to disadvantages caused by migration, it would be reasonable to expect changes in the job levels of black workers over time.

A government survey published in 1981 looked at changes in the job levels of white and black workers (according to country of origin) between 1966 and 1977.[4]

Percentage of black and white workers in various types of jobs[4]

	Great Britain	India	Pakistan and Bangladesh	West Indies		Great Britain	India	Pakistan and Bangladesh	West Indies
Non-manual	32.9%	37.1%	11.6%	8.0%		40.7%	34.3%	14.4%	11.6%
Skilled manual	40.3%	28.3%	22.2%	42.2%		39.9%	34.7%	31.2%	50.1%
Semi-skilled	18.3%	22.9%	34.9%	27.6%		13.7%	20.8%	38.0%	25.5%
Unskilled	8.5%	11.7%	31.3%	22.2%		5.7%	10.1%	16.4%	12.9%

1966   1977

Key: Non-manual   Skilled manual   Semi-skilled   Unskilled

The figures above show that there was little change over 11 years; in 1977 black people were still concentrated in manual jobs. Today many black people have been working in Britain for 10, 20 or 30 years, but have not moved into similar jobs to whites.

Other evidence gathered in the surveys quoted above makes it clear that **black workers are widely affected by discrimination in employment.** Further evidence shows that discrimination is not confined to black workers who settled in Britain; it also works against their children when they leave school.

Half a Chance: Youth unemployment in Nottingham[5]

In 1977–9, a survey was carried out in Nottingham to test levels of discrimination against young black people who have spent most, if not all, of their life in England. Jobs in the service sector (white collar) make up 50 per cent of all jobs in Nottingham, and 58 per cent of female jobs. While most of the parent generation work in manufacturing industries, surveys showed that many more black school-leavers hoped for service sector jobs. The survey was limited to service sector jobs. 161 advertised vacancies were selected from the local paper, representing both traditionally 'male' and 'female' jobs, and 'school-leaver' and 'adult' jobs.

Three letters of application were sent, or in a few cases telephone calls made. One of the applicants was white English, one of Asian origin and one of Afro-Caribbean origin; all were equally matched in terms of British exam qualifications, previous work experience, age and sex. All the letters sent were matched for content, style and handwriting ability. The only variable factor in the tests was the ethnic origin of the applicant. The person of Asian origin was identified by name, for example Balder Singh Virdee; the origin of the West Indian applicant was made clear in the letter, which said, for example, 'I came from Jamaica in 1965 . . .'. The native White applicant could be identified by name, for example John Clarke, and by the absence of any reference to overseas origin.

Of the 161 vacancies, 58 were invalid because none of the applicants were replied to, or all were rejected. The remaining 103 represent 206 test cases, as each involved an Asian and a West Indian applicant. The results were as shown in the table.

White applicant offered interview but not black	*48%*	*(98 cases)*
Black applicant offered interview but not white	*6%*	*(11 cases)*
All applicants treated equally	*46%*	*(97 cases)*

There was no difference in the level of discrimination against Asians and West Indians, 48 per cent in both cases.

The statistics from these surveys show that the Race Relations Acts have not stopped discrimination against black people in employment. Black people are still discriminated against in almost half their applications for jobs, simply because of their colour. The surveys showed that discrimination against young black people born and/or raised in Britain is just as high as for their parents. Also, the real level of discrimination may be much higher. These surveys don't show how many people would be discriminated against at the interview stage.

I was up in the manager's office at the time, and one of the Saturday boys came up to the office and said to the manager that they'd got two girls waiting, asking about a job. And the first thing he said, 'Are they black?' And he said 'Yeah'. You know, he said 'Well, tell them that we haven't got any vacancies here.' I mean, you know I was shocked. He just said that, and I was still there, and I just walked out.

Afro-Caribbean boy[6]

I've had a similar experience to him, because I went for a Saturday job one day, and the woman, I asked her if she had a job going. And there was actually a sign that said there was a job going. And she goes, 'Well, I don't mean to be prejudiced or anything, but we've already got a black person working here.' She just smiled and went back in the shop.

Young Afro-Caribbean woman, London[6]

Indirect discrimination in employment can occur in a number of ways: language tests that are not necessary for the job; culturally biased intelligence tests or entrance exams; dress or uniform regulations that some minority groups cannot comply with and which are not justifiable on other grounds; inflexible rules about holiday arrangements and extended leave. The example below illustrates how, in one organisation, direct and indirect discrimination were found to be interlinked in selection for promotion.

CRE *Employment Report* March 1984

INVESTIGATIONS
BRADFORD METRO
Wrong bus

The Commission for Racial Equality found evidence of both direct and indirect discrimination during its investigation of Bradford Metro, one of the operating districts of the West Yorkshire Passenger Transport Executive. A report of this investigation was published in June 1983.

The investigation started in 1979 after the Commission had received complaints from six Asian busmen alleging discrimination in promotion. The investigation looked into the reasons why only two of the 50 inspectors employed by Bradford Metro were black when over half the busmen, many of whom had over ten years' service, were of Asian origin. Bradford Metro cooperated throughout the investigation.

The Commission found that there had been direct discrimination as Bradford Metro were applying higher standards to black applicants than to white applicants for inspector posts. Indeed, the company admitted that they feared that there would be a backlash from white employees. In addition, they thought an Asian inspector would have more difficulty with the public and would therefore have to be better than a white inspector.

'I freely admit that I was looking for a superman', said the then District Manager.

The Commission also found that the written test used in the promotion procedure required a higher standard of English than was necessary for the satisfactory performance of an inspector's duties. As the test acted as a barrier to a disproportionately large number of Asian applicants, the report concluded that it amounted to indirect discrimination.

Action

Although a non-discrimination notice was issued in December 1982, Bradford Metro took action to ensure equality of opportunity earlier in 1982. For example, they reviewed their selection and training arrangements for inspectors, they introduced a record-keeping system to enable them to assess whether equal opportunities were being provided in recruitment and promotion, and they adopted a comprehensive equal opportunity policy.

The trade union concerned, the Transport and General Workers' Union, has also agreed to monitor the situation to ensure that no discrimination takes place.

The Commission has noted the response of Bradford Metro and the TGWU. It has also noted that four black inspectors are now in post and is confident that discrimination will be avoided in future.

Commenting on the report, Mr Peter Newsam, CRE Chairman, said:

'I welcome Bradford Metro and the TGWU's decision to take action to avoid discrimination. Any employer who employs a disproportionately small number of black employees, in any grade, should follow their example. If, like Bradford Metro, they find that their selection tests are acting as a barrier to black applicants, they should ensure that the tests are strictly related to the requirements of the job and do not result in discrimination.'

Institutional racism in jobs. Let's talk about hospitals for example. For years black people have been working in hospitals. If it was a natural process, if something inside of the hospital system was not blocking them getting to the top, I think it would not be possible for it still to be news when there is a black matron. Look on the railways. You see many railway porters, train drivers – ask yourself about middle management.

Ros Howell[6]

Housing

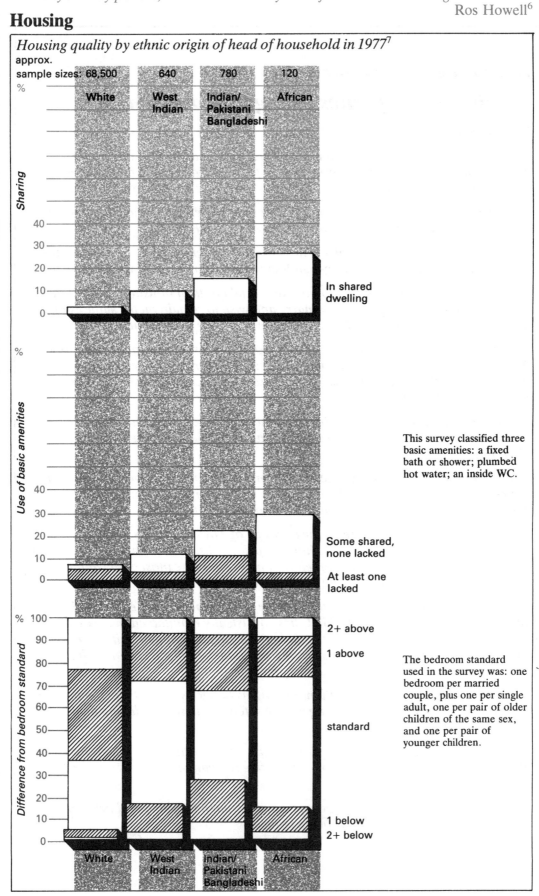

Housing quality by ethnic origin of head of household in 1977[7]

approx. sample sizes: 68,500 / 640 / 780 / 120

White / West Indian / Indian/Pakistani Bangladeshi / African

Sharing
In shared dwelling

Use of basic amenities
Some shared, none lacked
At least one lacked

This survey classified three basic amenities: a fixed bath or shower; plumbed hot water; an inside WC.

Difference from bedroom standard
2+ above
1 above
standard
1 below
2+ below

The bedroom standard used in the survey was: one bedroom per married couple, plus one per single adult, one per pair of older children of the same sex, and one per pair of younger children.

White / West Indian / Indian/Pakistani Bangladeshi / African

The figures above show that **a greater proportion of black people live in housing with poor amenities than white people**. The explanations for this are complex, but investigations show that a significant contributing factor is indirect discrimination in local authority housing policy[8], as the article below illustrates.

Long-standing tenants and relatives to lose priority

'Racist' housing rules changed to aid Bengalis

By a Correspondent

Bengali families living in the Spitalfields area of London are to be given a greater chance to rent more modern housing following a decision by the Greater London Council to change what it acknowledges is discriminatory policy there.

Under that policy, Bengalis received fewer than 10 per cent of housing built after 1964, despite making up 47 per cent of the area's households.

Now the rules are to be changed. The GLC is to scrap its policy of offering most of the newly-built property to long-standing tenants, almost all of whom are white.

Another change is the elimination of the special quota of housing stock offered to tenants' sons and daughters who marry and wish to remain on the same estate. This quota will now be offered first to families in severe housing need.

The GLC acted after receiving evidence from its housing chairman, Mr Tony McBrearty, and principal race relations officer, Mr Herman Ouseley. They concluded that the racial bias was not deliberate but a side effect of procedures which had worked fairly elsewhere.

They found that many Bengali families, though in the greatest housing need, were kept low on housing priorities lists because they had lived there a relatively short time.

Part of the problem has been the acute shortage of four- and five-bedroom flats which are in great demand by Bengali families. Stringent cost controls over new building has led to virtually no construction of large flats.

The GLC is putting pressure on the borough of Tower Hamlets, in which Spitalfields is located, to change its housing priority list. Borough policy is to offer the least desirable residences to homeless families. Because most of the homeless families are Bengali, this policy has been felt to be discriminatory.

One controversial policy likely to continue is the dispersal of Bengalis to estates in nearby Bow and Poplar. The GLC has consistently maintained that with a projected 40 per cent increase in the number of Bengalis living in Spitalfields over the next three years, as dependents arrive from Bangladesh, they can no longer be accommodated.

The Spitalfields Housing and Planning Rights Service says that moving the Bengalis to areas where they no longer have safety in numbers is laying them open to racial attacks.

On the Coventry Cross estate in Poplar, according to an unpublished survey, the organisation says more than four out of five Bengali families have experienced racial harassment.

There are reports of iron bars being thrown through windows and petrol being poured through letter-boxes and being ignited.

Guardian, 27.9.82

The flats are small and the stairway is badly lit. They are damp, the window frames are old and rotten and we do not have separate toilet and bathroom and there is no handbasin in the bathroom. The flats are the worst you can get in this borough.

Afro-Caribbean tenant.

The Council seems to pack black families in these flats. We were desperate for a flat so when they offered us one we thought it was heaven. We have asked to be moved but it has been in vain. The place is not nice. Do you know that when we got here we were the second black family on this balcony? Now all the flats except two of the 24 are occupied by black families.

Jamaican man.

Many of us feel that the authorities offer us these bad flats because few whites want them. It is bad when you concentrate blacks in one estate or area. What you then do is to stop whites from coming to such estates. Apart from that it seems once the Council has the poor blacks concentrated in particular estates then they refuse to improve existing facilities or add new ones.

Antiguan tenant.

You should have to change the colour of your skin to get a Council house in a nice and decent area.

Young West African couple.[9]

Another significant factor which limits housing choice for black families is the risk of racial attacks if they live in isolation from other black families. An extract from the *Guardian* below describes one such attack.

In Shadwell Gardens, by Cable Street, there is a large block of council flats. On the ground floor my interpreter from the Bengali Housing Association led the way into a small, bare flat inhabited by a Bengali widow with three children of six, eight and nine.

Last Saturday night they were watching television. They had just had the windows repaired from the last volley of stones. Fists started hammering on their windows. They turned the lights out and sat in fear.

They heard sounds in the kitchen: breaking glass, sounds of unknown things coming into their home. Peeking around the kitchen door, they saw rubbish being emptied from dustbins into their home. Then a stone came through the living room window. The widow gathered her children and ran out of the front door seeking protection from another Bengali family thirty yards across the court.

There were about thirty people waiting for them as they left their home. The bruises on the neck and face and legs of the widow and her children were still livid on the brown skin as they recounted how they had run a gauntlet of fists and kicks and curses of their neighbours.

Guardian, 6.6.77

I think it's very basic attitudes of people. I mean very basically attitudes of white people. To go into areas where there are hardly any Asians, and to walk into a situation where you are the only black face, and it seems as if everything comes to a standstill, and everybody's looking at you. And you sort of tend to have this extra sense in you, and you sort of feel the tension in people. I think it's a phenomenon that only people sort of in our position can really experience that.

Balraj Purewal.[6]

Education

In 1981 the government published the report of a Committee of Inquiry into the education of children from ethnic minority communities (known as the Rampton Report). Among other things the report discussed the main factors contributing to the 'under-achievement' of Afro-Caribbean children in schools. The Committee of Inquiry found that the **conscious and unconscious attitudes of teachers** towards black children was an important factor.

West Indian Children in Our Schools: Report of a Committee of Inquiry into the education of children from ethnic minority communities, HMSO, 1981.

Although genuine misunderstandings can sometimes lead people, both black and white, to believe mistakenly that racism lies behind certain behaviour or situations, we are convinced from the evidence that we have obtained that racism, both intentional and unintentional, has a direct and important bearing on the performance of West Indian children in our schools. [our emphasis]

The suggestions that teachers are in any way racist understandably arouses very strong reactions from the profession and is often simply rejected out of hand as entirely unjustified and malicious. Since a profession of nearly half a million people must to a great extent reflect the attitudes of society at large there must inevitably be some teachers who hold explicitly racist views. Such teachers are very much in the minority. We have, however, found some evidence of what we have described as unintentional racism in the behaviour and attitudes of other teachers whom it would be misleading to describe as racist in the commonly accepted sense. They firmly believe that any prejudices they may have, can do no harm since they are not translated into any openly discriminatory behaviour. Nevertheless, if their attitudes are influenced in any way by prejudices against ethnic minority groups, this can and does, we believe, have a detrimental effect on all children whom they encounter.[10]

. . . what we have is that a lot of people, thousands and millions of people, have been conditioned for hundreds of years, because this is something that has become part of our culture, to have certain attitudes towards foreigners, and particularly towards people who are black, whether they are foreigners or not. And the same people who have got those attitudes, of course, are running our institutions, are helping to create policies and practices in those institutions. And some of them inadvertently, and some very deliberately, write up their practices and policies in a way that excludes black people or prevents black people playing a positive and active role.

Dorothy Kuya.[6]

Black people are largely, by and large, excluded from the corridors of power in this country. At every level, decisions are being made from the view and concept of Britain as being a white society, and therefore all the decisions are being made from that kind of white norm.

Basil Manning.[6]

2.3 A misleading 'explanation' of racial inequality

Unless you yourself have been the victim of constant discrimination or have been close to someone who has, it is difficult to understand what it feels like to experience it daily because of the colour of your skin.

Ever since I can remember, and this is going way back, early sixties, from being very small I was always aware of being dark – black – and for a 6-year-old it wasn't very pleasant being called 'darkie' and 'monkey', not just by other kids and other people, but by your brothers and sisters as well. Because if you're dark then you're stupid – a fool –

and I wasn't stupid, I wasn't a fool, but I was quiet and different. I remember wanting to be white when I grew up because being black was something bad and awful and in all my dreams I was white and I'd go round in space from planet to planet in my spaceship doing good deeds and rescuing people.

West Indian/British man.[11]

Most black people, and I'm talking about West Indians and Asians, both my generation and my parents' generation are coming from a background where subconsciously they were taught to believe that things white and European were better. They were more civilised, they were more educated. And in fact I think that all black people that I know approach white people with positive expectations initially. The kind of black person who makes bitter statements about white people, you cannot imagine the rebuffs and the unhappiness he's suffered at the hands of white racists.

Sandra Macdonald.[6]

There is a tendency on the part of many white people to disbelieve, or to try and ignore, the extent of racial discrimination in this country. White people often try to explain away the difficulties faced by black people as 'cultural problems'.

'Cultural problems'?

There are numerous examples of literature which describe ethnic minority cultures in a way which makes them seem bizarre or backward, which emphasise minor practices, and which imply that poor health among black people is somehow caused by the nature of black culture. For example, there has been much publicity about the fact that *some* brands of surma, a type of Indian eye make-up, contain lead. The implication is that people are foolish to go on putting this make-up on their children.[12] On the other hand there are many practices in Western culture which are harmful to health – for example, smoking, working with carcinogenic chemicals, eating large quantities of fatty and sugary foods – but this does not cause white people to describe their own culture as 'bizarre' and 'backward' in the same way. This issue is discussed in detail in Chapter 4.

2.4 Discrimination, health needs and health care

Very few people can be said to be entirely without prejudice of one kind or another and in this country, due in part at least to the influence of history, these prejudices may be directed against West Indians and other non-white ethnic minority groups. A well-intentioned and apparently sympathetic person may, as a result of his education, experiences or environment, have negative, patronising or stereotyped views about ethnic minority groups which may subconsciously affect his attitude and behaviour towards members of those groups. . . . We see such attitudes and behaviour as a form of 'unintentional' racism.[13]

It is important for health workers to recognise that racial discrimination *is* a part of the black experience in Britain. It is an everyday reality which is likely to affect health and health care in various ways. Health workers should be aware that this experience also affects, consciously or unconsciously, the expectations of black people when they come into contact with institutions such as the National Health Service, whose administrators and managers are predominantly white. It may also affect the way black people react on an individual level to white people in positions of authority, such as health professionals.

State of health

Racial discrimination **indirectly** affects black people's state of health, because **it helps to create or reinforce** the kind of **disadvantages** in employment, housing and education that have just been described earlier in this chapter. (Chapter 3 looks in more detail at the link between discrimination and other economic, environmental and social pressures that are likely to affect health.)

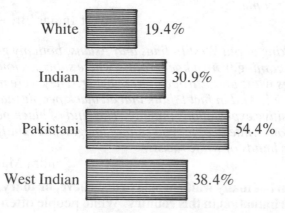

Proportions of black and white people in semi-skilled and unskilled manual jobs in 1977[4]

White   19.4%

Indian   30.9%

Pakistani   54.4%

West Indian   38.4%

People doing manual jobs face greater health risks than people in white collar and professional jobs. This diagram shows that a high proportion of black workers are concentrated in semi-skilled and unskilled manual jobs. Health risks are increased by discrimination which keeps a high percentage of black people in poorer housing and lower-paid, unpleasant jobs.

Discrimination **directly** affects health in two ways. Firstly, the subtle and unthinking forms of discrimination encountered daily can be just as **emotionally and psychologically painful** to a black person as blatant prejudice. Secondly, **fear of violent discrimination**, in the form of racist abuse or attack, **is also likely to affect the physical and mental wellbeing** of members of black communities, particularly those in a weak or vulnerable position such as the elderly and the isolated.

Access to health care

The Black Report on inequalities in health strongly argues the need to **improve the distribution of health service resources in order to match greatest need with most effective care.**[14] It suggests there is unequal access to health care for two main reasons:

- There is **less provision in some localities** (for example, inner city areas) than in others in relation to the size of population and need for services.

  *Differences in sheer availability and, at least to some extent, in the quality of care available in different **localities** provide one channel by which social inequality permeates the NHS. Reduced provision implied greater journeys, longer waiting lists, longer waiting times, difficulties in obtaining an appointment, shortage of space and so on.*[15]

- The way in which existing services are organised is **not always appropriate** for the nature of the population they serve.

  Class differentials in the use of the various services which we have considered derive from the interaction of social and ecological factors. A second channel is provided by the structuring of health care institutions in accordance with the values, assumptions and preferences of the sophisticated middle class 'consumer'. Inadequate attention may be paid to the different problems and needs of those who are less able to express themselves in acceptable terms and who suffer from lack of command over resources both of time and of money.[15]

Evidence suggests that, as a particularly disadvantaged section of the population, **ethnic minority groups are likely to experience unequal access to health care for the same reasons as other disadvantaged groups.** In addition, although the health services do not of course set out to discriminate against ethnic minority patients, **it is likely that certain existing policies, practices and attitudes are indirectly discriminatory** in that they can result in ethnic minority patients receiving less favourable treatment than others.

The discussion below focuses on specific examples of:

- health service policy;

- professional practice;
- the attitudes and expectations of health workers.

2.5 *Health service policies*

Health service policies determine the way services are organised, and structure the way in which the individual health professional works on a day-to-day basis. The policies of institutions also influence the attitudes of people working within them. The policy of a Health Authority towards ethnic minority health needs is bound to have some effect on the practice and attitudes of the health workers it employs.

I trained as a student midwife in a hospital where there were no paid interpreters, because the Health Authority did not feel there was any need. Part of my work involved taking the medical history of women attending the ante-natal clinic for the first time. Quite often I simply couldn't do the job properly because the patient spoke hardly any English. Most midwives found this kind of experience very frustrating, but we understandably took the view that it was the patient's responsibility to learn English because, given our own resources, it seemed the most obvious solution. I realised after talking to English language teachers that it isn't a very feasible solution at all. If you calculate the cost of setting up classes to teach, in a short period, what is a rather specialised English to a few women, the money could be used far more effectively to employ interpreters who could provide a service for the majority of non-English-speaking women who come to the ante-natal clinic. But it's difficult to convince other colleagues when the Authority itself doesn't recognise there's a need, even in principle.

Midwifery sister

There are a number of areas in which existing policies may indirectly result in ethnic minority patients receiving less favourable treatment, for example:

- introduction of health charges for overseas visitors;
- aspects of health worker training;
- organisation of medical records;
- allocation of resources to screen for specific illnesses;
- interpreting resources;
- hospital arrangements for religious needs;
- hospital catering arrangements.

Introduction of health charges for overseas visitors

With the introduction in November 1982 of new regulations for charging overseas visitors, **it is inevitably patients who look or sound 'foreign' who are more likely to be challenged than others.** Once health care becomes linked to an investigation of the individual's legal status, people may be deterred from seeking treatment. This could be detrimental not only to the individual's health but to the health of others he or she comes into contact with.

 For more information about this issue, see Notes at the end of this Chapter[16] and the section on health charges for overseas visitors in 3.4.

medication and rehabilitation. If health workers are not aware of such conventions and do not take them into account, **patients may not be able to comply with the regime prescribed for them.** Unless Health Authorities openly acknowledge their importance, staff are unlikely to take them seriously. Training is discussed in more detail in Chapter 12.

Organisation of medical records

A number of ethnic minority groups in Britain (for example, the Chinese, Indian, Pakistani, Vietnamese and Turkish communities) have **naming systems** which are different from the traditional British pattern. Yet many hospitals, clinics and GP surgeries with a high proportion of patients from these groups have no policy for coping with such differences in the filing of patients' medical records. This means that patients from these groups often experience a **disproportionate amount of delay and confusion** when attending clinic and surgery appointments and serious mistakes can occur over drugs and treatment.

Allocation of resources for screening specific illnesses

Health Authorities vary widely in their **policy on screening for diseases which particularly affect ethnic minority communities**, such as sickle cell disease and thalassaemia. For example, some authorities automatically screen all patients of Afro-Caribbean origin for sickle cell disease, while others screen only on request. There is often no coherent policy on follow-up counselling after tests have been carried out. As a result, diseases that particularly affect minority groups may be less well managed and treated. This issue is discussed in more detail in Chapter 9.

Interpreting resources

Most health care requires communication between health worker and patient. **A lack of interpreting resources can mean that health workers are unable to perform certain crucial tasks effectively**; history taking, making a diagnosis, counselling, giving advice and instructions about treatment cannot be done properly if the practitioner cannot communicate with the patient. In areas with a large non-English-speaking population, a significant proportion of patients will clearly **benefit less** than others from health service provision if properly trained interpreters are not available.

Hospital arrangements for religious needs

Most hospitals set aside a room or chapel for use by Christian patients for prayer or worship. **There may be nowhere for patients of other faiths to pray in private.** This means that devout patients who are not Christian are often denied a valuable source of support and comfort in their illness.

Hospital catering arrangements

Many ethnic minority patients are unable to eat food from the standard hospital menu, either for religious reasons or because they are completely unused to a western diet. The diets of Jewish, Muslim, Hindu and Rastafarian patients, for example, are directly affected by religious beliefs. In addition, elderly and more conservative members of other ethnic minority groups may only be familiar with their own traditional foods; the hospital menu may be their first contact with a conventional British diet. **Patients who cannot eat properly in hospital are likely to take longer to recover: long-stay patients may develop problems of undernourishment.** A few hospitals are beginning to recognise this area of need and some now provide Asian diets as a standard part of the hospital menu. But many hospitals serving areas with a large ethnic minority population do not provide diets which conform to religious requirements, and do not have a clear policy on the bringing of food into hospital by patients' relatives. In some hospitals bringing food in for patients is actually discouraged, which means that some patients can virtually starve during their stay in hospital.[17]

Food in hospital is discussed in more detail in Chapter 8.

2.6 *Professional practice*

The day-to-day practice of individual health workers is influenced, at least in part, by administrative policy. For example, a records clerk cannot be expected to cope with 40 medical records marked 'Mrs Begum' without confusion and error, if there is no policy to provide training in understanding Asian naming systems and an appropriate filing system to cope with the practicalities.

But individual health workers do have some degree of autonomy in the way they organise their work. To be effective, **the health worker's advice or action has to fit in with the material circumstances, beliefs and way of life of the family or individual she is working with. Lack of flexibility in individual practice can work to the disadvantage of ethnic minority patients in various ways.** Five specific but very different areas of practice are discussed below:

- psychiatric diagnosis of ethnic minority patients;
- communication skills;
- working with interpreters;
- giving family planning advice;
- asking for passports to check personal details.

Psychiatric diagnosis of ethnic minority patients

A recent study suggested that the high rate of admissions for schizophrenia and psychosis in Afro-Caribbean men may be due to the fact that **psychiatrists are more ready to diagnose psychosis or schizophrenia in members of some ethnic groups than in others.**

We have seen that non-Europeans were initially believed to have bizarre and incomprehensible mental illnesses. Is it possible that high rates of schizophrenia really mean little more than poor communication between patient and doctor? Perhaps the mental patient does not have a distorted relationship with reality so much as an inability to present his experiences and difficulties to the psychiatrist in a form the latter can understand?[18]

Communication skills

Health workers do not always make allowances for patients who do not speak 'middle-class' English, or who speak English as a second language. Health staff may not recognise that some patients have difficulty not only in communicating their problems to the health worker but also in understanding the health worker's own style of communication.

Language and communication skills are discussed in detail in Chapter 5.

Working with interpreters

The health worker can damage her relationship with non-English-speaking patients if she does not take care to establish a good relationship with the interpreters she works through. **If the interpreter is made to feel inadequate by the health worker because he or she lacks professional status**, this can create problems which are passed on to the patient.

The interpreters here are very good, though there are not enough of them. . . . But it has been suggested that the health professional will talk down to the interpreter because she is not a professional. And inevitably the talking down spreads through the translation. And all this is to an elderly lady who was living in India when the British were expelled, who has a lot of hidden aggression, and does not take kindly to being patronised. . . .

Often I will have a grandmother in here with a baby and she will ask if there is an Asian health visitor she can ask about feeding, and when I say there is no Asian health visitor, but she can use an interpreter, she will say, oh no, leave it.

Asian GP[19]

Making effective use of interpreters is also discussed in Chapter 5.

Giving family planning advice

Some ethnic minority women feel that health workers show more concern about reducing the birth rate in ethnic minority families than about other equally important health issues that affect their lives, such as hazardous working conditions and damp housing. Some women also feel they are rushed, without proper discussion, into using family planning methods that they don't particularly like, and subsequently stop using. Women with strong religious convictions on the subject find the approach of some health professionals distressing, and even offensive.

When I was in hospital two days after the birth of my fourth child I had a visit from the family planning nurse. She came into the ward, walked straight up to me and said in a loud voice 'Now then, dear, it's time you started thinking about family planning, isn't it?' I felt embarrassed and offended. Why did she single me out? Why didn't she speak to me privately? I hadn't asked about it and I certainly didn't want to discuss it in those circumstances, so I just pretended not to understand her. I thought it would be easier than making a fuss by refusing outright to talk about it. It happens to my people all the time, but most women are too shy or too polite to show they're offended.

Bangladeshi woman

Asking for passports to check personal details

Queries or confusion over the correct name or date of birth of an ethnic minority patient can sometimes arise, even though his or her eligibility for treatment is not in doubt. **The health worker may ask to see the patient's passport as the simplest way of checking she has the correct details, without realising how upsetting and offensive such a request can be.** To a black person it can appear that the health worker is suspicious and wants to check up on the patient's legal status in this country. This can destroy the patient's trust and confidence in the health worker making the request, and may deter some people from seeking help in the future. There are plenty of alternative forms of identification that the health worker could ask to see.

2.7 *Health workers' attitudes and expectations*

The health worker's private expectations or opinions of a particular patient should not directly affect the practical care or treatment she provides, but they inevitably affect the quality of her relationship with the patient. To be effective she needs to gain the patient's trust and confidence in her ability to help him get well. **If the health worker appears to have a negative attitude towards the patient's religion, culture, language, or skin colour, that confidence is easily undermined.** The patient may feel that the health worker is trying to ignore his own beliefs, or regards them as worthless; it may appear that the health worker is trying to impose her own beliefs and practices, or make radical changes, for no apparent reason. Patients who sense, rightly or wrongly, a negative attitude are likely to lose confidence in the health worker, possibly with serious consequences:

- **they may avoid or delay seeking treatment;**
- **they may discount the health worker's advice or instructions;**
- **recovery may be inhibited.**

What impression do health workers convey to ethnic minority patients?

Below are some examples of ways in which the health worker may unthinkingly convey a negative attitude towards ethnic minority patients. All the quotations are taken from real incidents.

- **Using the term 'immigrant' to refer to all black people**, even those born here; describing ethnic minority patients in terms such as 'these people'.
  You see, these people all seem to live in these overcrowded conditions.
  (Community midwife to student midwife, in front of an English-speaking Bengali woman)

- **Making fun of the patient's first language** or expecting him to speak English when he clearly finds it difficult.
  Stop that! You must speak English in this hospital.
  (Ward sister to two women speaking in Punjabi)

- **Behaving towards someone who speaks little English as though they are deaf or stupid.**
  You . . . no . . . come . . . last . . . time . . . YOU NAUGHTY GIRL!
  (Midwife to ante-natal clinic patient)

- **Making derogatory comments about the patient's lifestyle.**
  You can't go on with arranged marriages if you live in England.
  (Medical social worker to Asian teenager)
  You see, even your baby prefers our food to yours.
  (Health visitor to Pakistani mother)

- **Joking about problems relating to skin colour in a way that suggests they are not being taken seriously.**
  The sister told the doctor my baby was slightly jaundiced and he just said 'Oh, I thought all Chinese babies were jaundiced . . . ha ha . . .' I thought he was very rude.
  (Chinese woman)

- **Making derogatory comments about the patient's own health beliefs and practices,** even though the patient derives benefit from them.
  This herbal stuff is all mumbo-jumbo you know. . . . Throw it away.
  (GP to Vietnamese patient)

Health care can only be effective if it fits in with the choices available to the patient. Bearing in mind that the options available to ethnic minority families facing economic and social disadvantage are likely to be limited, the health worker has an obligation to identify and suggest solutions in a way that is sympathetic and non-judgmental.

Developing an open-minded approach

It is easy to label people whose behaviour does not fit in with professional expectations as 'problem' or 'inadequate' patients, when the real problem may be a lack of knowledge, or misunderstanding, on the part of the health worker. The checklist below questions some of the common assumptions about ethnic minority families.

- Who is the term 'immigrant' used to describe?
- Is it a term that has positive or negative associations in your own view?
- Is it an appropriate term to describe black people who were born and have grown up in Britain?
- What is your reaction to patients who can't speak English?
- Who should take responsibility for communication with patients who do not have English as their mother tongue?
- Is it up to the patient to make his own interpreting arrangements?
- Should the health authority provide an interpreter service?
- What do you think about patients using their own first language in hospital or in the clinic?
- Do you expect ethnic minority patients from different backgrounds to adapt to 'British ways' or to maintain their own traditions?
- Bearing in mind that patients' level of confidence and self-esteem affects their ability to seek help and communicate with health staff, how do you recognise in practical terms those aspects of cultural identity on which that confidence is based?
- How do patients' own health beliefs and practices affect their state of health and the appropriateness of the health care they are given?
- How do you take patients' beliefs and practices into account in your professional approach?

- How do you respond when other staff or patients make derogatory comments about ethnic minority patients?

2.8 *Practical action*

This chapter has focused on several examples of health service policy, professional practice and professional attitudes that can work to the disadvantage of black patients. Direct and overt discrimination is easily identifiable, but **more research and analysis is needed to identify the areas in which indirect discrimination may be unintentionally operating** in the delivery of health care. The questions below suggest a starting point.

- **What aspects of health service policy with which you are familiar may result in ethnic minority groups receiving less favourable treatment?** For example, what aspects of the way primary health care services are organised in the inner city areas might deter ethnic minority patients from using those services?

- **What aspects of current professional practice in your own field may work to the disadvantage of ethnic minority patients?** For example, is the weaning advice given by health visitors to ethnic minority women based on 'English' norms or on patients' own traditional diet?

- **To what extent do health workers' expectations of ethnic minority patients as a group influence their professional relationship with individual patients?** For example, what comments or actions might unintentionally distress or give offence to ethnic minority patients?

Below is a summary of action points based on some of the issues raised in this chapter. Bear in mind that these action points are intended as examples only.

Policy

These points should be borne in mind when reviewing current policy:

- All aspects of **basic and in-service training** should take account of the multiracial nature of the British population. **Course curricula** should be reviewed using this criterion and changes made where necessary (see Chapter 12).

- Receptionists, records clerks and registrars should receive proper **training in the naming systems of all ethnic groups** and should learn effective ways of eliminating confusion and duplication in medical records (see Chapter 15: Training materials).

- Where none exists already, Health Authorities should adopt a **standardised policy on screening for illnesses** that particularly affect ethnic minority groups, and on follow-up and counselling services.

- **Paid and trained interpreters should be provided** where necessary (especially where loss of information, or misunderstanding because of language difficulties might have serious consequences).

- In hospital, **facilities for worship should be provided** for all patients, not only Christians (for example, a quiet room for prayer open to patients of all faiths).

- The **range of diets on the hospital menu** should include dishes that are acceptable and appropriate to the religious and traditional dietary conventions of ethnic minority patients who find 'western' food unacceptable.

- Where no suitable hospital food is available arrangements should be made or improved to **encourage friends and relatives to bring appropriate and acceptable food in to patients.**

- **Community Health Councils and patient participation groups** in multiracial areas should include **proper representation of the ethnic minority communities** in the area. Representatives may need to be actively sought and specifically invited (see Appendix 1).

- In hospitals, clinics and health centres serving a sizeable non-English-speaking population, **signs should be provided in appropriate minority languages.**

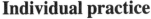

Individual practice

Bear in mind these points in day-to-day practice:

- **Make allowances** for patients who don't speak English very well. Be flexible in your own style of communication.

- Take care to **establish a good rapport with the interpreters** you work with. In the long term using an interpreter may save time, but initially it is essential to **allow more time** to develop mutual trust and confidence (see Chapter 5).

- **Don't press family planning advice on a patient** if it is not asked for and not welcome. If there are strong medical grounds for family planning advice, the reasons should be made explicit to the patient, and to other members of the family if appropriate.

- **Never ask to see a patient's passport** unless it is offered. Ask for an alternative form of identification (NHS card, driving licence) if necessary.

- Try to **develop an awareness of the social, religious and cultural conventions that are likely to influence patients' choices** about health and health care (see Chapter 7).

- **Your role**, the service you provide and your relationship with other staff patients come in contact with **may need careful explanation** to patients who are unfamiliar with the NHS or who speak little English.

Notes

1. See for example:
   Coard, B., *How the West Indian Child is Made Educationally Sub-Normal in the British School System*, New Beacon Books, 1971.
   Rampton, A. (ed.), *West Indian Children in our Schools: Interim report of the Committee of Inquiry into the education of children from ethnic minority communities*, HMSO, 1981.
   Runnymede Trust and the Radical Statistics Race Group, *Britain's Black Population*, Heinemann, 1980.
   Simpson, Alan, *Stacking the Decks: a Study of Race, Inequality and Council Housing in Nottingham*, Nottingham and District Community Relations Council, 1981.
   Smith, David J., *Racial Disadvantage in Britain: The PEP Report*, Penguin, 1977.
   Smith, David J., *Unemployment and Racial Minorities*, Policy Studies Institute, No. 594, February 1981.
2. *Racial discrimination*, Cmnd 6234, HMSO, 1975, p. 3.
3. Smith, David J., *Racial Disadvantage in Britain*, Penguin, 1977, pp. 75–77.
4. This quote is taken from *Ethnic Minorities in Britain*, Home Office Research Study, No. 68, HMSO, 1981. The diagrams first appeared in *Racism in the Workplace and the Community*, Open University Continuing Education Pack, 1983.
5. The quote and diagram are taken from *Racism in the Workplace and in the Community*, Open University Continuing Education Pack, 1983. They first appeared in Carter, S. and Hubbock, J., *Half a Chance: Youth Unemployment in Britain*, Nottingham and District Community Relations Council, 1980. The extract 'The only variable factor . . . reference to overseas origin' appears in the original report only.
6. These quotes are taken from a transcript of the tape-slide production *The Enemy Within*, Ikon Productions, British Council of Churches, 1981.
7. The diagram and quote are taken from the Department of Environment, *National Dwelling and Housing Survey*, HMSO, 1979, table 8 but the diagram originally appeared in the Runnymede Trust's and the Radical Statistics Group's publication, *Britain's Black Population*, Heinemann, 1980.
8. For examples, see:
   Ouseley, Herman *et al.*, *The System*, Runnymede Trust and South London Equal Rights Consultancy, 1982, Chapter 9: Housing Services.
   Runnymede Trust and the Radical Statistics Race Group, *Britain's Black Population*, Heinemann, 1980, Chapter 4: Housing.
   Simpson, Alan, *Stacking the Decks: a Study of Race, Inequality and Council Housing in Nottingham*, Nottingham and District Community Relations Council, 1981.
   Smith, David and Whalley, Anne, *Racial Minorities and Public Housing*, Vol. 1, Broadsheet No. 556, Political and Economic Planning, 1975.
9. These quotes are taken from Morrison, L., *As They See It: A Race Relations Study of Three Areas from a Black Viewpoint*, Community Relations Commission (now the Commission for Racial Equality), 1976, p. 59.
10. Rampton, A. (ed.), *West Indian Children in our Schools: Interim report of the Committee of Inquiry into the education of children from ethnic minority communities*, HMSO, 1981, p. 12.
11. This quote is taken from 'Personal experiences of multi-ethnic Britain' in Husband, C. (ed.), *Race in Britain: Continuity and Change*, Hutchinson, 1982 p. 175.
12. *Black People and The Health Service*, Brent Community Health Council, 1981, p. 13.
13. Rampton, A. (ed.), *West Indian Children in our Schools: Interim report of the Committee of Inquiry into the education of children from ethnic minority communities*, HMSO, 1981, p. 12.
14. Townsend, Peter and Davidson, Nick, (eds), *Inequalities in Health: The Black Report*, Penguin, 1982.
15. Townsend, Peter and Davidson, Nick, (eds), *Inequalities in Health: The Black Report*, Penguin, 1982, p. 89.
16. Regulations governing the charges for overseas visitors have changed several times since the original proposals were drawn up. The administration of the regulations has proved so unwieldy that there is considerable pressure within the NHS to abolish them.
   For a detailed critique of the regulations see: *From Ill Treatment to No Treatment*, Manchester Law Centre Immigration Handbook No. 6, 1982.
17. O'Brien, Maureen, *Hospital Food for Ethnic Minority Patients*, Haringey Community Health Council, 1981.
18. Littlewood, R. and Lipsedge, M., *Aliens and Alienists: Ethnic Minorities and Psychiatry*, Penguin, 1982, p. 108.
19. This quote is taken from 'Giving an Asian community a better health service', an interview with an Asian community health officer and GP, in *Medical News*, Vol. 14, No. 47, 9 December 1982.

More information

'Cultural problems' see
4 **Culture: a misleading explanation of health inequalities**

The connection between migration, discrimination and disadvantage, see
3 **Migration and health**

Screening for specific illnesses, see
9 **Patterns of illness**

Hospital catering arrangements, see
8   **Foods and diets**, especially
8.8 **Food in hospitals and institutions**

Communications skills, see
5 **Communication**
Interpreters, see
5.6 **Practical action: improving communication across a language barrier**

Family planning advice, see
6   **Working with families and individuals**, especially
6.4 **Family planning**

Health workers' expectations and professional practice, see
  7.1 **Concepts of health**
  7.2 **Expectations and experience of the health services**
  7.4 **Working with different health beliefs and practices**
  8.7 **Practical action: giving nutritional advice**
  10.4 **Practical action** (individual practice)
  12.3 **Professional values**

Health service policy, see particularly
10 **Responding to need**
11 **Ethnic minority staff in the National Health Service**
12 **Health worker training and professional values**

Finding out about local needs, see
14 **Local needs: guidelines for doing your own research**

Materials on racism and cross-cultural communication see
15.3 **Training resources for health workers and other professionals on working in a multiracial society**

Further reading

See the reading list in Chapter 16
16.2 **Racial inequality and health**

See also relevant publications in
16.1 **Why is a multiracial approach necessary?**
16.3 **Migration and health**
16.4 **Culture: a misleading explanation of health inequalities**

3 Migration and health

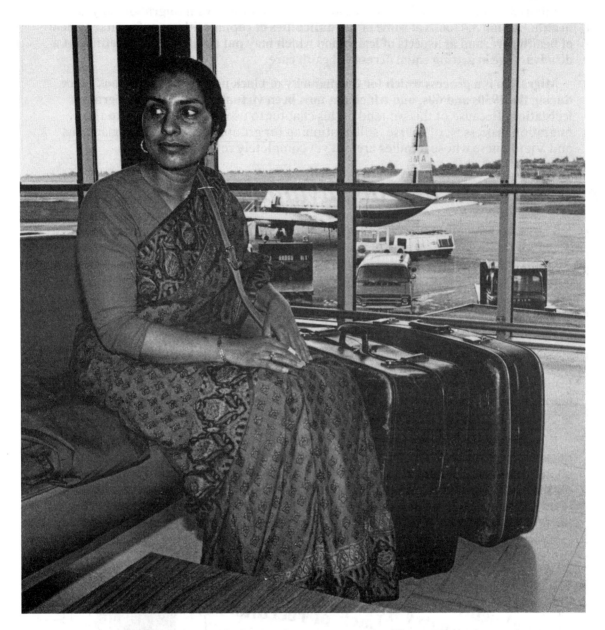

Introduction

This chapter looks at some of the economic, environmental and social pressures facing black migrants* and settlers* in Britain. It is in many ways an arbitrary exercise to try and separate the effects of migration and settlement on the health of black people living in Britain from the effects of racial discrimination and disadvantage. For this reason there is an inevitable overlap between the issues discussed in the last chapter and those discussed in this one, but the focus is somewhat different. The first part (sections 3.1–3.3) looks at how the disadvantages resulting from migration may affect health. Section 3.4 looks at some of the difficulties of coping with an unfamiliar system of health care, and at aspects of legislation which may put ethnic minority settlers at a disadvantage in getting equal access to health care.

Migration is a process which for the majority of black people in Britain took place during the 1950s and 60s, and which has now been virtually halted by immigration legislation. Because of this we tend in this chapter to use the past tense. But the migration process is, of course, still continuing for groups such as the Bangladeshis and Vietnamese whose families are not yet completely reunited in Britain.

3.1 *Migration and disadvantage*

There are problems inherent in leaving one's homeland which put all migrants at a potential disadvantage on arrival in a new country. But a great deal depends on the circumstances in which migration takes place and on how migrants are received by the population of the country where they settle. In Britain, because great social importance is attached to skin colour, the disadvantage is enormously increased by racism*.

In the 1950s and 60s, migration to Britain from the colonies and ex-colonies was encouraged for economic reasons. **British employers, such as London Transport and the NHS, actively recruited workers from the Caribbean and the Indian sub-continent.** London Transport opened a recruiting office in Barbados in the 1950s because of the labour shortage in Britain. **Poverty and high unemployment in the sending countries provided the impetus for people to take up the invitation to come and work here.**

But although their labour was welcome, attitudes towards newly arrived black migrants were ambivalent. There was no initial action by the government to counteract disadvantages or help people settle in and find their feet. For example, there was no formal provision in the early days to help non-English-speaking workers learn the language, and legislation to prohibit acts of racial discrimination was not introduced until 1965.

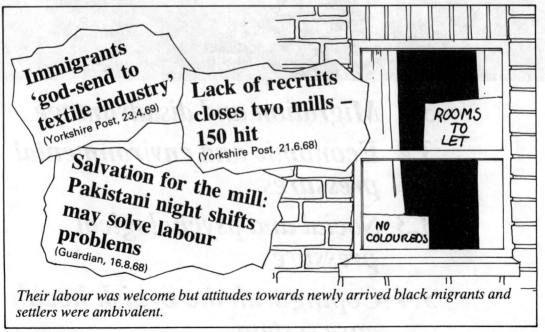

Immigrants 'god-send to textile industry'
(Yorkshire Post, 23.4.69)

Lack of recruits closes two mills – 150 hit
(Yorkshire Post, 21.6.68)

Salvation for the mill: Pakistani night shifts may solve labour problems
(Guardian, 16.8.68)

ROOMS TO LET

NO COLOUREDS

Their labour was welcome but attitudes towards newly arrived black migrants and settlers were ambivalent.

* See *Notes on Terminology, p. 3*

3.2 Economic and environmental pressures

Newly arrived black migrants and settlers were (and still are) faced with specific disadvantages.

Dislocation and loss of informal support systems

Migrants lose the support of their own family and community networks and find themselves excluded from the networks in their new country. This means that they have no way of learning how the systems in their new country work; they do not get to hear through the normal word-of-mouth channels about better job opportunities, or better housing options; they cannot draw on the informal help of friends and relatives in finding ways to improve their situation. In Britain the effects of this dislocation have been made worse by widespread prejudice and discrimination on the part of employers and landlords.

Poor working conditions

The stimulus for immigration in the 1950s and 60s was the shortage of labour in **certain sectors** of the economy. **Most of the vacancies were in manual industries and occupations, mainly in unskilled and semiskilled jobs for which it was difficult to recruit other workers because of unsocial hours, unpleasant working conditions and relatively low earnings.** A high proportion of migrant and settling workers got jobs in heavy industries where morbidity and mortality rates are historically high because of health and safety hazards. Many migrants ended up working long hours for low pay, and often on permanent night shifts.

Differences in hours worked and wages received between British born and immigrant workers in the early 1970s.[1]

	Average hours per week	Average wage per week	Average hourly rate
British-born	48.7	£27.90	58.2 pence
Immigrant	53.8	£30.90	58.3 pence

Percentages of white and black male workers in shift work in the early 1970s.[1]

Key:
- Day shifts
- Night shifts
- Permanent nights

Vulnerability to unemployment

According to Department of Employment figures, **unemployment among ethnic minority communities increases disproportionately when the general level of unemployment is rising**.

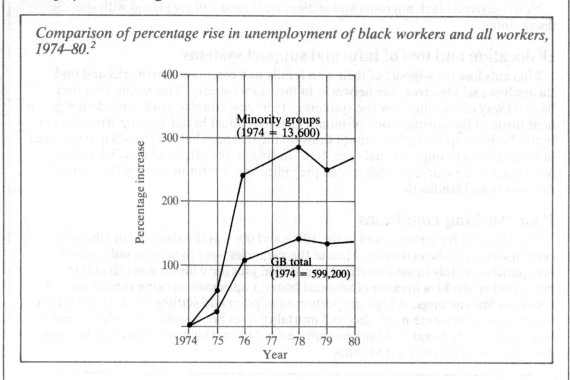

Comparison of percentage rise in unemployment of black workers and all workers, 1974–80.[2]

A report published in 1980 outlined several factors which may be responsible for this increase.[3] Some are clearly linked to the effects of migration, but others are linked to discrimination and affect British-born black people as well as migrants and settlers.

- There are increasing numbers of black young people leaving full-time education and entering the employment field at a time when job prospects for young people generally are adversely affected by the cutbacks in recruitment during the present recession.

- The shorter average length of time in employment of black workers makes them vulnerable to 'last in, first out' rules at times of redundancy. Many black workers found jobs in the older manufacturing industries such as textiles and steel, where other workers would not accept the poor conditions; it is this sector of the economy that has been worst hit by the recession.

- There have been greater percentage increases in unemployment in the regions – for example, the South East and West Midlands – where most black people live.

- Racial discrimination by individual employers and in recruitment and selection procedures means that, faced with a plentiful supply of labour, managers will hire white in preference to black labour.

- Lack of appropriate skills and qualifications, including knowledge of English, on the part of recent immigrants from the Indian sub-continent.

Poverty and inner city deprivation

Low-paid jobs meant that newly arrived migrant workers were often forced to take cheap low-quality housing that was not acceptable to other people. This kind of property is usually located in inner-city areas, where there is already a high density of population, putting heavy demands on limited education, health and welfare resources. Inner-city populations also suffer from environmental problems such as lack of play space and other social amenities, traffic pollution and accidents, and poor shops. Thus, black migrants and settlers on coming to Britain share many of the disadvantages facing other semiskilled and unskilled manual workers: low income, poor working conditions and high rates of unemployment, low quality housing, poor nutrition, and restricted educational opportunities.

Racial discrimination

As we have seen in the previous chapter, it is not solely the process of migration that produces these disadvantages. **Racial discrimination in all areas of life severely limits the opportunities available to black families to change their situation.**

The effects on health of these cumulative disadvantages are clear. A wide range of evidence in the Black Report clearly shows that ill health and premature death are unequally distributed between social groups, and that poverty is one of the major causes of ill health. **A lack of the basic necessities – adequate housing, diet, clothing and fuel – is directly damaging to health.** This is clearly illustrated by the Court Report, a 1976 government survey which looked at the health problems of children in low-income families.[4] The report points out, among other things, that a child born to parents in socio-economic group V (unskilled working class) is four times as likely to be dead at the end of the first year of life as a child born to professional parents.

A doctor in Peckham, south London, estimates that four of the patients who attend his surgery each day come, wholly or partly, because of their housing problems. Sometimes the issues are straightforward; they are suffering stress because of overcrowding, noise, lack of play space for the children, damp, cold, poor maintenance of the flat. At other times the cause is less tangible. They bring their children with illnesses which are really an expression of their own distress. They speak of the 'bad environment', of vandalism or the fear of physical attack. They are angry and frustrated by the apparent intransigence of the housing department. They seek the panacea of the 'doctor's letter' that they imagine will magically get them a transfer or a home.

'Housing can play an enormous part in their ill-health', says the doctor. 'And no matter what the medical indications are, I think it is the patient's subjective assessment of the distress caused by housing which matters. If you have a number of personal, social and economic difficulties to start with, the agony caused by housing problems can literally drive you round the bend. You'll probably never get an academic study to prove it but the link between housing problems and stress is glaringly obvious.'

ROOF March/April 1982

3.3 Social and psychological pressures

As well as a lack of the basic necessities, black migrants and settlers often have to cope with considerable social and psychological pressures:

Culture shock

For people who have moved from a rural third world village, living in a Western industrialised inner-city environment can be a shattering experience.

Lack of support and immigration restrictions

The initial move often meant separation from the rest of the family and community, and **isolation from the practical help and emotional and psychological support that family and friends could offer.** Immigration restrictions meant that people often faced the additional strain of several years' waiting and uncertainty before permission was granted for their spouses and children to join them in Britain.

A story (translated from Gujarati) told by an elderly Asian who has fallen victim to rigid immigration control:

I came to the UK in 1964 from India to earn my living. I came on my own, leaving my wife and baby daughter back home, because I intended to settle first – to find a job and proper accommodation so that when at a later stage I invited my family to join me here, I could offer them a certain amount of comfort.

On my arrival, I found it very difficult to obtain a job and the environment as a whole unfriendly and hostile. As I was determined to stay on and make my living here, I took up a job in a restaurant. In the year 1968, I decided to call my family over to join me as I thought I will be able to give them good accommodation and a happy life.

Unfortunately, during this time, when I was coming back from work one evening, I was attacked by several hooligans and the beating I took was so severe that I ended up in hospital partially paralysed. Since then, I have never been well enough to go back to work.

I have lived with a hope that one day I will be all right and will be able to return to work, and call my family to join me here. This dream of mine till today has not materialised. Since the last three years, I have been feeling very depressed and broken because my health has given in and I have become bedridden and I have been frantically trying to bring my family (wife and young daughter) to join me so that I could be looked after by them, but it seems that the Government does not wish for me and my family to be happy.[5]

This situation is perhaps felt even more acutely by refugee groups (East African Asians, Chileans, Vietnamese), who were forced to migrate and have had to sever ties with their homeland.

White attitudes to black migrants

For many black migrants, **the British way of life represents an alien and sometimes threatening culture** which discounts their own values, beliefs and way of life and appears to regard people from other cultures with different lifestyles as inferior and backward, needing to change 'for their own good'.

Adapting from one culture to another can be compared to learning to eat with your left hand. But for ethnic minorities, adapting to a racist culture is like learning not to eat at all. And there is no dispute about the depth of racial discrimination in this country.[6]

Emotional and psychological effects of racism

We discussed in Chapter 2 some of the ways in which racial discrimination and prejudice contribute to the material disadvantages facing migrant families in Britain. **Black settlers have also had to suffer the emotional and psychological effects of coping with overt and covert racial prejudice and discrimination** as a normal part of everyday life in this country. The resulting sense of isolation can lead to loneliness and depression or to frustration, resentment and anger.

One group particularly affected by loneliness and depression are non-English-speaking women. The reason is often a complex interrelationship of all the pressures we have just outlined.

I get angry with white people who say, 'Oh, the women are isolated because they don't speak English' or 'Their husbands won't let them out of the house.' That's a superficial understanding. The real reasons go much deeper. Women who haven't grown up in an extended family can't understand what it's like for a woman to come to Britain and be suddenly and permanently separated from all her women relatives and friends back home. The loneliness can be terrible. That and the shock of finding yourself in an alien and hostile society. Maybe her husband doesn't like the idea of her going out on her own . . . that's partly because he knows that she's very vulnerable. Who will protect her from abuse or come to her help if she's attacked? All right, it doesn't happen every day, but it's a constant fear for Asian families in this area. Wouldn't all that wear you down? It's not surprising women get depressed.

From what health visitors in this area tell me, a lot of immigrant women suffer from depression and some get quite ill. But I don't think medical help can make much difference unless the professionals begin to acknowledge the real causes. A lot of GPs believe that women must automatically be better off over here than they were back home and don't understand their unhappiness. Materially some women are better off perhaps, but a telly and a fridge don't make up for the loss of your family and they certainly don't cure racism.

Asian community worker

Frustration and powerlessness

The kind of pressures we have described are heightened for black migrants (and their British-born children) by the knowledge that **they are a vulnerable (and often disliked) minority denied the economic or political power to effect real change in their situation.** A sense of powerlessness contributes to the depression and despair of the non-English-speaking women described above. It is also responsible for the frustration, resentment and anger in young people that gave rise to the recent riots in Britain's inner city areas. In his report on the Brixton riots of 1981, Lord Scarman concluded:

The evidence which I have received . . . leaves no doubt in my mind that racial disadvantage is a fact of current British life. It was, I am equally sure, a significant factor in the causation of the Brixton disorders. Urgent action is needed if it is not to become an endemic, ineradicable disease threatening the very survival of our society.[7]

Mental illness

It might be expected that the kind of social and psychological pressures faced by black migrants and settlers would result in a higher incidence of mental illness among ethnic minority communities. **Psychiatric medicine in Britain has only recently begun to look at the relationship between migration, racism and mental illness**, although more research in this field has been done in the United States.[8] In Britain, **some work has been done on the importance of cultural factors in psychiatric diagnosis, but in general this is still an area which is little understood by the majority of psychiatrists.** Because of the highly complex and sensitive nature of the issues involved, it is an area which really requires a book in itself. There is not enough space in this handbook to do proper justice to the subject, but several relevant works have recently been published which readers may find useful.[9]

3.4 *Coping with the British health care system*

We have looked at some ways in which migration can affect physical and mental health. What difficulties do black migrants face in getting access to health care and in coping with an unfamiliar system of health services?

Lack of information about the health services

People who have only recently arrived in Britain and/or don't speak English very well may find it difficult to find out what health services are available and how the NHS works. Even migrants and settlers who have been in Britain for some time may never have been given clear information about where to go for any support or help they may need and what benefits they are eligible for. This is the kind of information one picks up through informal networks such as family, friends and workmates. A recent initiative to improve this situation is discussed in 10.2.

Communication difficulties

Non-English-speaking patients may be unable to communicate with health staff, and there may be other barriers to communication because of the differences in health workers' and patients' expectations. These issues are explored in Chapter 5.

Cultural variations and awareness of health staff

Many aspects of health service provision are culturally specific. For example, hospital diets, washing and bathing facilities, and arrangements for religious observance are generally geared to the needs of the white British population. This can present problems to migrants and settlers whose norms and values are different.

The way that British institutions organise health care has grown up to fit in with Christian practices; for example, we try to send patients home over Christmas, Christian chaplains make regular rounds of hospital wards, and Christian services are held on hospital premises. When patients in hospital wish to make confession, to receive communion, or to baptise their babies, ward staff generally understand what to do, and, equally important, are immediately sympathetic to requests. Health workers know the significance of prayer books and crucifixes, and how to avoid causing unnecessary offence when preparing Christian patients for surgery. They may be less confident when, for example, a child comes into hospital with a leather pouch attached to his arm, or a Sikh patient protests when being shaved for an operation. Non-Christian patients often find it more difficult to get help in fulfilling their religious duties merely because these duties are unfamiliar to staff. This increases patients' feelings of isolation and unhappiness.[10]

The effects of government legislation

Immigration legislation and court judgements may indirectly result in migrants and settlers being reluctant to seek treatment when they need it.

Immigration status

Recent court judgements have extended the definition of 'illegal entrant' to cover anyone who, on entry, failed to disclose material facts, even though they were not specifically asked to do so at the time and did not realise they were relevant. This means that **the individual's status can be redefined as 'illegal' at any time**. If a person has worries, however ill founded, about his or a relative's legal status, he may be wary of any form of official intervention that might lead to investigation. This may deter some people from seeking treatment, because it will involve questioning, and from disclosing important information to health staff.

A health visitor involved in the resettlement of Vietnamese refugees thought this might explain her own experience:

It was noted that the families tended to withhold relevant information about their health. Nevertheless, after a number of visits, when they seemed able to trust me, more details of past medical history were revealed voluntarily. Whether, initially, they had an erroneous fear of being deported if they disclosed unfavourable information about their health is hard to say.[11]

Health charges for overseas visitors

The introduction of health charges for visitors to Britain who have been here less than 12 months (now revised to 6 months) means that people who look or sound 'foreign' are likely to be questioned in greater detail about their status. **The complexity of administering the regulations means that some people may be subjected to lengthy delays and uncertainty while their eligibility is checked, and then faced with large hospital bills they cannot pay.** This uncertainty, coupled with a fear of being unable to pay, may deter some migrants and settlers from seeking treatment altogether, even though they may be perfectly entitled to free treatment.

Inquiry ordered after foreigners escape Clarke's health charges

By Andrew Veitch
Medical Correspondent

The Government's controversial scheme to raise £6 million a year by charging overseas visitors for hospital treatment appears to have flopped. The Health Minister, Mr Kenneth Clarke, has disclosed that it produced only £374,459 in the first six months. He has ordered an investigation into why health authorities failed to obey his instructions.

The figures, given in a written answer to the shadow health minister, Mr Frank Dobson, show that 69 authorities raised no money at all from the scheme, and many others earned less than £100. Paddington topped the list with £36,664 while Mid Essex produced just £4.

Mr Dobson yesterday described the scheme as ludicrous. 'In order to raise this pathetic sum the Government has breached the principle that anyone falling ill is entitled to free treatment.' he said.

'They have caused harassment to black and brown British residents and have imposed an enormous extra burden on hard working hospital staff.'

The scheme was introduced in October last year despite criticism from doctors, who described it as racist, and administrators who said it would cost more to administer than it would yield in charges: on average each health district has had to print 300,000 extra forms.

Health workers in several hospitals attempted to boycott the scheme, and it was opposed by immigrant organisations.

Mr Clarke added, in his reply, that the figures for the first six months were likely to be untypical because some authorities had failed to start the scheme on time, and they were winter months when there were fewer overseas visitors.

Guardian 18.11.83

The 1981 Nationality Act

This Act has serious implications for the **registration of babies** born to ethnic minority parents who are migrants or settlers:

Throughout history, any child born in Britain (except to parents who are foreign diplomats) has automatically become a Citzen of the UK and Colonies with full rights of residence in the UK. Under the new law children born in Britain whose parents are not permanently settled in Britain do not automatically acquire British citizenship.

A child who does not become a citizen at birth will be entitled to be registered as a British citizen when either parent becomes a British citizen or legally settled in Britain, or at the age of ten, provided that the child has not been outside the UK for more than 90 days in any of the first ten years of his or her life. This clause means that some children will be born and may remain stateless. It also means that many parents will be asked to prove their residents' status when they register the birth of a child. This is likely to lead to a situation where people who look or sound 'foreign' are asked to prove their residence and legal status when registering their new-born baby.[12]

MIGRATION

Migration involves the transfer of a valuable economic resource – human labour – from the poor to the rich countries. The workers who migrate may have been unemployed in the country of origin, but this does not alter the fact that the community has invested considerable sums in their upbringing. Economists sometimes speak of 'emigration as capital export' similar to the export of other factors of production. It has been estimated that the upbringing, the price of survival till the age of twenty of a migrant, has cost the national economy of his own country about £2,000. With each migrant who arrives, an underdeveloped economy is subsidising a developed one to that amount. Yet the saving for the industrialised country is even greater. Given its higher standard of living, the cost of 'producing' an eighteen-year-old worker at home is between £8,000 and £16,000.

The use of labour, already produced elsewhere, means an annual saving for the metropolitan countries of £8,000 million.

To those who have machines, men are given.

Apologists for the system argue that the advantages are mutual. According to them, emigration benefits the under-developed country in the following ways:

1. *Emigration reduces population pressure. Young migrants marry later. Married migrants – absent from their wives – procreate less.*

45

2. *Emigration reduces unemployment and raises wages. Further, a shortage of labour in the migrant's country of origin will encourage mechanization.*

3. *The migrants acquire industrial skills to take home with them. Their experience in industry is educative.*

4. *The remittances the migrants send home improve their country's balance of payments. (In 1972 the remittances sent home by migrant workers in Germany totalled at least $3 billion.) These remittances help to supply capital for local industrial investment.*

Behind this curtain of argument, the distant reality remains unchanged:

1. *Migrants are the most enterprising of their generation.*

2. *Their labour is lost to their own country.*

3. *If local unemployment is reduced, it usually means whole areas losing nearly all their able-bodied men. Around the 'ghost villages' cultivation deteriorates further.*

4. *The moneyed classes in an underdeveloped economy have little interest in industrial or agricultural mechanization.*

5. *Migrants remain unskilled workers. They learn their new job in a few days.*

6. *When they return home, the factories have not been built.*

7. *The under-developed countries are in debt to the developed countries – hence their balance-of-payments problem. Migrants' remittances are deposited in banks who lend this money back to the developed countries. When the remittances are withdrawn from the banks, a large part of them is spent on the purchase of further commodities from the developed countries.*[13]

Notes

1. Smith, D., *The Facts of Racial Disadvantage*, Political and Economic Planning, 1976.
2. Department of Employment, *Gazette*, Vol. 88, no. 3, 1980.
3. Runnymede Trust and the Radical Statistics Race Group, *Britain's Black Population*, Heinemann, 1980.
4. *Fit For the Future: The Report of the Committee on Child Health Services*, Vol. 1, Cmnd 6684, HMSO, 1979.
5. *Point of No Return*, background paper on elderly Asians, Brent Indian Association, 1979.
6. Fatma Dharamshi, quoted in Amin, Geeta, *Some Aspects of Social Policy Affecting Asian Women in Britain*, paper presented to Asian Women's Conference on 'Our Role in Britain Today', 16 July 1977, p. 2.
7. Lord Scarman, *The Scarman Report: The Brixton Disorders 10–12 April 1981*, Penguin, 1981, p. 209.
8. Gaw, Albert, (ed.), *Cross-cultural Psychiatry*, John Wright (PSG Incorporated), 1982.
9. Littlewood, Roland and Lipsedge, Maurice, *Aliens and Alienists: Ethnic Minorities and Psychiatry*, Penguin, 1982. Rack, Philip, *Race, Culture and Mental Disorder*, Tavistock, 1982.
10. Henley, Alix, *Caring for Muslims and their Families: religious aspects of care*, National Extension College, 1982.
11. Lam, Emily, 'Health Visiting Vietnamese Refugees in Britain', *Health Visitor*, Vol. 53, No. 7, 1980, p. 257.
12. Henley, Alix, *Immigration in Britain: a chronological account of immigration into Britain with emphasis on Asian settlement from the Indian subcontinent and East Africa*, Draft manuscript, 1982.
13. Berger, John and Mohr, Jean, *A Seventh Man: Migrant Workers in Europe*, Penguin, 1975, pp. 68–72.

More information

Economic and social disadvantage, see

2 **Racial inequality and health**

6.3 **Racism and bringing up black children in Britain**

Coping with the British health care systems, see

5.2 **Communication difficulties for ethnic minority patients**

5.4 **Communication difficulties for people whose mother tongue is not English**

7.2 **Expectations and experience of the health services**

Further reading

See the reading list in Chapter 16.

16.3 **Migration and health**

See also relevant literature in:

16.2 **Racial inequality and health**

16.6 **Working with families and individuals**

4: Culture: a misleading explanation of health inequalities

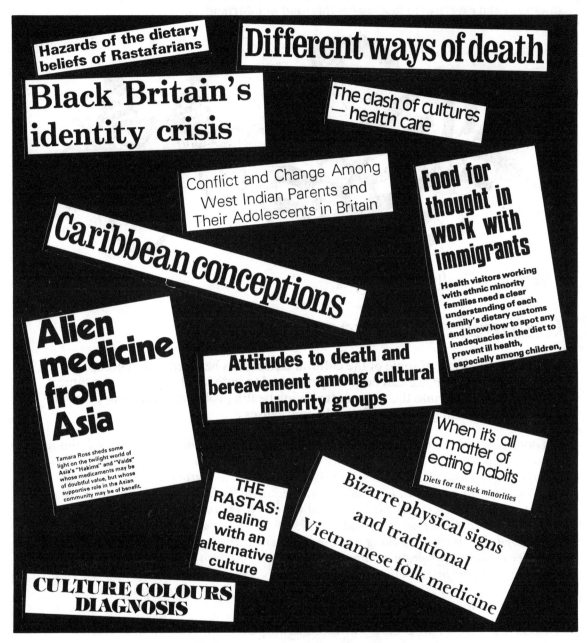

Hazards of the dietary beliefs of Rastafarians

Different ways of death

Black Britain's identity crisis

The clash of cultures — health care

Conflict and Change Among West Indian Parents and Their Adolescents in Britain

Food for thought in work with immigrants

Health visitors working with ethnic minority families need a clear understanding of each family's dietary customs and know how to spot any inadequacies in the diet to prevent ill health, especially among children,

Caribbean conceptions

Alien medicine from Asia

Tamara Ross sheds some light on the twilight world of Asia's "Hakims" and "Vaids" whose medicaments may be of doubtful value, but whose supportive role in the Asian community may be of benefit.

Attitudes to death and bereavement among cultural minority groups

When it's all a matter of eating habits

Diets for the sick minorities

THE RASTAS: dealing with an alternative culture

Bizarre physical signs and traditional Vietnamese folk medicine

CULTURE COLOURS DIAGNOSIS

4.1 Cultural differences

4.2 Stereotypes

4.3 Other social factors

4.4 The limitations of information in professional practice

4.5 Practical action

Introduction

When health worker and patient come from very different backgrounds, any information which helps the professional worker to see the situation through the patient's eyes is valuable. But it is important to always check this kind of information for its accuracy and relevance to individual members of the local community.

The first part of this chapter looks at the reasons for the variable quality and usefulness of available literature. In the last two sections there are some practical questions and exercises to help assess this kind of information.

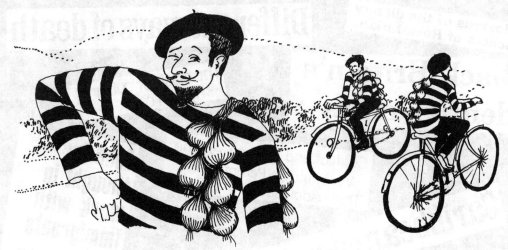

Be wary of cultural stereotypes

4.1 Cultural differences

An understanding of some of the cultural differences between social groups means that professional practice can be closely matched to individual needs. At the same time it is easy to fall into the trap of attributing health problems **entirely** to cultural differences, diverting attention from the real causes.

It's not only ethnic minority patients whose problems are labelled as 'cultural' although it probably happens more to them. I was struck by the case on a TV programme of an elderly English woman who when she visited a geriatric department as an outpatient was forcibly bathed against her will. She subsequently lodged a complaint, and when the interviewer asked her about it, she said she had been forced to sit in a bath, naked, by a male nurse, surrounded by student nurses . . . she said she felt degraded and humiliated. The interesting thing was the comment of the Nursing Officer who was interviewed for the programme after the complaint had been lodged. She felt the problem lay in the fact that the lady was extremely sensitive about her modesty . . . if they'd realised she was so sensitive, said the Nursing Officer, they might have done things differently.

This is the point . . . the problem was seen as the patient's unusual if not peculiar attitude, her extreme modesty, just as it is with many ethnic minority patients . . . I would suggest the problem lies more in the lunacy of a health care system that requires caring professionals to force patients into doing things against their will.

Community relations officer

'Inadequate culture'

Literature which explains the health problems of ethnic minority communities in terms of cultural factors fosters the misconception that the way of life of those communities is in some way inferior or less adequate than those of the majority, and therefore needs to be changed 'for people's own good'. Health workers may be mistakenly led to try and impose changes in the behaviour of patients where none is **necessary.** (This can damage or destroy the relationship between health worker and patient.) It can also mean that the real causes of problems are obscured or overlooked, so that health workers take inappropriate action or give wrong advice. A case in point is the issue of Vitamin D deficiency in the Asian community. Critics of the recent DHSS 'Rickets Campaign' argue that it generated a widespread belief that the root of the problem lies in the nature of Asian culture – more specifically, that the traditional Asian vegetarian diet is inherently defective and is the main cause of rickets. The real causes of rickets are not properly understood, but a recent report (see Box, below) makes it quite clear that the traditional vegetarian diet is not in itself a significant factor.

Vitamin D deficiency in the Asian community
*It is often assumed that the diets of British Asians tend to be low in vitamin D because many Asians are, to a greater or lesser extent, vegetarian. This assumption is highly misleading. Only about a quarter of British Asians eat a predominantly vegetarian diet. Meat does not anyway contain significant amounts of vitamin D, and fish, which does, is less commonly avoided. But even avoiding fish need not cause a problem. After all, if fish were left out of the average British diet, it would not make a vast difference to the total vitamin D intake. Most Asian vegetarians eat significant amounts of dairy products, although some (particularly women in some groups) avoid eggs. A few vegetarian Asians are vegans – that is, they exclude dairy products as well; it is clear that for these people several of the standard sources of vitamin D would be excluded. However, for other British Asians, their vegetarianism need present no problem, particularly if they eat large quantities of dairy products. Vegetarians can, of course, eat most brands of margarine, the food chosen for mandatory fortification, but it happens not to be a food commonly eaten in quantity by most Asian groups; Hindus in particular value butter very highly, especially for cooking. **For many Asians, the main reason for their lower than average vitamin D intake is not vegetarianism but the fact that it was margarine that happened to be chosen for fortification** [our emphasis].*

. . . So whether or not somebody eats fish is not necessarily important for their dietary vitamin D intake. This is not, however, the impression usually given in discussions of this question. They almost always start by listing foods naturally rich in vitamin D and go on immediately to point out that such foods may not be eaten by British Asians . . . omitting to mention that many non-Asians in Britain rarely eat them either.

. . . It would be less misleading to start instead by listing the foods that are the major sources of vitamin D in the average British diet. (Remember that about 60 per cent comes from margarine and eggs.) Given the information that way round, people could see immediately that, if Asians are getting substantially less than average vitamin D, it is not because of their vegetarian diets. Vegetarianism is quite compatible with eating margarine (if it is not made from unacceptable animal fats) and most vegetarians also eat eggs and dairy products. Indeed, vegetarians might be eating more than the British average of some sources, such as some commercial yoghurts.

. . . Finally, health educationists should recognise that vegetarian diets are commonly – and wrongly – thought to be nutritionally inferior to those that include meat, and that it is important for them to counter this assumption explicitly. They could emphasize that for a diet to contain no or very little meat is completely compatible with good nutrition. Indeed, reducing meat consumption can be a good way of eating less fat. Stressing such positive aspects of the vegetarian diet could help to dispel notions that British Asians who are vegetarian would be better off adopting eating habits more like those of the rest of the British population.[1]

Culture as a fixed and static state

Some materials give the impression that 'Chinese', or 'Asian' or 'West Indian' culture is static and inflexible; that there is little cultural variation among individuals within a particular ethnic group; that people do not adapt their lifestyle and behaviour to meet changing circumstances.

While changes in economic and social circumstances are easily visible, an outsider may be blind to the more subtle way in which individuals within a community change and adapt to cope with new situations.

Take the idea of 'culture conflict' . . . when Asian teenagers run away from home or when an Asian woman is having problems with her marriage, it's often put down to a problem of conflicting values between Asian and British culture . . . there is the idea that the sooner the Asian community abandons the extended family network and arranged marriages – the sooner all these problems will disappear . . . but will they? . . . What about white girls who run away from home, what about English women whose marriages break down. . . . What about white children living in care?

Their social problems aren't defined as 'cultural' by the professionals who sort them out – nobody points a finger at the nuclear family and says people have these problems because the nuclear family is a backward cultural form that should be done away with . . . nobody says the divorce rate among English people is so high because the system for choosing the marriage partner is defective and must be changed.

I'm not saying that Asian girls and women don't have to cope with contradictions in their lives – of course they do – but talking about a 'conflict' of cultures seems to imply culture is something rigid and inflexible, that people have to make a choice between two opposite and irreconcilable poles, which just isn't the case for most of us. It seems to me that pigeonholing problems as 'cultural conflict' is a way of setting black people's problems apart – it's ignoring the social realities.

Asian community worker

Growing up in an Asian family in Britain does not in itself cause stress. Many of the problems which do occur are not the result of conflicts caused by migration and the experience of great social change, but of external pressures. Living in inner city areas, where housing, schools and recreational facilities are poor, may give rise to tension and anxiety which are compounded by racial hostility. . . . The notion that young Asians are likely to suffer from culture conflict is a gross oversimplification of complex personal experiences.[2]

False generalisations

Bear in mind that talking about 'Asian', 'West Indian' or 'Chinese' culture is as useful as talking about 'British' culture; it is essential to specify which social group within a particular culture is under discussion. For example, does 'British culture' mean Scottish, Irish, Welsh or English? Upper, middle or working class? Black British or white British? Teenagers or the elderly? **The variations between social groups within one culture are enormous.**

The experience of an outside researcher may be confined to observation of a very small, unrepresentative group within a community. For example, if a British anthropologist spent a week at the holiday home of a middle-class French family, and then generalised about the social habits of the whole French middle class on that basis, how accurate would those generalisations be?

The extract below describing the British middle class is from a book written in 1966 for American readers and it shows how misleading generalisations can be when based on limited observation.

The middle and upper class Englishman . . . is brought up in a nursery shared with brothers and sisters. The oldest occupies a room by himself which he vacates when he leaves for boarding school, possibly even at the age of nine or ten. The difference between a room of one's own and early conditioning to shared space, while seeming inconsequential, has an important effect on the Englishman's attitude towards his own space. He may never have a permanent 'room of his own' and seldom expects or feels he is entitled to one. Even members of Parliament have no offices and often conduct their business on the terrace overlooking the Thames. As a consequence, the English are puzzled by the American need for a secure place in which to work, an office.[3]

4.2 Stereotypes

It is clear that **background information, if it is not used carefully, can act as a barrier** to understanding between health workers and individual patients. **People cannot be neatly pigeonholed into a particular cultural, national, religious or ethnic group.** For example, when someone gives their religion as Muslim or Catholic, it does not necessarily mean they are strict observers of that religion. Someone who says they are Catholic may or may not use the pill, someone who says they are Muslim may or may not eat meat from the hospital menu.

An Iranian woman on our ward had 'Muslim' down on her admission form, so the ward sister just assumed she would want a vegetarian diet. After about four days the poor woman asked in desperation why everybody else got meat except her. She wasn't a strict Muslim at all . . . in fact she said she wasn't really anything. . . . She'd given her religion as Muslim the way a lot of English patients say 'C of E' even though they're not at all religious and never go to church. . . . But when they ask you on admission what your religion is most people say what they think they're expected to say.

Student nurse

There is as much diversity in attitudes, expectations and behaviour among the Asian, West Indian, Cypriot or Chinese population in Britain as there is among the indigenous white population. The fact that such variations are less obvious to the outsider makes it even more important to question assumptions and check first with the patient.

'Bizarre' or 'backward' cultures

An outsider is always in danger of misunderstanding or wrongly interpreting the unfamiliar cultural patterns of another community. For example, **beliefs and behaviour which have a sound logical basis may strike the outside observer as irrational or absurd. From this lack of understanding, negative stereotypes easily develop.** An American Professor of Nursing demonstrated how the commonplace can seem bizarre to the uninitiated, in a parody which was an account of the nursing profession in the United States as it might be seen by a foreign anthropologist.

THE GNISRUN TRIBE

The Gnisrun* tribe is the largest health professional group in the United States. It claims nearly 850,000 members. They are a rather unusual tribe in that they are sex-slanted with nearly 93 per cent of their membership female, and predominantly White Anglo middle-class Naciremas*. Only recently have they vigorously enticed males and minorities to enter their sacred tribe. The few males who gained membership early into the tribe were predominantly administrators or caretakers of the emotionally ill in large institutions. . . .

The Gnisruns are primarily matrilineal groups with matriarchal leaders. They tend to be patrilocal if married, or neolocal if single. Apartment dwelling is their dominant choice of living. All of these tribal members claim matrilineal descent to their founding leader known as Florence Nightingale. There is no question that 'Florence' is their tribal leader and cultural heroine. Periodically, the members reaffirm their tribal allegiance by ceremonial acts in sacred places such as schools of nursing, hospitals, and public gatherings. They also display Florence's few and rare books in which one finds her sacred credos. These credos guide and reaffirm the tribe in their cultural behavior, the essence of Gnisrun tribal goals, and their cultural history. The heroine's statues and other sacred paraphernalia are becoming more and more highly treasured items since her death in 1910. Indeed, her artifacts and other effects are being feverishly collected in several sacred Gnisrun temples in Nacirema land.[4]

---

* 'Gnisrun' and 'Nacirema' are of course 'Nursing' and 'American' spelt backwards.

4.3 Other social factors

Writers who focus exclusively on 'culture', often ignore other key factors which have an important bearing on health:

- The generally **low social and economic status** of migrant and settler communities and its effect on health.

- **Racial discrimination** and its social and psychological effects on black communities, particularly as a barrier to seeking health care.

- **Experiences and needs shared with the white population**, especially shared disadvantages such as poor housing, unemployment, ill health, etc.

- **The lack of flexibility** in the organisation of the health services provided.

An understanding of these factors is as important as an understanding of culture if the interventions of health workers are to be appropriate and effective.

4.4 The limitations of information in professional practice

There are two further reasons why health workers need to be very careful about using unadulterated 'cultural background' information as a basis for their professional response:

- Local needs vary according to local circumstances, and the particular background and history of the local minority population. **General information is almost certain to need adaptation and additional research to make it locally relevant.** For example, the experiences and needs of third generation British-born blacks in Liverpool are likely to be very different from those of the first generation Ghanaian population in Birmingham.

- Some inner-city communities are made up of a large number of different ethnic groups. **It would be foolish to expect health workers to absorb detailed information about the cultural background of each group in the area.** In this situation, the most appropriate course of action might be local research to identify specific needs, followed up by in-service training to review practices and services that might be 'colour-blind' or 'culture-bound', and to develop strategies for improving communication with ethnic minority patients and clients.

4.5 Practical action

Health workers need an understanding of their patients' background but the available literature should be subjected to critical scrutiny. There are two simple ways of achieving this.

- **Develop a critical approach when reading about 'culture'** – for example, try to find parallels within your own culture to compare with statements you read about cultural patterns that you are unfamiliar with.

| How accurate is this information? | |
How useful is it in working with individual patients?	
Christians go to church on Sundays	Muslims pray five times a day
Catholics wear crucifixes	Sikhs wear turbans
Scotsmen wear kilts	Indian women wear saris
The British eat bacon and eggs	West Indians eat salt fish
Italians speak European	Punjabis speak Indian

- **Check anything you read about a particular culture with people you know from that background.** Talk to a cross-section of people so that you can build up a well rounded picture of the variety and range of views and lifestyles within that community.

Checklist: assessing cultural background information

- Is the material dealing with the culture of an entire society? Of a particular **social class** or **caste?** Of a particular **age group?** Of a particular **area of the country**? Of a small localised group, for example a **village** or an **extended family group?**
- **Is it made clear** what section of the population the information applies to?
- Does the information include broad or simplified **generalisations?**

  Analyse one or two examples. Are they at the level of:
- The British eat fish and chips (**a generalisation and not very useful**).
- Over 40 per cent of British families eat fish and chips, on average once a week (**a bit more specific but doesn't give much insight**).
- Most countries have their own variety of cheap fast food. The British version is traditionally fish and chips. Fish-and-chip shops are mainly located in working-class areas and provide a cheap and nutritious convenience food for the working-class population. Since the 1960s other foods have gained ground in the take-away market, notably Indian and Chinese food and more recently hamburgers, pizzas and pasta. (**A useful insight into the reasons for a particular 'custom', and how that custom is changing over time.**)
- Does the material describe cultural patterns that are **unfamiliar** to you?

  Analyse one or two examples.
- Does the writer simply **describe** patterns of behaviour?
- Are they described in a way which makes them seem **absurd** or **bizarre?**
- Does the writer discuss the underlying **reasons**, or suggest possible **explanations**, for unfamiliar patterns of behaviour?
- Is it clear whether the patterns described are **ideal** or **actual norms**? In other words, is the writer describing what people **say** they do, or what they **actually** do?
- Is culture seen as a **fixed** state or a **dynamic** phenomenon? Does the writer consider **changes that are taking place over time**, and **changes that occur when people move to another country**, or **come into contact with another social group**? Is this aspect discussed or ignored?
- Does the author make **value judgements** about the cultural patterns described? Does the author's attitude strike you as **positive? neutral? negative?**
- Does the information analyse the situation of minority cultural groups in Britain **purely** in terms of culture and cultural differences? Does it make any reference to important **economic and social factors** (for example, unemployment and racial discrimination?)
- What specifically have you gained from the information? **Has it confirmed or challenged cultural stereotypes?** Has it increased your understanding of the reasons why people believe what they do and act how they do? Or has it just described the surface without giving you any deeper insight into other people's way of life?

Notes

1. Sheiham, Helena and Quick, Alison, *The Rickets Report*, Haringey Community Health Council, 1981, p. 16, p. 34, p. 35.
2. Ballard, Catherine, 'Conflict, Continuity and Change', in Khan, V. (ed.), *Minority Families in Britain: Stress and Support*, Macmillan, 1979, p. 128.
3. Hall, E. T., *The Hidden Dimension: Man's Use of Space in Public and Private*, Bodley Head, 1966, p. 130.
4. Leininger, M., *Transcultural Nursing: Concepts Theories and Practices*, Wiley Medical, 1978, pp. 268–269.

More information

For more information about cultural variation and the need to develop health care that is appropriate, acceptable and effective, see:

5 **Communication**

6 **Working with families and individuals**

7 **Health beliefs and practices**
8 **Foods and diets**

Health education and rickets and osteomalacia, see
 9.5 **Rickets and osteomalacia**
13.2 **Health education and ethnic minority communities**

Professional training, see
12 **Health worker training and professional values**

Finding out more about local communities, see
14 **Local needs: guidelines for doing your own research**

For sources of more information about particular cultural differences, see
15 **Sources and resources**

Further reading

54

5 Communication

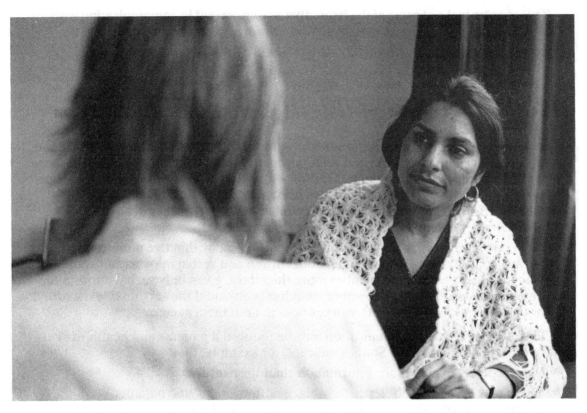

Introduction

Health workers and others are increasingly aware of the importance of communication in health care: most health worker training now includes some practical work on communication skills. There are more and more in-service training courses on communication and related topics. It is also becoming recognised that health workers may need to learn special skills to ensure effective two-way communication across barriers of language and culture.

This chapter looks at some of the issues that are important in communicating with ethnic minority patients and suggests ways of improving communication across the language barrier.

5.1 Health worker–patient communication

Several recent British research studies have looked at gaps in health worker–patient communication and have suggested ways in which it could be improved. Most of these suggestions apply equally to communication with patients whose first language is not English. **The way in which health workers present advice or instructions has a significant effect on how much patients remember and whether they act on the information they receive.** Research evidence[1] suggests that:

- Most patients forget 50 per cent of what their GP said within five minutes of a normal consultation. Patients given both written and verbal information about diagnosis and treatment remember more than those given only verbal information. Patients are less likely to remember what has been said if they are anxious, worried or under stress, and the health worker does not put them at ease.

The effectiveness of communication may be reduced if patients and health workers have different expectations. Studies indicate, for example, that:

- Most patients expect more information than they receive.
- There may be a wide difference between health workers' and patients' interpretation of common medical terms. Health workers may confuse patients if they use jargon and technical terms.
- Patients often have different views from health workers about the importance of health risks, the inevitability of disease, and the desirability of certain treatments.

Middle-class patients are more likely than working-class patients to communicate effectively with middle-class health professionals.

The greater the gap in terms of class, experience, background and expectation, the more likely communication is to be difficult, and the greater the responsibility of the professional health worker to take action to overcome this.

5.2 Communication difficulties for ethnic minority patients

It is often assumed that there are no communication problems between health workers and British-born ethnic minority clients, since both parties speak fluent English. However, this is not necessarily true. Problems may arise because of differences in:

Class

Ethnic minorities are concentrated particularly in unskilled and semi-skilled jobs and are therefore likely to experience the same problems in communicating with middle-class professionals as other working-class people.

Expectations and culture

There may be major gaps in terms of experience, culture and expectations between client and professional. Although neither party may be aware of these differences at a conscious level, they can easily give rise to misunderstandings on both sides, for example, about what is being agreed, and about the attitudes and intentions of the speakers.

Because I wear western clothes and speak with a Birmingham accent everybody assumes I must think and feel like an English woman too. But I don't. A lot of my attitudes and beliefs are Indian. I agree with my parents on a lot of things, moral issues particularly. And the way I behave is much more like an Indian woman than an English woman. But they assume that I think and behave just as they would. They don't really understand me. Sometimes I feel we just talk past each other.

Young Asian woman

*Whenever I go to see someone new at that office to try and sort out my housing situation the first question they ask me is 'When did you come to this country?' Now I don't know why they keep asking this, I've been here 25 years now and I'd like to feel that I belong here. It doesn't make any difference to this housing problem I've got now. Maybe they don't know what else to say, so they ask that. But every time it's like a slap in the face you know. Every time I think, Oh hell they're never going to accept me, or any of us. My kids were born here and **they** get asked that. I don't know why, but every time I feel just full of hopelessness. I look across the desk at them and I think, how would you feel if every time you were in a mess or needed help somebody just asked a suspicious question first? In a country where you know how most people feel about you. I don't think they have any idea what that question always does to me. It makes me feel they don't **want** to help.*

Afro-Caribbean man

Health workers and patients may have different beliefs about, for example, what causes illness or pain, what behaviour is appropriate in response to pain or stress, and about what can be discussed with whom.

The more expectations differ, the greater the risk of misunderstandings and the greater the need for professionals to step back and question their own assumptions, as in the examples below.

- **Beliefs about causes of illness and pain.** For example, the French equivalent to an 'upset tummy' is *"crise de foie'* (liver trouble). Would a British health worker recognise it as the same problem?

- **Variations in patterns of illness between ethnic groups.** For example, an Asian woman suffering from osteomalacia might complain of aching bones. Would her symptoms be recognised for what they are?

- **Beliefs about effective remedies**. In a number of third world countries injections are believed to be the most effective form of medication. The French and Italians believe that suppositories are most effective. The British prefer to take their medicines orally. If a Vietnamese patient was unwilling to take tablets and kept asking for an injection, would his concern be understood? Should the health worker try, as far as possible, to provide medication in the form the patient wants?

- **Conventions about what can be discussed with strangers.** For example, in some communities, it is not generally acceptable to discuss personal, emotional and psychological problems with strangers even if they are professionals. How useful is it to refer a Chinese patient with this traditional viewpoint for psychiatric consultation?

- **Conventions about what can be discussed between men and women.** For example, an Asian woman might find it unacceptable to consult her male GP over a gynaecological problem or to have to use her husband as an interpreter on this kind of matter. What alternative provision could she be offered?

- **Responses to pain.** For example, the traditional British response to pain is the 'stiff upper lip'. There is a common misconception that certain ethnic groups 'have a lower pain threshold', but there is no scientific basis for this belief. People from different cultures respond in different ways to pain, and have different ways of coping with it, but this does not diminish their need for sympathy or support.[2] It may in fact increase it. How should the health worker respond to patients who express pain more openly?

Racial prejudice

Communication can also be affected by conscious or unconscious racial prejudice. A well intentioned and sympathetic doctor or nurse may still have stereotyped or prejudiced expectations of certain groups of patients. These can become a major barrier to communication. The health worker too easily sees and hears what she expects to see and hear; the patient cannot get his real self or wishes into the picture at all. Misjudgements are inevitable. How should conscious or unconscious prejudice be tackled?

5.3 Forms of English spoken in the Afro-Caribbean community

Many health workers do not understand the differences between the English spoken in the West Indies and 'standard' British English. They may not be aware that **Afro-Caribbeans in Britain may speak different forms of English depending, for example, on age, class, experience and personal choice.**

- Some people speak Creole or patois, but tend to use it only within their own community. (Some linguists consider Caribbean-forms of patois to be a dialect form of language; others consider them to be languages in their own right. The type of patois spoken in the Caribbean varies from island to island. The main influence may be French, Spanish or English depending on which was the dominant power in the colonial period.)

- Many younger black British people are developing a style known as 'Black English' or British Jamaican (based on Creole).

- Others speak mainly in the local or regional British dialect.

Most people use more than one of these forms, choosing the style to suit the occasion.[3] A very few, but especially some of the older generation and new arrivals, speak exclusively in Creole. They may have particular difficulty in communicating with health workers who expect them to use standard English.

5.4 Communication difficulties for people whose mother tongue is not English

People who did not grow up speaking English face the greatest and most obvious communication problems with English-speaking health workers. In addition, people who speak little English are often confronted with intolerance, blame, hostility or insults.

Yes, I know a few don't speak English, but the more intelligent ones do, don't they?

General practitioner

Recent estimates state that there are over 200,000 adults resident in Britain who speak English only slightly or not at all. The majority of these are of Asian origin, but there are also substantial numbers from Cyprus, southern Europe, North Africa, and south-east Asian countries.[4]

The table shows what percentage of men and women of Pakistani, Indian and East African Asian origin spoke English fluently, fairly well, slightly or not at all in a study published in 1976. (The figures for those of Pakistani origin include a small proportion of people of Bangladeshi origin as well.)

Ability to speak English in minority communities, 1976[4]

Percentage who speak English	Pakistani		Indian		E.A. Asian	
	men %	women %	men %	women %	men %	women %
Fluently	28	8	43	22	56	33
Fairly well	29	11	28	15	21	34
Slightly	35	36	19	36	14	22
Not at all	8	41	7	24	5	19
Not stated	1	2	4	3	3	1

Many health authorities and individual health workers take the view that all communication difficulties would be resolved if everybody learnt to speak English. This is based on the assumption that it is possible for every individual to do so. There are many reasons which make it impossible or impracticable for people to learn English.

There's a lot of blame attached to people who can't speak English, and of course it is very very frustrating for health workers. They can't do their job properly and the reason is the patient's inability to speak English. But sometimes I feel that if they themselves had ever tried to learn another language, as adults I mean, or if they'd ever taught English and seen what hard work it is to learn a foreign language, they might be a little more tolerant. After all, let's face it, the person who really suffers is the patient who can't speak English. And if they could they would. So many of my students really try but find it very difficult. And the dice are loaded against them in learning terms: many of them have never had the chance to go to school before, they have small children who take up all their time and energy, they have homes to run; they get too tired to think let alone learn, they don't most of them know any English people who'll give them the time they need to have even a little conversation, a little positive feedback on what they're learning, they face hostility, they get laughed at or sworn at or shouted at because they don't speak English. None of that is likely to help them learn, is it? It's a vicious circle really. And I don't think blaming people helps. They get enough hostility without getting it from people who are supposed to be caring for them. As I said, they would if they could.

Teacher of English as a Second Language

The Commission for Racial Equality suggests that there will be a sizeable non-English-speaking population in Britain for the next 30 or 40 years.[5] The reasons for this were analysed in a survey carried out between 1972 and 1975 by Political and Economic Planning (PEP).[4] The survey found that:

- **When migration took place in the 1950s and 60s there was no English language programme** to provide non-English-speaking immigrants with the language skills they needed to help them settle in Britain.

- **Existing language training schemes only reach a small number of people.** In many areas there are one- or two-year student waiting lists for language classes, and no finance available to expand provision.

- **Younger people are likely to be more fluent than older people.** Even so, the PEP Report found that a quarter of the Asian population aged 16–24 spoke English slightly or not at all.

- **It is the older generation that faces the greatest language difficulties.** People who came to Britain after young adulthood tend to have the most limited English. In 1976 two-thirds of the Asian population aged 45 or over spoke English only slightly or not at all (see table above).

- **Short exposure to English as a young person is far more effective than a longer exposure when older.** Non-English speakers do not necessarily become more fluent in English the longer they spend in Britain. Those people who came to Britain as young adults in the 1950s and 60s but received no language training at that time, and those who came in middle age are never now likely to achieve real fluency in English, even if there were suitable classes available.

- **People living in areas where their own community is well established are less likely to be fluent in English** than those who live in mainly white areas. There is a clear link between language ability, occupational status and area of residence. For example, the PEP Report found that Asians with limited English tend to do manual jobs and live in areas of high Asian concentration. Whatever the starting point in this chain of relationships, the correlation suggests a closed circle of disadvantage for non-English speakers from which it is difficult to escape.

Other factors which can make it difficult for someone to learn a foreign language are:

- Lack of contact with English speakers.
- Lack of educational opportunity in the past.
- Lack of confidence.
- Age.
- Availability of English-speaking relatives and friends.

Lack of contact with English speakers

Non-English-speaking members of minority groups often have little or no social contact with native English speakers, largely because they are **not often readily welcomed in** English-speaking social circles.

An Asian woman came to my parentcraft classes last year and she could speak a little English but the other women in the class didn't make her feel at all welcome – they made comments in front of her and things – she only came twice.

Community midwife

Lack of educational opportunity in the past

Some non-English speakers who have come to Britain from a rural background have had only limited schooling. They are not likely to have the study skills that make it easier to learn a language. They often lack the confidence to attend formal education establishments. If they do attend, the teaching materials and methods used may be unsuitable. Most English teaching materials are written for people with a European education and background.

Lack of confidence, fear of not being understood

Many people are shy, embarrassed or nervous about trying to express themselves in a foreign language, especially in formal situations and in contact with 'official' people.

Quite a lot of the women who come in here do speak a little English, just please and thank you and good morning and so on. But when they get here they are so nervous and unsure of themselves that they daren't open their mouths. They say they are worried that people will laugh at them or that they will get the words all muddled up. So they feel less conspicuous and safe if they don't say anything.

Hospital interpreter

Age

People's ability to learn a new language generally decreases dramatically after puberty and continues to decrease.

We run English classes for older women twice a week here. In fact they act mainly as a social forum. Most of the older women just can't get their tongues round the new sounds. And what they painstakingly learn one week they've forgotten the next.

English teacher

My family came to England just after the War. I was eleven, my brother was nine. Neither of us spoke any English. He now speaks fluent accentless English. Mine is fluent but I've still got quite a strong Polish accent.

Polish man

Availability of English-speaking relatives and friends

When you know you are not very good at something difficult it is natural to ask someone who is good at it to do it for you. People who know that their English is not good often rely on more fluent friends and relatives to speak for them on important matters.

My husband goes out to work so he speaks English much better than me. I speak very little English and I am very shy about it. So when I have to go anywhere I always try to take him with me and he can do all the talking. I would feel a fool speaking my bad English when he can say the things so much more clearly for me. Especially when it's really important and the people are so busy and in such a hurry always.

Punjabi woman

5.5 *How the message is put across*

The way in which a message is put across crucially influences how well it is understood, particularly when health worker and patient come from different cultures and so may interpret tone of voice and non-verbal signals differently.

Non-verbal signals

Health worker and patient may misinterpret each other's intentions if the non-verbal signals they use are based on different conventions. For example there may be differences in the meaning people attach to:

- **eye contact or lack of it**
- **facial expressions**
- **head and body movements**
- **gestures**
- **touch**
- **physical distance from the other speaker**

In some cultures, looking people in the eye indicates honesty and straightforwardness, in others it is seen as challenging and rude.

At one point I was working as an interpreter in a reception centre. I used to translate during medical check ups. Once the doctor asked me, 'Why won't some people look me in the eye? Are they afraid of doctors?' It was difficult to explain to her that for our people it's just being respectful, looking down. I think she wanted me to tell people to stop doing it because it irritated her, but I felt it would have made things worse – people would get very embarrassed because they would think it was rude not to look down if it was their way of showing respect.

Vietnamese interpreter

In some cultures 'yes' is indicated by nodding the head, in others by shaking it. Movements and gestures such as shrugging the shoulders, tossing back the head or making a fist can have very different meanings. In some cultures it is unacceptable for members of the same sex to touch each other in public; in others it is unacceptable for members of the opposite sex to do so. Comfortable physical distance between speakers varies in different cultures, as does the degree of eye contact acceptable at different distances. All these conventions are culture-bound and largely unconscious. It is important to beware of making inappropriate judgements about personality or intentions on the basis of them. If possible, always check out any judgements you make with the person concerned or with other people from his/her community.

Conventions of courtesy

Words and gestures associated with politeness and good manners also vary from culture to culture. Each culture and society has certain rules of polite behaviour. Children are taught these while they are still very young. In Britain, for example, the words 'please' and 'thank you' are extremely important.

I've noticed with my son how automatically I teach him to say please and thank you. If he asks for something I always add please, and so on. I started that even when he could hardly talk. And I notice, he's four now, that when we go shopping or on a bus or something, if he talks to anyone and forgets to say please and thank you they always say it for him. It's obviously terribly important for English people. And people get terribly insulted if please and thank you aren't said.

English mother

In many Asian languages, the words please and thank you are not normally used except on very formal occasions. **Gratitude and polite requests** are expressed in other ways, for example by a range of polite and familiar verb forms (not unlike 'tu' and 'vous' in French), and forms of address. This makes 'please' and 'thankyou' unnecessary redundancies. Such differences can lead to misunderstanding and resentment. People who speak English as their second language may unintentionally give the impression of being abrupt or rude because they don't use please and thank you so much. In turn, they themselves may see the liberal sprinkling of 'please' and 'thank you' as rather superficial and meaningless formalities, compared with the richness of their own language.

My mother speaks Hindi. Her English isn't very good but she can follow what we're saying O.K. She thinks that compared with Hindi, English is full of politenesses that don't mean anything . . . 'please' . . . 'thank you' . . . 'sorry'. . . . When we did something wrong as kids and said 'sorry' in English, she would reply in English, 'don't say sorry, say apologise'. As she pointed out to us, people will barge past you in a queue and then turn round and say 'sorry' and it's absolutely meaningless . . . they don't really mean it at all.'

British-born Indian woman

Different cultures and societies also have different norms about, for example, **meetings, greetings, farewells**, how you show that people are welcome and so on. Failing to observe these can give real offence.

When I did my holiday job in Germany I had to shake hands with everyone in my department every morning and evening. There were about eight of us in the department, and every morning and evening we all shook hands with each other and said good morning or goodbye. If I hadn't done it they would have thought I was very unfriendly and off-hand. It wasn't a stilted gesture; I came to regard it as a sign of friendship and harmony towards my colleagues.

English engineer

When I visit Asian households I always feel it's very important to accept the cup of tea I'm offered. I don't know why it is, I just feel in my bones that it matters, that even with those families where people don't speak much English and I can't really talk to them, if I didn't stay for that cup of tea they'd be really hurt and upset.

English community midwife

Paralinguistic features

In addition to physical signals, every language has its own set of unconscious linguistic conventions which speakers use to signal their meaning and to understand what other people mean. These conventions are sometimes referred to as **paralinguistic** or **non-verbal** aspects of speech. They include variations in:

- **tone of voice**
- **pitch**
- **stress**
- **speed**
- **loudness**
- **rhythm**

When we speak, all these elements combine to contribute to the overall shape and sense of what is said. We use them, for example, to emphasise a point; to indicate logical connections between pieces of information; to correct or contradict; to imply what is not specifically stated, and to convey our overall emotion or attitude.

To see how they work, try saying this sentence, **'This patient says he's been waiting for an hour'** in three different ways:

- **as a straight statement**
- **as a question**
- **indicating that you don't believe him**

Try how many more ways you can say the same sentence with slightly different meanings and implications. Listen to the way you do it. In English we can indicate a good deal more than the bare meaning of the words, and particularly a good deal more about our own attitudes, views and feelings, by changing our tone of voice, stress, loudness, pitch and so on.

Different languages use these kinds of conventions in different ways to convey attitude and meaning. They are as important a part of language as words and grammar. English, for example, uses stress to signal emphasis or new information, e.g. 'Did *he* change the baby's nappy?' 'We saw a *blue* doubledecker bus in London today!' Speakers of other languages may not recognise that stress is signalling a special meaning or may use stress to signal something different.

In some languages an increase in normal speed may be used for emphasis; in some languages, including English, emphasis is indicated by slowing down.

Each language also has its own natural intonation or 'tune'. Raising the voice in English may be associated with intense emotion, such as anger or excitement; in other languages it may be used simply to emphasise or to contradict.

This is why speakers of English often stereotype Italians or Spaniards as excitable or overemotional; intonation that indicates normal speech in Italian or Spanish if used by English people would show great excitement or emotion. Germans may be thought heavy and pedantic by native speakers of English. Again, the intonation of normal German speech would, if used by an English speaker, indicate a ponderous rather heavy train of thought.

In general the differences in the 'tunes' and other paralinguistic features increases the further apart the languages are. Western European languages are fairly similar. Northern Indian languages often have different paralinguistic features from Western European languages.

The paralinguistic features of a new language are the most difficult thing to learn. People almost always carry over the intonation of their mother tongue, and may never master the new intonation fully. People who have learnt English as a second language and speak it fluently may retain an intonation which to the native English ear sounds odd, irritating, abrupt or even rude.

If someone who speaks English as a second language seems abrupt or rude consider whether it is likely that they intend to be before reacting as if they are. Unfortunately one's reactions to what seems like rudeness, aggressiveness or abruptness are almost automatic; it is difficult not to become angry and hostile in response. In most cases, however, people who speak English as their second language do not intend to be rude or seem impolitely demanding, particularly when they are in the position of patients. If you can, try to suspend judgement and presume that people who depend on you for service are unlikely to wish to anger or alienate you. It is far more likely that they are not aware of and perhaps cannot help the impression they are giving.

The unpopular patient

A study published by the Royal College of Nursing called The Unpopular Patient *looked at factors that might influence nurses' enjoyment or lack of enjoyment in caring for particular patients.*

Nurses felt that the patient's personality was the most significant factor. In describing people they enjoyed caring for, most nurses referred to patients being fun, having a good sense of humour, being easy to get on with, and friendly. Some preferences related to how well nurses knew the patient, but actual nursing needs had little influence on popularity.

The study summarised the characteristics of the most popular patients:

- *they were able to communicate readily with nurses;*
- *they knew the nurses' names;*
- *they were able to joke and laugh with the nurses;*
- *they co-operated in being helped to get well, and expressed determination to do so.*

63

It was found that foreign patients tended to be more unpopular with nurses than UK patients, perhaps because foreign or non-English-speaking patients lack the characteristics of the popular patient. They cannot communicate fluently, they do not therefore get to know nurses and they cannot join in jokes and verbal banter on the ward. This suggests that nurses may in certain cases wrongly interpret a patient's behaviour and attitude as indicators of an 'awkward' personality, when they are in fact due to language difficulties and lack of confidence.[6]

5.6 Practical action: improving communication across a language barrier[7]

There are five main practical ways in which health workers can improve communication with people who speak little or no English or who speak English as a second language:

- **reducing stress**
- **simplifying your English**
- **checking back properly**
- **using a qualified interpreter**
- **learning the client's language**

Reducing stress

Emotional and physical stress have a clear effect on language ability, even in one's first language. For second language speakers this effect is much more marked; even people who normally speak fairly good English often find that it disappears when they are ill, worried, frightened or tense. In order to enable the best possible communication, try to reduce the stress on the client as much as possible. Here are some suggestions:

- **Allow more time than you would for an English-speaking client.** Even if time is short, try not to look at your watch or show other signs of impatience. That will only increase the stress on your patient and reduce even further the amount you get out of the short time available to you.

    If you really are short of time it may be helpful to say so at the beginning and to tell the patient when you can see him again at more leisure.

    Do not expect patients from other ethnic groups always to pick up what you think are very obvious signals that, for example, you are in a hurry or that you think the consultation is over, e.g. giving the patient a prescription or standing up to say goodbye. Non-verbal signals vary from culture to culture; people under stress do not always pick up the signals other people are sending. If you have something important to say try to say it directly, though sensitively, rather than hoping the patient will pick it up.

- **Give plenty of non-verbal reassurance.** If the patient doesn't understand verbal reassurances you need to make much more use of non-verbal signals – smile, touch where appropriate, gestures of encouragement, and a sympathetic manner.

    People who are nervous about their ability to cope with a difficult situation may be extremely sensitive to signs of irritation, tension, etc. Try to avoid making someone nervous of you even before they meet you:

When I go somewhere where I have to queue, you know, like the post office or something, I always look at the people behind the counter to see who looks friendly. Because my English is not very good and some people get very impatient and even sometimes rude when you do not understand them the first time or when they do not understand you. Sometimes I stand in one queue and then if I think someone else is more friendly I go to another queue and start again. But it always makes me very nervous to think what will happen when I come to the front of the queue and have to ask for what I need.

Gujarati woman

- **Try to communicate some information about what's going to happen next even at a very simple level.** NEVER maintain total silence or give the impression of ignoring the patient.

I've noticed that some of the doctors do internal examinations in complete silence, particularly, though not only, if a woman doesn't speak much English. And the tension, it's terrible, you could cut it with a knife. The woman lies there feeling humiliated and nervous and nobody says anything, you don't hear a sound except the instruments and breathing, and the longer the silence goes on the worse the tension gets. Which of course makes it much worse for the woman. I try to keep talking, just to have the sound of a voice, even if I know the woman doesn't understand much English I say a few words, tell her it won't be long now, ask her if she's OK, just to show a bit of common humanity really. Sometimes I hold her hand. Of course it's difficult with some doctors, they think I'm stepping out of my place.

Family planning nurse

If the patient has to undergo an uncomfortable or embarrassing procedure, it is essential (and only fair) to give some warning, by making a simple drawing or using mime if no other means are available.

- **Get the patient's name right.** There is often confusion in recording names of patients from different cultural backgrounds. This can cause delay and frustration when records can't be found, and being continually misaddressed can be irritating and upsetting. Find out about the naming systems of ethnic minority patients and make sure the patient's name is down correctly and in full. The name that the patient uses himself may be different from the 'official' name on records. Make a note of it and address him by the name that he recognises.

- **Try also to pronounce the patient's name correctly.** To have one's name consistently mispronounced can be both irritating and depersonalising. If the way a patient says his name sounds very different from the spelling, make a note of the correct pronunciation and stress in brackets beside the name.

Razia Begum	(razia baygum)
Harbans Kaur	(harbans kor)
Erol Tuncay	(erol tunjay)
Lew Sapieha	(lef sapiayha)
Nguyen Thi Hoa	(new-en tee hwa)

In one of the ante-natal clinics where I work they call out the women's names from the files and if the women don't come forward after the second call, they put the file right back to the bottom of the pile. And quite often the way they pronounce the names is completely unrecognisable, and so the women don't go forward and they may wait hours and hours never realising that their names have been called several times.

Clinic worker

- **Keep fuller case notes. This avoids subjecting the patient to repeated unnecessary or complicated questioning.** Repeated questioning by different people going over the same ground can be a nerve-racking and demoralising experience for someone struggling to communicate in English.

- **Try and ensure that the patient sees the same staff as far as possible.** The difficulties of developing a relationship with a patient are more acute when there is a language problem. Getting to know particular members of staff helps to reduce stress and means that communication becomes easier for the patient, who doesn't have to keep re-explaining his situation to strangers.

- **Try and find out whether the patient has any specific fears or worries.** English-speaking relatives or friends may also be able to tell you whether the patient has any particular worries. If the patient is staying in hospital, suggest that an English-speaking relative writes down during visiting time any questions that he wants to ask the doctor.

- **Write down any important points clearly and simply on a piece of paper for the patient to take away.** Under stress, any patient may become so distracted that he can't listen to what is being said to him. Written information to take away helps the patient recall verbal instructions or advice. If someone cannot read it for himself, he will probably be able to find a friend or relative who can.

Simplifying your English

These suggestions should, of course, all be used judiciously. A fluent English speaker would be insulted if addressed in slow and simple sentences. Be aware of what each patient knows, doesn't know, or has learnt, and adapt your language accordingly. The first three points, and the last three, apply to all your conversations.

- **Speak clearly but do not raise your voice.** Talking loudly to a non-English speaker as if he were deaf is a natural reaction, but it is very disconcerting for the listener.

- **Speak slowly throughout.** Try not to speed up as you get more involved in your subject.

- **Repeat when you have not been understood.** If you have said something as simply as possible and it has not been understood – try repeating the *same* sentence again. Don't change the words. If you do, you are giving the patient a whole new task. If you repeat the words you used the first time, they may begin to make sense.

- **Use the words the patient is likely to know.** If there are several words which mean the same, use the simplest and most common: 'start' and 'finish', not 'commence' and 'terminate'. Try to avoid using words that are, for example, used only in connection with health. It is all too easy to slip into jargon without being aware of it. Pick up and use the words the patient uses himself, that way you can be sure you are using familiar language.

- **Be careful of idioms.** The meaning may not be at all clear to your patient: don't say 'fed up', 'start from scratch', 'spend a penny', 'red tape'.

- **Simplify the form of each sentence.** Every language has different ways of saying more or less the same thing. For example, there are many ways of asking somebody to bring some water.

  > Can you find me some water please?
  > Would you mind getting some water?
  > Could you possibly bring me some water?
  > Would you mind me asking you to bring me some water?
  > Have you got some water I could use?
  > I'd like some water please.
  > I think I'll need some water.
  > Could I have some water please?
  > Fetch me some water please.
  > I shall need some water.
  > Will you fetch me some water please?
  > Pop out and get me some water, could you?
  > Etc., etc.

  For somebody who is learning English, these different forms are unnecessarily complicated and difficult. Choose simple forms and use them consistently. This is easier to understand and will provide the patient with a good clear model to copy.

- **Use the simple forms of verbs: active, not passive.** 'The doctor will give you a blood test', not 'You will be given a blood test by the doctor.'

- **Don't speak pidgin English.** It does not help people to learn to speak English properly, it is not easier to understand and it can sound condescending. 'You should go to the doctor on Monday' said slowly with emphasis on the important words is no more difficult to understand, and is far less ambiguous than, 'You doctor Monday.'

- **Give instructions in a clear, logical sequence.** Even if the patient does not understand the words 'first' and 'then', he is likely to do things in the correct order if that is the order in which he heard them. Say 'First sterilise the bottle. Then rinse it.'

  Do not say: 'Rinse the bottle after you sterilise it',
  or 'Don't rinse the bottle until you have sterilised it',

or 'Before you rinse the bottle, sterilise it.'
The words, 'before', 'after', 'until', which indicate the order in which to do things, are fairly complicated and are often misunderstood.

- **Simplify the total structure of what you want to say in your mind before you begin.**
  If you are giving instructions or explaining something, break your topic down into clear, logical stages before you start. Don't try to simplify it as you go along, but look at what you want to explain and work it out clearly and simply in your own mind before you begin.

  Simplifying is not the same as condensing. If you condense what you say, you make it *more dense* and often more difficult to understand. You avoid the natural repetition which we all use to help us follow a conversation. **A longer simplified explanation is easier to follow than a condensed one.**

- **Stick to one topic at a time.** Pause between topics, check that you have been understood, and signal clearly that you are moving on to a new topic.
  'Now I want to ask you about . . .'
  If you keep consistently to this form your patient will soon understand what you are doing.

- **Be careful when you use examples.** People may become confused between your example, which you think is helpful, and what you are actually trying to convey.

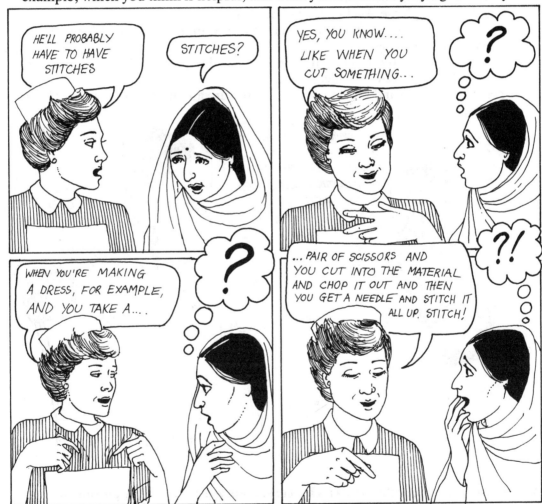

- **Use pictures or clear mime to help to get the meaning across.** When you find there are words that you often have difficulty with, cut out or draw some clear explanatory pictures and stick them on cards. Bring them out whenever you need them. For example, a cardboard clock face with moving hands can show time; simple and clear pictures of male and female bodies can be used for showing where it hurts. Many excellent pictures and models can be found in toy shops. Note that photographs or realistic drawings are easier to understand than signs and symbols. Having a picture to look at or something to handle may also help to ease the tension of a difficult conversation.

- **Judge how much people are likely to remember.** The effort of concentrating in order to understand can affect the memory very badly. Even people with no language problem only remember one or two points from each session. It may be useful to leave a simple note for the patient to read after you have left.
- **Be aware of your language all the time.** Listen to yourself speaking and judge whether what you are saying is as clear as you can make it.

Checking back properly

Develop a regular pattern of checking that what you have said so far has been understood. Do not move on to another point until you have checked that the earlier point has got through. If it is clear that the patient does not understand even at an early stage, stop and reconsider. There may be no point in ploughing on. You may need to revise your plans for this conversation or to go and find an interpreter.

There are various simple ways of checking back.

- **Try not to ask 'Do you understand?' or 'Is that all right?' You are almost bound to get 'yes' for an answer.** 'Yes' is often the first word one learns in a foreign language, and can very easily mean:

    Yes, I'm listening but I don't understand.
    Yes, I'm listening but I don't agree.
    Yes, I want to please you but really I don't agree.
    Yes, I know you want an answer and I want to help, even though I haven't a clue what you're talking about.
    Yes, I'm listening but I'm too tired and confused to take in what you're saying even though I know you mean well.
    Yes, I'm listening and I feel under great pressure and if I say 'yes' you might go away.

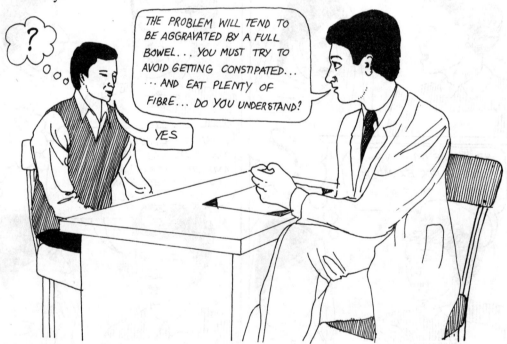

- **Try also to avoid questions to which a correct answer is 'Yes'.** Try putting the question differently. For example, phrase the question so that the correct or required answer is 'No'. There is a good chance that the person who answers 'No' has understood the question.
- **Ask the patient to explain back to you what he is going to do.** If the instructions are complicated, ask several simple questions rather than one long one. Don't accept a (possibly uncomprehending) repetition of what you have just said.

The following eight extracts are from conversations between a health worker and a mother with a young baby. In which of these has the health worker checked that the mother understands?

CHECKING BACK

1   Health worker   *Do you drink a lot of milk?*
     Patient   *Milk, yes.*
     Health worker   *Good.*

2   Health worker   *Is baby eating any solids yet?*
     Patient   *Yes.*
     Health worker   *That's nice.*

3   Health worker   *Take one of these pills after breakfast and one before you go to bed. Do you understand?*
     Patient   *Yes.*

4   Health worker   *Get baby weighed first and then go to see the doctor. Then come to see me. Now what are you going to do?*
     Patient   *Baby weighed.*
     Health worker   *Yes, and then what?*
     Patient   *Go and see doctor.*
     Health worker   *And then what?*
     Patient   *See you.*

5   Health worker   *Is baby still vomiting?*
     Patient   *No.*
     Health worker   *Has he been sick again?*
     Patient   *No.*

6   Health worker   *Does baby have tins? Baby tins?*
     Patient   *Baby tins.*
     Health worker   *Well I think that should be all right for him at the moment.*

7   Health worker   *You're giving him oranges are you? Good. Plenty of fruit juice? Fruit juice? Good. And he's getting his milk OK?*
     Patient   *Yes.*
     Health worker   *Good. Well he's a fine little boy isn't he?*
     Patient   *Yes.*

8   Health worker   *Are you taking any pain killers – aspirin, Panadol, Hedex or something?*
     Patient   *Aspirin.*
     Health worker   *Well that should take the pain away.*

Answers:
1 Not checked – mother may be merely repeating the word 'milk'.
2 Not checked – 'yes' doesn't necessarily indicate a positive reply.
3 Not checked.
4 Checked – mother is asked to repeat the instruction.
5 Checked – the answer 'no' to both questions indicates that the mother has understood.
6 Not checked – 'baby tins' may be just repetition.
7 Not checked.
8 Not checked – 'Aspirin' may be the only one the mother has heard of, or may be just repetition.

Using a qualified interpreter

Where people do not speak very much English you will have to use an interpreter to ensure that they receive good health care and that they fully understand what is happening and any choices they have to make. It may also be necessary to use an interpreter with patients whose general English is fairly good but who do not know the specialised words used, for example, in an ante-natal clinic or a surgery, and with people whose English is badly affected by the stress of the situation. A good deal of energy and concentration are required to sustain any kind of conversation in a foreign language; people who normally speak some English may find the effort too great when they are ill, or may tire and lose concentration very quickly. Interpreters may also be invaluable in interpreting cultural differences and explaining whether, for example, a course of action suggested by a health worker is likely to be acceptable, or suggesting alternatives.

Using an interpreter is not simple. A poor interpreter may cause more problems than he or she solves. It is hardly ever acceptable to use children to interpret for their parents.

Under no circumstances should children be expected to interpret medical details for their parents. This practice is unsatisfactory, unprofessional, unethical, uncivilised, and ought to be totally unacceptable. Consultant psychiatrist[8]

I have seen what happens when children are used to interpret for their parents. In some cases it totally distorts the family relationships. Children get power and knowledge they should never have over their parents. Parents have to rely on their children, they are helpless, powerless; the children may use, I mean misuse, their power.
Portuguese interpreter

They think we don't mind. Of course we do. And of course we would very much like the hospital to provide someone who could interpret for us. There are many things my son should not know at his age and they ask him all these questions to ask me and explain to him all these things. And he knows I am embarrassed, and of course some of the things I cannot tell him, even if I think they are really important, like some pains that I get, or bleeding. But I am not going to tell a boy of his age: I am worried about how all this will affect him later. But what else can I do when it is left up to me?
Cypriot woman

A husband or wife may also be undesirable as an interpreter. Patients may not wish to tell their spouses everything that they wish to tell the health worker. There is also the danger that an adult family member will not translate directly but will be reticent about some things, add an explanation, or put his or her own interpretation on the facts.

Using a member of the family for anything beyond the translation of simple factual questions or instructions can be unreliable and upsetting. In the same way the use of unqualified interpreters, however well-meaning, can cause major problems for both health worker and patient. Where it is possible to predict that they will be needed regularly, qualified interpreters should be employed to improve the service offered to patients who speak little or no English, to save the time and increase the effectiveness of professional health workers.

This is nonsense. Every time I see a patient who doesn't speak English I have to spend three or four times as long with her as with my other patients. And I don't really achieve anything. It can't cost more to employ a competent interpreter than to waste my time like this.
Hospital doctor

Points to think about when using an interpreter

- **Have you checked that the patient and the interpreter speak the same language?** If there are dialect variations, do they speak the same dialect?

- **Have you checked that the interpreter is really fluent in the patient's language?** You may be able to do this by getting someone else who speaks both languages to listen to the interpreter at work.

If it seems that the interpreter does not understand the patient or is not interpreting exactly, it is important to find out why. You may need to find another interpreter.

- **Is there any reason why the patient might be embarrassed by the interpreter?** For example, a patient may accept a health worker of the opposite sex because professional status is respected. But the interpreter should be of the same sex as the patient, and is more likely to be accepted if he or she is older and married.

  If the patient is embarrassed, what can you do to make things better?

- **Might the patient be prevented from telling you certain things because of his relationship with the interpreter?**

  The patient will not answer all your questions truthfully if he does not trust the interpreter. Be careful whom you use to interpret anything that the patient would not want widely known. Would you, for example, want to communicate intimate, personal details about yourself through your next door neighbours?

- **Is there any reason why the interpreter might be reluctant to interpret everything the patient says? Or might worry about your reaction? How can you prevent this?**

  The interpreter may come from a background very different from that of the patient. She may feel ashamed of the patient's behaviour, and embarrassed about her own culture as a result. This can affect the translation you get.

  An interpreter is also likely to react in this way if you show impatience, or if you treat her – because she, too, is a member of a minority group – as in some way responsible for how a particular patient behaves.

  The interpreter may become defensive and try to hide things about the patient or about her culture if she thinks you will disapprove, or she may distance herself from the patient and be chiefly concerned to show you that she does not share the attitudes of such people. In either case, communication between you and your patient is disastrously affected.

- **What can you do to help the interpreter develop a good working relationship with the patient?**

  Introduce the interpreter. Give her time to talk briefly to the patient and explain her background, before she starts interpreting. She may like to reassure the patient about her trustworthiness. She may wish to remind the patient to speak slowly and to allow time for the translation.

- **Are you communicating directly with the patient as much as possible? Are you making as much use as you can of whatever English he speaks or understands?**

  Most people understand more of a foreign language than they can speak. You may be able to speak directly to some patients who do not speak very much English, and only use the interpreter to translate whenever the patient does not fully understand. The patient may also be able to check that what the interpreter translates back to you is completely accurate.

  Speak directly to the patient as much as possible. Look at the patient and not at the interpreter when you are speaking, even if the patient cannot understand you. Sit facing the patient.

  If the patient does not understand very much English, express your sympathies for him through the interpreter, just as you would if you could communicate directly. When the interpreter is interpreting, she is speaking for you or for your patient. While she is speaking, behave as you would if you yourself were speaking to the patient, or if he were speaking to you. Look at the patient, notice reactions, give reassuring nods and smiles, and use the time to study the patient.

- **Are you behaving abnormally towards your patient because you are using an interpreter?**

  While the patient is in the room, do not discuss him, or anything you do not want him to know, with the interpreter. The patient may understand a good deal of what you say to the interpreter and may become confused, anxious or offended.

  How can you maintain as good as possible a relationship with your patient when you are using an interpreter?

- **Are you making things as easy as possible for the interpreter?**

  Speak clearly and slowly, use simple words and keep the style of what you say straightforward. Give the words in the way you would like them translated. If you don't, the interpreter will have to translate your message into simple English in her head first, before translating it into the patient's language.

  Give simple but full explanations, just as you would to an English-speaking patient. But pause frequently to allow the interpreter to translate. Do not make too many demands on the interpreter's memory by giving her long chunks of speech to translate.

- **Does the interpreter understand the purpose of your questions and of the whole session? How can you help with this?**

  A lot of what you say cannot be translated directly into another language. The interpreter may be able to put things in a way that makes more sense than a direct translation. She is more likely to be able to convey the meaning of your message if she knows exactly what your aims are. She is also more likely to be able to help ensure that the whole session goes well. Ideally, health workers and interpreters should work as a team, advising and helping each other where necessary.

- **On the other hand, if the interpreter is not translating exactly what you and your patient are saying to each other, she may be adding or substituting her own views and interpretations. How can you prevent this?**

  You may have an amateur diagnostician between you and your patient. The interpreter may be tempted to re-interpret what the patient says as well as to translate it. Her own attitudes may influence her translation. This is more likely when the interpreter is close to the patient.

  The interpreter may identify either with you or with the patient. She may be blamed by either of you for what she translates, for not making things clearer, or for not being more helpful. She may sometimes be in the difficult position of knowing that the response of one of you is wrong, or that the advice she is being asked to translate is inappropriate. Being a meticulous and neutral mouthpiece is a very difficult job.

- **Does the interpreter tell you when and why she is having difficulty in translating? How can you make sure that she does tell you? What can you do to help?**

  The patient may not understand certain medical or anatomical terms, even in his own language. The interpreter may have to give a lengthy explanation to the patient in order to get an answer to your question. She may find it very difficult to make the patient understand exactly what is being asked. It may also be difficult for the interpreter to translate what the patient is saying. He may have a strong regional accent, may be using colloquial terms the interpreter does not know, may speak too fast or may meander because he is muddled or reluctant to answer. The interpreter must trust you enough to tell you when things are getting difficult.

- **Are you putting too much of a burden on the interpreter? Is she doing some of your work for you? How can you reduce the pressure on her?**

  It is tempting when one is hard pressed to delegate part of one's role to an interpreter; for example, to leave her to give instructions or an explanation to a patient and to go off to see someone else. This puts pressure on the interpreter; she is being asked to do part of your job, and the patient will not trust her 'medical' authority.

- **Are you maintaining as good a relationship as possible with your interpreter? What kind of relationship are you aiming for?**

- **Are you allowing enough time for your interview?**

  Allow two or three times as long for a conversation when you are using an interpreter. She needs time to listen to what is said, to assess it and to translate it. Remember that language ability often fails under stress; this is true for the interpreter as well as for the patient. Do not look at your watch or otherwise show impatience. Try not to interrupt while the patient and the interpreter are conversing. Try not to cut down your explanation because you are short of time.

Is there anything you or your interpreter can do beforehand so that the time you spend interviewing can be used as effectively as possible?

- **If you have a regular interpreter available, is there any way you can arrange your interviewing or visiting schedule to make the best possible use of her?**

- **Are you getting the interpreter you need and deserve? If not, what can you do about it?**

  The interpreter who can best serve your needs:
  is fluent in both English and the patient's language;
  has some training in interpreting;
  has some medical knowledge, and knowledge of how the health services work;
  accompanies you every time you visit the patient;
  is acceptable to, and trusted by, the patient;
  is sensitive to both your needs and those of the patient;
  takes a neutral role;
  puts the patient at ease;
  has a good memory and pays careful attention to detail;
  can translate fine shades of meaning;
  tells you when she has difficulty in translating what you have said, and explains why;
  is aware of cultural expectations or attitudes – yours and your patient's – and can explain things to both of you when needed;
  can tell you a good deal about the patient from her own observation after the interview.

The health worker and the interpreter should be a working pair who each contribute to the other's understanding. The health worker remains in control of the progress and direction of the conversation, while the interpreter uses her own understanding to give additional insight into the patient's problems. Time, mutual trust and cooperation are required to achieve this kind of relationship.

Health staff with access to interpreters can benefit greatly from training in how to make the most effective use of interpreting resources. People who regularly interpret for patients, on a paid or voluntary basis, are also likely to be far more effective if they receive some training in medical interpreting.

Learning the client's language

This is the most difficult of all the options: learning a new language is hard for adults; most health workers lead busy lives and do not have the time to attend regular classes or to practise a new language; the more different a second language is from one's first the more difficult it is to learn; French is relatively easy for English speakers to learn, Bengali or Vietnamese are far harder.

Nevertheless it may be possible to learn the basic phrases and a few vital words in the client's language. Several Education Authorities now run short courses for professionals working with linguistic minorities. These either teach simple word-related sentences and phrases, or combine cultural information with the language learning part of the course. Here is a sample course. This was taught by an English language teacher and a Bengali community worker working together and was designed for health visitors.

Bengali Life and Language Course, Camden[9]		
The programme was as follows:		
Week	Life	Language
1	Foreground: Bengalis in Camden and Islington	Greetings and partings Asking for and giving names
2	The naming system and family relationships	Identifying self Kin terms and dates of birth
3	The role of the mother and of the father. Childcare and play. The role of women	Talking about family Days of week, numbers Asking how many

4	The role of women (cont.) Family planning	Asking about age Asking when is husband's day off
5	Education	Greetings, the weather Locating address and phone number of children's school and husband's work Asking what time husband comes home
6	Diet. Breast feeding	Vocabulary of food items Asking what child eats and drinks. How much/many Advising on food and bottle-cleaning
7	Health issues in general, immunisation, school health Religion	Asking about health and illness. Appointments
8	Expectations of children's development and behaviour. ESL provision	Dosages and frequency Advising about English classes

Each week the participants also had a language handout in cartoon form, written in an English orthography. They were not taught to be literate in Bengali. Two examples of these handouts can be seen below.

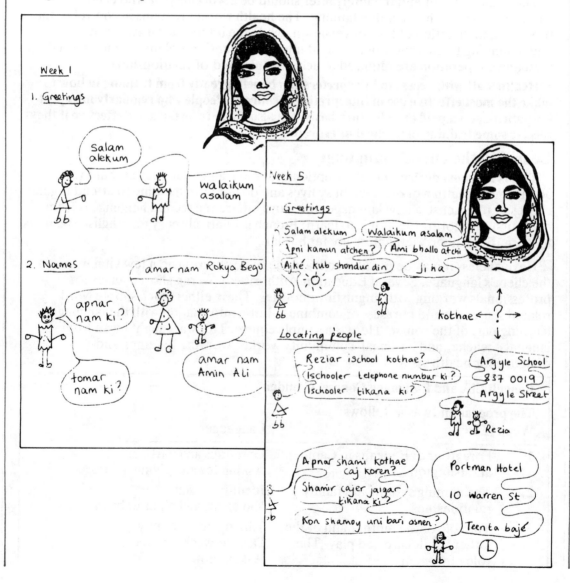

If this seems too difficult, you may at least be able to compile a list of key words and phrases to carry around with you. Examples from one such list, to do with food and dietary advice, are given below.[10]

DISCUSSING DIET: SOME USEFUL PUNJABI WORDS		Language Sheet: PUNJABI 1	

N.B. See Guide To Using The Language Sheets for a key to pronunciation.

Sikhs:	hello & goodbye	sat sree akaal	yes	haã
			no	nãhi/nehi
Muslims:	hello	asalaam alaykum	not	nãhi/nehi
	goodbye	khodaa hafiss/ rap daraka		
Hindus:	hello & goodbye	nãmastay		

MEAT*	maas/meat		
beef	gaa da maas	minced meat	keema
chicken	kooker/moorga	goat meat	bakri da maas
kidney	goorda	mutton	bed da maas
liver	kalayji	fish	machli

FRUIT	fal/phal		
apple	say/apple	water melon	tarbooz
banana	kayla	orange	santra
grape	angoor	orange juice	santra da ras
lemon/lime	nimboo/limoo	pineapple	ananas
mango	aam	raisins	kishmish
sweet melon	karbooja	dried fruit	sooka fal/sooka phal

VEGETABLES	sabzi/sabji		
cabbage	band gobi/gand gobi	lettuce	salad
carrot	gajar	onions	ganda/piaaz
cauliflower	fool gobi/pool gobi	peas	matar
coriander leaves	hara dania	potato	aloo
cucumber	keera	pumpkin	payta
eggplant	bataun/vataun	sweet potato	shakarkandi
fenugreek leaves	meti	spinach	paalak
green leafy veg.	haria sabjia/saag	salad	salad
green pepper	shimla meerch	tomato	tamaatar
ladyfingers/okra	bindi	white radish	mooli

* Many Punjabi Hindus and some Punjabi Sikhs are strict vegetarians and do not eat meat or eggs. Beef is particularly strictly prohibited and pork hardly ever eaten even by non-vegetarians. Punjabi Muslims do not eat pork. All other meat is permissible to Muslims provided it is 'halal'.

Language Sheet: PUNJABI 2

PULSES			
black gram	maahaa/urad	kidney beans	rajma
chickpeas	chana	lentils	massoor
cow peas	lobia/rajma	pigeon peas	arhar
green gram	moongi	chickpea flour	bayssan

CEREALS			
barley	jau	semolina	rawa/sooji
bread	bread/dabal roti	wheat	kanak
maize	maki	wheat flour	meda
millet	bajra	wholewheat flour	atta
rice	chaawal		

DAIRY PRODUCTS			
butter (UK type)	butter	egg white	ande di safedi
milk	dud	egg yolk	ande di jardi/zardi
dried milk	sooka dud	boiled egg	ooble anda
egg	anda	omelette	ande da poora/amlet
eggs	ande	yoghurt	dahee

NUTS			
almond	badaam	peanut	moong fali
cashew	kajoo	pistachio	pista

SPICES & HERBS			
cardamom	elachi	cumin	jeera/zeera
cinnamon	dalchini	garlic	tom/lassan
green chilli	hari meerach	fresh ginger	taaza
red chilli	laal meerach	dried ginger	soond
cloves	long	mustard seeds	rai
coriander	dania	turmeric	haldi

75

Notes

1. See two useful short reviews of recent research into practitioner–patient communication:
   Nuffield Working Party on Communications with Patients, *Talking with Patients – a teaching approach*, Nuffield Provincial Hospitals Trust, July, 1980.
   Ewles, Linda and Shipster, Pieter, *One to One: a handbook for the health educator*, East Sussex Area Health Authority, 1980.
2. For a useful summary of research in this field, see:
   Wolff, B. B. and Langley, S., 'Cultural Factors and the Response to Pain' in Landy, *Culture, Disease and Healing*, Macmillan, 1978, pp. 313–319.
3. Sutcliffe, David, *British Black English*, Basil Blackwell, 1982, Chapters 5 and 6.
4. Smith, David J., *The Facts of Racial Disadvantage*, Penguin, 1977, p. 55.
5. *Fact Paper 4: The language barrier in employment,* Commission for Racial Equality, 1978.
6. Stockwell, Felicity, *The Unpopular Patient*, Royal College of Nursing, 1972.
7. The following section has been adapted from Chapters 12 and 14 of *Asian Patients at Home and at Hospital* by Alix Henley, The King's Fund, 1979.
8. Rack, Philip, *Unpublished paper*, 1980.
9. Naish, Julia, *Report on Bengali Life and Language: a course for health visitors in Camden and Islington*, Camden English Language Scheme, 1981.
10. Henley, Alix, *Asian Foods and Diets*, DHSS/King's Fund, National Extension College, 1981.

More information

Communication difficulties and unfamiliarity with health services, see
3.4 **Coping with the British health care system**
7.1 **Concepts of health**
7.2 **Expectations and experience of the health services**

Giving advice, see
6.4 **Family planning**
7.4 **Working with different health beliefs and practices**
8.7 **Practical action: giving nutritional advice**
13 **Health education**, especially
13.3 **Written materials**

Professional training in communication skills:
10.2 **Improving access to existing services: 'Beating the Language Barrier' course**
12.2 **In-service training for working in a multiracial society**

Useful visual aids and resources, see
15 **Sources and resources**

Further reading

See Chapter 16
16.5 **Communication**
and relevant literature in
16.13 **Health education**

Part 2: Health needs and expectations

Part 2: Health needs and expectations

Professional expectations are likely to differ significantly from those of patients from different social, cultural or religious backgrounds. Variations in people's expectations and way of life have important implications for health workers who are concerned with the practical health needs and health care of individual black patients. Part 2 looks at four areas in which the expectations and health needs of patients from ethnic minority communities may be different from those of the ethnic majority.

Chapter 6: variations in **family life;** ways in which health workers can develop their understanding of different family systems; the importance of supporting and working with rather than against different ways of doing things.

Chapter 7: health beliefs and practices within different communities; different ideas about health, illness and health care; practical ways in which health workers can learn more about traditional health systems and work positively with them.

Chapter 8: foods and diets of different communities; some of the economic, social and cultural factors which influence dietary traditions; what health workers need to know to help them give appropriate and acceptable dietary advice, and to ensure that ethnic minority hospital patients are properly catered for.

Chapter 9: variations in patterns of illness between different ethnic groups in Britain; some examples of illnesses specifically affecting ethnic minority groups; the need for consultation with the community concerned on issues surrounding the management of certain illnesses.

6 Working with families and individuals

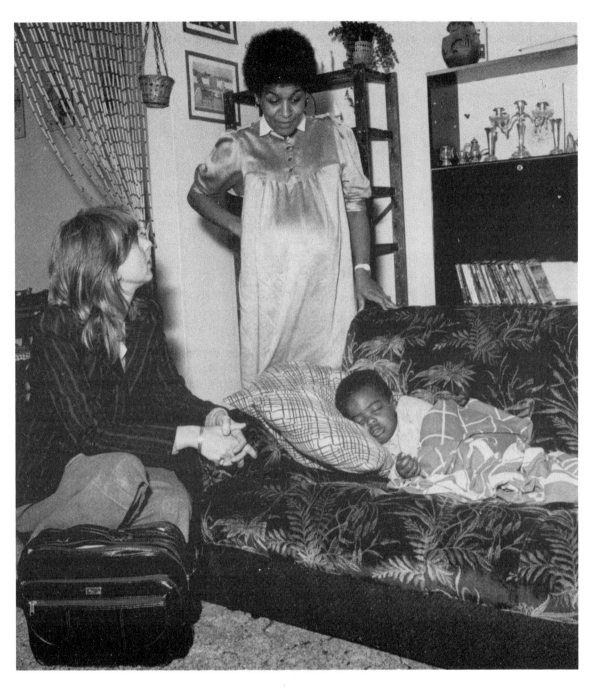

Introduction

An understanding of family life is essential to the health worker if health care is to be effective. This chapter begins by looking at family life in different communities in Britain. The family and family relationships can influence health and health care in a number of ways, and subsequent sections discuss three specific aspects that health workers need to be sensitive to: different ways of bringing up children; the effects of racism on children and family life; differing attitudes to family planning.

Health workers need to be wary about imposing their own cultural expectations on families and individuals who live in a different way. Throughout the chapter there are questions for discussion which health workers can use to gain a more complete understanding of their own cultural beliefs and ideas about family organisation.

6.1 *Different family systems*

I just went to that – what do you call it – social welfare or something, but I don't want to go there again. It's a strange place. I get the feeling they don't want to see me. I had to wait a long time. Then they took me to this tiny room where an English officer – a boy young enough to be my son – spoke to me. I couldn't explain myself properly. I don't think he understood – you know us women, we have such different problems, our family ways, only our own people can understand.

Asian woman[1]

The way in which the Western nuclear family is organised and is developing is only one of many possible ways. It is the result of a multiplicity of interlinked factors: economic, historical, political, religious, climatic, cultural and so forth.

Although no two British families are completely alike, certain values are generally accepted, and certain assumptions form part of majority British cultural and social norms. These then define and influence the way that health and other services are organised in Britain, and the way that most health workers approach individuals and families. If such norms are not compared with other family systems during professional training, health workers expectations of 'normal' family relationships may be based on very culture-specific values.

As a result families in Britain with different structures and different cultural norms and assumptions may find that health and other services are offered in such a way that they cannot use them or are alienated by them. The assessments that health workers make of minority group families and their needs, and the service they offer, may be wrong or irrelevant.

This does not only affect ethnic minority families. The barriers between professionals and clients from different classes in Britain have long been acknowledged, but those faced by people of minority cultures are often greater. Most professionals are sensitive to cultural differences between classes and recognise a responsibility to make professional practice appropriate to the lifestyle and needs of working-class families. There has been less willingness to recognise the needs and rights of ethnic minority communities in this respect. Some people still feel that ethnic minority ('immigrant') communities must adapt to the services offered in Britain or do without. If the Health Service is to fulfil its intended role, that of enabling, supporting, caring for and helping, it must respond sensitively and positively to all its clients or patients as they are. The way services are organised must not cut out, intentionally or unintentionally, families and individuals who do not present themselves in a predefined way because their way of life is different from the majority norm. Health workers must **work with** families of different kinds, making use of their strengths and taking care not to ignore or undercut a family's chosen way of doing things. They must **work with** individuals, respecting the priorities and values they live by, not imposing additional pressures of rejection and ignorance. For most people their family provides a vital and lifelong source of support and security. This must be sustained, not undermined.

The family's the most important thing in the world. If you've lost that you've got nothing.

Young Asian man

Working within other family systems

Each of us has a personal set of beliefs about families and the way they should be: about, for example, the size and shape of a 'normal' family, the emotional relationships it should contain, and the kind of support our family can be expected to give; the rights and responsibilities of different family members; how much independence and freedom of action family members normally have, and how much they must abide by other people's decisions.

We are not always aware of our own beliefs until we encounter people whose family systems and values differ sharply from our own. We tend to regard our own values as universal and to expect other people to see things in roughly the same way. There is however a danger that we will regard other systems as deviant rather than just different, or as flawed versions of our own system rather than as independent systems with their own internal logic. There is a danger that we will see them as problems, and work against or despite them rather than with them.

Questions to think about

Because our views are to a large extent defined for each of us by the culture and society in which we grow up it is difficult or impossible to detach ourselves from them.

- What are your own beliefs about families and how they should be? What kind of family did you grow up in?
- What do you think a family is for?
- What does it consist of? How many people?
- How many people do you define as your immediate family? What kinds of relatives do you include? How many people in your family do you feel a responsibility for?
- Is there a chain of authority within your family? How important and firm is it?
- Who has authority over whom in your family? Until what age? Why? How far does anyone have the right to enforce their authority?
- Does anyone have ultimate authority over you?
- Which is the most important relationship in a family? Husband and wife? Parent and child? Brother and sister?
- At what age do you think a young person should be independent of his or her family? What do you mean by 'independent'? In what decisions should older family members still be allowed to have a say?
- How important is your family's reputation to you? What would harm it? Do you avoid doing certain things to protect its reputation?
- How close would you want to live to your parents?
- When you are old do you expect to live with your children? With other relatives? Alone at home? With other people of your age? Or go into an old people's home?

The family is the unit through which values and priorities are learnt and handed down and through which we learn most of our deeply felt ideas about our roles and duties in life. People brought up in different family systems are therefore likely to have very different expectations of acceptable family behaviour, and different values and priorities. For instance, it is not true that 'a mother is a mother all over the world'. Mothers in different cultures have different roles and practical responsibilities and different ideas about what makes a 'good' mother, what are desirable motherly qualities and behaviour, and what a mother's duties are.

To work effectively, therefore, in a multi-cultural society, we first have to be aware of and analyse our own preconceptions and deeply held cultural beliefs about how families and individuals should behave. It is important that we do not impose them inappropriately on other people who believe in and live their lives according to a different system.

For a lot of white women women's lib. is about the freedom to work, to have an existence outside the family and the home, to wrest their independence from men. But black women have always had to be self-supporting, to fight their own cause, go out to work, to be independent. For us women's lib. is about somehow freeing ourselves from the oppression of those *things.*

Young Afro-Caribbean woman

Things got so bad at home after they found out about my boyfriend that I thought I was going to have a breakdown and I went to the doctor for some pills. He's a nice man and really kind to me. He told me that leaving home was the best thing that I could do and he lent me £5 so that I could move to a hostel straight away. I had three sleepless nights there and then I went back home. I couldn't stand being alone. I missed my family terribly in spite of all the rows. I knew that by sleeping away from home I might be getting myself into real trouble for the future. Who's going to want to marry a girl who has run away? When I tried to explain to my doctor why I'd gone back he thought that I was barmy or that my parents had threatened me. He's never been quite the same to me since. He just didn't get it.

Sikh girl[2]

The assessment of strengths, aspirations and adaptability must include a good understanding of the special socio-economic pressures on immigrants and their descendants and on minority groups. For example, black parents' observation of the job market and experience of discrimination convinces them that their children must do as well as possible in school. Their pressure on them is therefore rational; too often it is dismissed as unrealistic. Such pressure often proves effective. Despite ample evidence of the importance of parental involvement in children's education white social workers (and teachers) frequently dismiss black parents' efforts as counterproductive. The costs are exaggerated; the gains ignored.[3]

In general, Western cultures emphasise individualism and individual self-development. The happiness and the needs of an individual come before the happiness and the needs of his or her family, particularly parents and older relatives. Where there is a tension between the two an individual has the right to place his or her wishes first. People should not 'sacrifice' themselves to the wishes or demands of other family members. British social customs, educational systems and institutions all reflect these basic values.

Even though within British society there are many variations from the outline given above and many types of family and many views of what a family should be, most people believe ideally in the rights of the individual over the family, and patterns of behaviour and assessment tend to mirror this.

Some minority communities in Britain find this shocking, and threatening to their own values and conventions, though, like majority British culture, patterns of family life in minority cultures are changing over time and contain a good deal of variation. For most young black people, growing up in Britain is a process of synthesis – combining certain majority beliefs with those of their own community and culture.

[Studies of ethnic minorities in Britain] illustrate the successful adaptations and negotiations of families wrestling with two traditions. Although there are casualties and some unavoidable conflicts, which tend to hit the headlines and to be the daily fare of social workers, the prevailing picture is one of energetic exploration of the virtues and gains of differing value systems and styles of life. Some commentators argue that this produces 'the best of both worlds'. Common sense should have convinced us that long established traditions of mutual support which have survived the onslaughts of poverty, natural disaster and oppression would be more than equal to the stresses of migration.[3]

What I feel a lot of people seem to do when they come across an Asian or a Cypriot family where there's a problem between a girl and her parents is to put it all down to 'culture conflict' and then side with the girl because they see her as wishing to adopt and identify with white British culture. They start to line up on the girl's side and dash around trying to rescue her from her oppressive parents and all that. And most of the time they make it much worse; they persuade the girl to do terribly final things, or she knows they're terribly final, and they widen the gulf between her and her parents; and the poor parents, who thought the social worker was supposed to be helping them, find themselves cast in the role of villains. Every family has conflicts between the generations, and it's bound sometimes to be worse among minority families because parents and children have such different influences and expectations, but when white kids have fights with their parents we don't rush in and help to tear the family apart, do we?

English social worker

Views about the relationships between families and individuals are bound to vary between communities. There may be some striking differences between the expectations of minority communities in Britain and those of the majority.

- **The centre of the family** may be the mother; the grandmother; the biological parents; the grandparents; or the wider extended family.

- Family members and the family unit may be far more important in people's lives. **People may have far greater family responsibilities:** their priorities and values may be closely tied up with those of their family. Decisions may be made by the whole family rather than by individuals. The welfare of one member may be seen as dependent on the welfare of the whole family and all its members.

- **There may be a formal hierarchy of responsibility and authority.** It may be the duty and responsibility of older family members to make all major and many minor decisions. If older family members are living elsewhere they may still be referred to for most important decisions, many of which might be considered entirely personal and individual in British cultures.

Even though my parents are back in Pakistan we always ask them and discuss it with them if we are going to take any big step, or about the children. Like when we bought this house, or even, you know, about my daughter's school. If it's any big decision, anything big, we'd always ask them. The only problem is, so far away you know, it takes a long time, and also it's difficult to discuss it properly in letters.

Muslim man

- **People may consider themselves to be a part of a large family network all their lives.** Marriage, for example, may not necessarily mean the setting up of a new and independent unit, in which a young couple moves finally out and away from the authority of their own parents. A married couple may remain physically and emotionally very much part of the extended family unit. They may still regard older family members as having ultimate responsibility for decisions affecting their welfare.

- **Individual freedom or self-interest may not be a goal to be aimed for.** Individualism may be seen as undesirable, or selfish, as a sign of coldness and lack of proper human feeling. Children may not be brought up to see individualism as a desirable goal; they may grow up with the view that self-interest and self-reliance at the expense of caring about the family are not moral virtues. Adults may not see their interests as autonomous or independent from the family's interests. In many families nobody is 'independent', everyone has a responsibility towards other family members; everyone always has the right to look to older members for emotional and physical support; everyone always has the duty to give emotional and physical support to anyone who is younger or in need. Obligations to other family members may be expected to override personal self-interest.

You bring up your children. We live with ours.

Asian mother

- **The family unit may be large.** It may contain three or four generations and several adult married couples. Children may be brought up by all the adults together, and particularly by the elderly women. They may regard all the adult members of their family as parents. Older family members may have final authority over them rather than their biological parents.

'I have many mothers,' said a Ghanaian doctor during a discussion on family relationships, crystallising in a few words the difference between the western style, closed, nuclear family, where the concentration of relationships is between husband,

wife and children, and the far more open, traditional, extended family, still the norm in West Africa in spite of inevitable changes resulting from the pressures of modern urban living and the impact of western technology.[4]

Within the same generation of adults there may be a clearly defined structure of family responsibilities. Older brothers and their wives may have responsibility for younger brothers and their wives and children. Men may have responsibility for women. Respect for the advice and authority of older adults or of men within the family may be very important. Older children may have authority over and expect respect from younger brothers, sisters and cousins.

Even when the family is split up into nuclear units, close bonds of support, love and responsibility may be maintained between the units. In some families it is a normal alternative for children to be brought up by other relatives, uncles and aunts, or by grandparents instead of by their parents.

A very basic illustration of the kind of misunderstanding that arises can be seen if one looks at the concept of fostering. Although the same term is used in Britain and West Africa, the meanings ascribed to it are very different. In our society, fostering is resorted to reluctantly when there is some kind of breakdown in the normal family arrangements – it is definitely second best. In West Africa, it is a normal part of extended family life; relationships with wider family members are very important and children may move around a great deal during childhood. Fostering is usually kin-fostering but children also go to stay with friends, perhaps so that their education can be furthered. West Africans come to Britain thinking of fostering as a perfectly usual and acceptable practice. They often do not realise that being fostered in a British nuclear family represents a very different set of experiences for the child than being fostered at home in West Africa and that it can have profoundly different consequences for that child's development.[5]

- **The roles and ambitions of men and women may be the same or may be very different.** Men and women within a family may have different responsibilities and areas of authority. They may have different and separate spheres of interest and influence.

  In some communities the women may take most of the responsibility for children and bring them up alone. They may value and take pride in their own strength and independence and turn mainly to their own mothers and to other women for support and companionship.

  In some communities men may be responsible for taking decisions; women may not be expected to act on their own, but to seek consent from an appropriate male relative first.

- **The honour and reputation of the family may be a major concern of all its members.** If one member gets a reputation for, for example, meanness, ill temper, bad behaviour, promiscuity, or criminal behaviour, this may affect the reputation of the whole family and the lives and futures of all its members. The family may be very concerned to prevent one member from ruining the lives of all the others. Restricting the self-interest of one individual may seem a small price to pay in overall terms.

- **The maintenance and support of the family may be seen as everybody's most important duty.** The family may be seen as the permanent source of all the love, support, companionship and happiness that anyone will need and as the centre and focus of each person's life.

At home the family structure is different. You have got mother and father, who maybe have got their mother and father. Grandparents take an interest in the children, and you would no more think of cheeking your grandmother than flying in the air. Here it is totally different, because your family is scattered further apart. The family involvement in the West Indies is totally different from family involvement here.

Afro-Caribbean woman[6]

- **The position of elderly family members varies a good deal.** In some families old people are the most important people and also the centre of power and authority;

in others their needs and wishes are subordinate to those of younger members; they may be given care and attention but have little authority. Some elderly people expect to live with their families and be supported by them; others wish to retain their independence as long as they can.

There is a widely accepted myth that the Asians in this country are able to care for their old as well as their young under one roof because of the extended family system. This may have been the case elsewhere but here the immigrant Asian population is frequently faced with housing problems and other economic structures which make it impossible for children to shoulder their traditional responsibilities towards their parents.[7]

- All parents very much want their children to marry someone with whom they will be as happy as possible. The degree of overt or covert influence and control that parents may exert may vary a good deal. **In some communities marriage may be seen as a permanent bond between two families rather than two individuals**; it is felt to be essential that the experience of older, wiser members of the family is brought to bear in choosing a suitable partner; **in some communities marriage may be seen as an intensely personal exclusive union between two people. In some communities marriage may not be particularly important, or may be a step taken fairly late in life to confirm and celebrate an existing relationship.**

How do possible differences like these affect the health worker? Check that you are working with the grain of people's lives and values and not against it.

More questions to think about

Do you and your client have different ideas about:
- the importance and role of the wider family?
- what kinds of decisions he or she can make?
- who else should be involved or consulted?
- who has final authority in this matter?
- his/her responsibilities and those of other family members?
- the dignity and rights of individuals?
- his/her wishes, priorities and hopes?
- the respect due to older family members?
- marriage and motherhood?
- what makes a good marital relationship?
- acceptable male and female behaviour?
- appropriate topics for discussion between men and women?
- desirable parent–child relationships?
- the kind of behaviour that is considered responsible or irresponsible?
- the consequences of particular actions and decisions for the person you are talking to and their family?
- the responsibilities of different family members or of the whole family when one member is ill or needs special care?
- the appropriate amount of practical and emotional family involvement when someone is ill?
- appropriate topics for discussion with different people?
- the need to protect people's reputations and what might harm them?

Your effectiveness as a health worker will be badly flawed if you are imposing views or values on your client that he does not share or agree with. Where you are not sure that you and your patient or client are thinking along the same lines it may be necessary to check by asking an explicit question.

Ethnic minority clients are the most direct source of information, but a source that is usually neglected. Ask people about their wishes and values and experiences. If there are problems to be sorted out, find out how they see them and what solutions they would suggest. Provided that people feel you are genuinely interested and that you respect and will value their wishes, opinions and feelings, they are generally glad to discuss their views with you.

A note of caution

Culture is a factor; yes it's a really important factor. But I think in some cases social workers use culture, or culture conflict, as a diagnosis too readily. Because first of all people's culture is changing here, a lot. For all sorts of reasons, including their economic position and the way of life they have to live here. And then when they call it all culture, they sometimes don't bother to go on to look below that, into what's really happening: how the people feel, what has happened up to now, that kind of thing. Everybody is an individual, not just a lump of culture. But they don't go into the issues as they normally would. They kind of say – 'Well, it's culture and we can't do anything about it; and they also see it almost always as a direct clash between British ways and the family's ways. And I think usually they see the British ways as better. And secondly, I feel very strongly about this, if they just look at the cultural things they ignore something that is a crucial experience for black people here; conscious or unconscious racism by white people. And obviously that's going to affect black people's reactions and behaviour; there is no black person living in this society who isn't deeply affected by racism. And you mustn't leave it out when you are working with minority groups.

Asian community worker

Possible conflicts between client needs and professional practice

Here are some examples of how traditional British expectations or provision may work against the needs of ethnic minority clients or patients:

- Health workers tend to work in a **one-to-one relationship** with adult clients, giving advice, for example, to a young mother-to-be about her diet or her routine. These may sometimes be things about which a client may have to consult older women in the family, or about which they decide, though she may not feel able to discuss these with them. Unless they too are involved in the discussion and the decision-making process they may oppose the health workers' advice or give conflicting instructions.

- It is not part of the **traditional role of some women** to make major decisions. For example, in Pakistan and Bangladesh the consent of a male guardian is always required for an operation on a woman. Some (but not necessarily all) Asian Muslim women in Britain may wish their husband or guardian to be consulted before they agree to any operation for themselves. Hospital authorities may need to take this into account when getting consent forms signed. It is essential to find out about and take into account the decision-making structure of the client's family.

- British hospitals usually restrict **visiting** to two adults at a time and only at certain times. This may cause real distress to relatives from an extended family, all of whom are likely to feel that they must visit and comfort the patient and many of whom may have come long distances to do so. To be told to come back tomorrow may unintentionally be very cruel.

  Hospitals in most Third World countries do not impose restrictions on visiting, but rely on family members to stay with patients and perform basic practical and nursing chores such as providing food for and washing the patients. The constant presence of one or more family members, often sitting quietly and just giving comfort by being there, may be tremendously reassuring to patients who are already frightened and unhappy in an alien hospital setting. Where possible this should be permitted.

- In many societies **men and women** lead largely separate lives. Men support men and women support women at times of need. Pregnancy and childbirth, for example, are often regarded as entirely female matters and may not be discussed in front of men. In such situations it is clearly inappropriate to use a husband, a son or another man to interpret for a woman about female matters. (The use of children or unqualified strangers as interpreters in personal matters – except in real emergencies – is never acceptable.)

A woman going into labour may wish to have her mother, sister or another woman with her during the birth, as is the norm in many countries, rather than her husband. Each couple will differ on this issue. It is important to check beforehand whom a woman would prefer to have with her. Patients should not be urged to bring their husbands if neither husband or wife are happy at the prospect.

In some communities husbands may not visit new mothers after their delivery. Sisters and other female relatives may come instead. Some couples are adopting the British custom and husbands are now choosing to stay with their wives during and after delivery. But the absence of a husband among visitors to a newly delivered mother in a maternity unit does not necessarily indicate that something is wrong. It is important to be sensitive both to general cultural difference and to variations within cultural patterns.

- In many communities the **decision-making** within a family is more formal than most British health workers are used to. For example, the father of a sick child may want to consult his older brother or his father before making a major decision regarding treatment. It may be important to acknowledge this by speaking directly to whichever family members have final responsibility for a decision.

- **Girls and young women** are regarded as extremely vulnerable in many societies. Members of the family may feel it is their duty to protect unmarried daughters and sisters, and to ensure that their reputation is spotless. Boys and girls may be segregated from puberty to prevent any encouragement to premarital sexual activity. The reputation of a whole family and of all its members may be ruined if one of its daughters is thought to be unruly or promiscuous. Older brothers and male relatives may have a particular responsibility for young women and may act as chaperones if a girl wishes to go out. In Britain many Asian families, for example, feel that their daughters' morals are threatened by what they see as the generally lax moral standards of wider society, and by pressure from their peers to have boyfriends and to go out to discos, youth clubs and parties. Some families may become particularly strict because of the increased dangers in Britain, recognising the additional pressures their daughters are under and wishing to protect them. Health workers from a different background may regard this as repressive and as depriving a young women of her normal and natural freedoms. Such judgements are very much influenced by one's own culture and beliefs and must be made with care. A confrontation with parents over the way they wish to bring up their children is likely to be extremely counterproductive for everyone concerned.

*When a girl or woman is seen to behave in a manner which is considered fitting to her age and sex, she is said to have shame or sexual chastity. When attempting to articulate their understanding of sexual shame to me, Cypriots usually had recourse to examples. These varied according to whether the speaker was a young London resident, an elderly villager, someone from Nicosia and so on. There was a consensus of opinion on one fact: a girl anywhere who was found to have lost her virginity before marriage would be said to have lost her virtuous reputation and her sense of shame. On the other hand, a girl, whether married or not, would come to be described as having shame or virtue if, over time, she was seen to avoid those situations and activities which would earn her the reputation of being shameless. Thus in London, if she was **never** found talking to unrelated boys on the street; if, apart from family outings, she did **not** spend time out of the house at weekends and in the evenings; if her friends were known to be chaste; if she was seen to behave modestly at all public gatherings; and so on. Because it is a case of continually avoiding doing what is wrong rather than positively doing what is right, a virtuous reputation takes some time to acquire.*[8]

- The higher proportion of **single-parent families** and families where parents are not married in the Afro-Caribbean community has its basis in the destruction of the African family system in the West Indies by white slave-owners during the period of slavery, and in the economic problems of the colonial period after the abolition of slavery. The brutal relationships imposed by slave-owners upon their slaves are described in this extract by Dilip Hiro:

Under slavery, marriage was meaningless because the 'husband' could not protect his 'wife' from the sexual demands of other men. Any attempt to protect his 'wife' from being ravished by the white master meant stiff punishment. By law, the slave had no rights; nor could a free man plead for him. Subject women were the exclusive 'property' of the master for whom they performed three major functions: labour; the breeding of slaves; and his sexual gratification.

There was a popular notion among the masters that a slave woman would breed more and better if she were mated with different men. The male slave's function, therefore, began and ended with being a sexual inseminator. As the slave children too were the master's property and could be separated from their mothers at his whim, there was no such thing as a 'slave family'. The end-result was the total destruction of the conventional family system.[9]

After slavery ended many men were forced to go overseas to find work; either to other Caribbean islands or to Panama and North America. In a situation where men were unable to get work, women and girls could not afford to rely on men for their security. In most Afro-Caribbean families, therefore, girls are traditionally brought up to be self-sufficient and independent.

In a white man's world black women have it easier than black men.[10]

In white capitalist Britain the black man is still at the lower end of the social scale. He is more likely to be unemployed, more likely to be in low-paid work or shift work. White employers often see black men as a physical threat, aggressive, violent, etc. They won't employ them. So black women often find it easier to get work and to support themselves. In a way the slavery and neocolonial patterns are being re-enacted in Britain, with the same effects on relationships and on how men and women see their roles and opportunities.

Afro-Caribbean health worker

Marriage in West Indian society is generally highly respected as a serious responsible step and the confirmation of a lifelong association. As in traditional British culture, a husband is considered responsible for the support of his wife and children. Marriage may therefore be entered into only when the couple know each other thoroughly and often only after they have lived together for several years. They may already have children. Marriage is also traditionally a large and expensive celebration and is therefore a major expense for which a couple may save for several years.

As in British society, class also influences people's view on this issue. Middle-class Afro-Caribbean couples may be more likely to share the values of white British middle-class couples with regard to marriage and children born outside marriage.

Like an increasing number of white British couples, most Afro-Caribbean couples who live together have a stable relationship and are married in all but name. They accept shared responsibility for children. Within some sections of the Afro-Caribbean community the social stigma and reputation for instability, traditionally attached by white British society to cohabiting couples with children, generally do not apply.

Young people of Afro-Caribbean origin in Britain will obviously be influenced by the values of both their parents and the West Indies, and by those of majority British society. In Britain the proportion of young Afro-Caribbean men and women who get married is increasing and is higher than in the West Indies. Nevertheless girls are still generally regarded as self-sufficient and responsible for their own actions. If an unmarried girl has a child she will expect and be expected to take some responsibility for supporting and looking after the child herself. She will also, in most cases, receive help and support from her own parents and from the father of the child.

Some West Indian people, when they came to this country, were affected by white people's reactions and judgements and so they got married. There are a lot of factors really, it's very complicated. For example, there may be more stigma attached to an unmarried girl getting pregnant in this country, her parents may feel she's let them down, gone back to the old ways. After all the effort they made to come here. Then there are the class differences. But then a lot of working-class West Indians joined the pentecostalist churches and they are very strict about sexual morality. And now sometimes their children, the next generation, are alienated by that and so they've gone back to traditional West Indian values, or possibly adopted white British values.

Afro-Caribbean community worker

Young single Afro-Caribbean mothers in Britain often face real difficulties in their contacts with welfare services and professionals. British society's attitude to the single mother is still largely punitive, and children born outside marriage are seen as the result of deviant and irresponsible behaviour. One child can be forgiven as an accident, but two or three arouse real disapproval which may not be hidden by health workers or other people. Many single Afro-Caribbean mothers, like single mothers from other groups, face poverty, inadequate housing, and the lack of formal child care provision. The extended family may not be available or able to provide the kind of support that would have been provided in the West Indies.

The West Indian tradition is to give your baby the father's surname. And if you have children with different fathers each has its own surname usually. Here that's seen as irresponsible, feckless, brazen, all those things. And young women are really made to feel bad about it. At hospitals and so on the receptionists and other staff really make you feel disapproved of.

Afro-Caribbean woman

6.2 *Bringing up children*

There are few explicitly stated concepts about children or principles of childrearing which would be agreed to by most people in this country.[11]

Beliefs about childrearing are usually bound up with beliefs about life itself. They are culturally transmitted and culturally learned. They are held without question.[4]

Ways of bringing up children, and the values that parents try to instil in them, will depend on the parents' own upbringing, their values, and the circumstances in which they live. **What is meant by a 'good child' varies from culture to culture and from class to class.**

Our young people, seeing the way that their counterparts in this country behave, try to pull away from their parents. Consequently, there is a battle going on between parents' discipline and what they want to go after. At home there was no question of that. You did as you were told. . . . Here it is different, because you have a child of a West Indian parent who is thinking in the West Indian way, mixing with children who have got parents who were born here – English parents – and they see that these children have got more freedom than they have, and they are pulling that way, so consequently there is a struggle going on in the home. The next thing we find is that the children decide 'I am not sticking to this, so out I go.'

Afro-Caribbean woman[6]

Socio-economic factors

Culture is of course partly the product of economic and other circumstances. In white middle-class families, for example, with a fair amount of living space and money for books and toys, a 'good' child may be energetic, enquiring, active, voluble and outgoing. In low-income white working-class families living in smaller, noisier accommodation with little space and parents under stress, a 'good' child may be the quiet one in the corner who causes no trouble and is hardly noticed. **Economic circumstances, housing and environment all have a major influence on culture, and affect the way that children are brought up as much as they affect the lives and values of the whole family.**

For some ethnic minority families the constraints of an unfamiliar industrial inner-city environment and poor housing may seriously restrict their ability to bring up their children as they would wish.

The kind of open-air rural childhood they may have had, for example, is no longer possible, and their children may miss out on the space and natural playthings that they took for granted.

Over there we'd leave all the doors open and our friends would just walk in and out as they wanted. But here in England people keep their doors shut all the time.

The one thing we really miss here is the space. Just the other day I was saying to the children, 'Are you going to pull the house apart?' They don't have enough room to play about. We children used to spend most of our time outside.

Afro-Caribbean woman[12]

There is no question that the quality of life in rural Bangladesh is far and away better than it is for Bangladeshi families in inner-city Britain. Families over here are caught in a trap not of their making. Men can only get work which is pitifully badly paid, or they have spent years saving to bring their families over and then find themselves suddenly made redundant. Some white professionals believe that our families live the way they do by choice . . . that it is an improvement on life in Bangladesh to live one family to a room in a damp broken down terrace and only able to afford a paraffin heater for warmth in winter. Believe me this is no improvement. How can anyone believe people live in this way out of choice?

Bangladeshi community worker

Parents may be afraid to let their children play outside in concrete areas littered with glass and dirt, or on streets where cars rush past. They may worry that their children will be harassed by young white racists. Racial harassment has been suggested as a contributory factor to rickets in young Asian children; their mothers are afraid to let them play outside in the sun.

For families where children and childcare are usually shared between several adults the loss of the extended family may cause real difficulties for a mother on her own. A young first-time mother may never have expected to have to cope with a baby or a toddler alone. She may have grown up knowing that her own mother, her mother-in-law or her sisters-in-law would look after it and that when there were problems she would be able to turn to them for help and support. Without family support in Britain she may be isolated and desperate, unaccustomed to looking outside the family for help and support, possibly cut off by language from health workers and other caring professionals, and with small children totally dependent on her.

Although the options open to parents will often have been drastically reduced by their economic circumstances in Britain, each family will still try to bring up its children according to its own beliefs and values. Families from different cultures may therefore differ a good deal in what they consider desirable and right. This places a responsibility on health workers, whose role is primarily to support and help families in the way they wish to bring up their children and organise their lives.

The health worker's influence

Ethnic minority mothers in Britain are often aware that some health workers disapprove of and disagree with their ways of bringing up their children. This may affect their confidence in themselves as capable mothers. Any mother will welcome discussion about her family and her children, but this must be in the context of support of her own views and wishes. Families have the right to bring up their children in the way they know best. A confident relaxed mother will produce confident relaxed children. A worried, distressed mother, aware that 'the authorities' disapprove of her as a mother, will too often pass her tensions and worries on to her children.

It wasn't until I had my own child that I realised how susceptible you are to other people's comments and disapproval. I'm a trained doctor but when I had my first baby I lost all my self-confidence. I suddenly realised how my unthinking remarks must sometimes have affected other women.

English doctor

90

It's funny you know. Because you know they are watching you all the time, they don't really trust the way you are looking after your kids, you start to get really worried yourself. You start to think, well, maybe they're right to be worried, maybe our way of bringing up kids is wrong, maybe I am a no-good mother. It's funny what it does to you.

Middle-aged Afro-Caribbean mother

For many families the intervention of the state and its institutions in intimate family matters, such as the bringing up of children, is threatening. What role does each of the caring professionals who visit their home have? How far are they friends and confidantes? How far are they an arm of the law? On what criteria is the family being judged? Visiting health workers and other 'officials' may need to give a clear explanation of their role and functions. They will certainly need to work at developing a relationship of mutual trust, and to show mothers very clearly that their judgement and childrearing methods are supported and respected, not judged as deficient or inferior.

Different ways of bringing up children

Questions to think about:

Which of the possibilities below correspond most closely with your own ideas on bringing up children? How do your ideas differ from those of people of other cultures with whom you work? How can you find out what your clients' ideas and wishes are?

- Who should bring children up?
  Their mother? both parents? several female relatives? an older woman? a whole family or community?

- Who has authority over children in your family?
  A child's own mother and/or father? the parents' own older relatives? any adult?

- How do you show children love and affection?
  By hugging and physical contact? by discipline? or through physical care and cleanliness?

- How do you discipline and control children?
  By physical punishment? by withdrawing privileges? by withholding affection? by scolding? or by imposing unpleasant tasks and penalities?

- Do you discipline children fairly firmly when they are young but give them increasing freedom as they grow older? or do you allow them total freedom when they are young but increasingly control and discipline as they reach their teens?

- Should children be educated consciously from a very early age? Should they pick things up as and when they are able? Is a routine essential for their security and discipline? or should they be cared for, fed, bathed and so forth whenever they need it and it is convenient? Is your family consciously child-centred? or are children regarded as just part of the family?

- How do you think children should behave towards their elders? Should they show respect? How? Should they talk and join in when older people are present? Should they remain politely silent?

How can you find out the views and values of the families you work with? How can you support them?

Are your interventions in the way they bring up their children justifiable and necessary, or are you imposing your own cultural and social preconceptions?

I was talking to a health visitor about the Pakistani families she works with. She said 'Children aren't allowed to be children so much in their society, are they?' I asked her what she meant by that.

Asian community worker

6.3 Racism and bringing up black children in Britain

Children pick up the attitudes of the society in which they grow up. Research in Britain and in America has shown that children distinguish racial groups from an early age (two or three years old) and within the next four or five years have learnt the racial values of the society in which they are growing up. In Britain this means that black children often pick up negative white attitudes towards black people, such as the prejudiced belief that whites are 'intellectually superior', 'more civilised' or 'cleaner'.

Children find it very difficult to identify with a socially rejected group. Some black children have been shown to exhibit a strong preference for the dominant white group, and a tendency to devalue their own group. There is well documented experimental evidence of black children rejecting black dolls because they are 'ugly' or 'bad'; and of choosing a white rather than a black doll when asked which doll looked most like them. There are cases of black children trying to bleach or scrub themselves white because again they wish to reject their black skin and identity.[13]

These attitudes are likely to be reinforced as children get older, by the messages they receive in the media, by racist gibes at school or in the street, by negative or embarrassed references to their parents, origin, culture and backgrounds in the classroom.

I had a discussion with a small group of Gujarati women about the problems they were having with their teenage children. Much of what the women said showed how their children had picked up the negative attitudes of white society towards them and their community. For example, some of the children were embarrassed and refused to go shopping with their mothers because their mothers did not speak very good English; there was a girl who kept forgetting the lunch her mother prepared for her to take to school because it was Indian food and who finally lied to her mother that she was not allowed to take food to school; there were children of 14 and 15 refusing to bring their English friends to their own homes but going often to their English friends' houses; there were Asian girls in home economics classes who told their teacher that they never ate Asian food at home; and children who brought English friends home but behaved very strangely and only spoke English while their friends were there, pretending not to understand a word of Gujarati.

Asian community worker

To counteract this, black families and communities are increasingly making moves to reassert their own identity. There are, for example, a growing number of groups set up to teach and maintain aspects of minority group culture, such as black dance and music groups and cultural workshops; there has been, in the past few years, an increase in Afro-Caribbean and Asian youth clubs and schemes, and black women's groups. Young people are also demonstrating their sense of pride and identity in their dress; Sikh boys grow their hair and wear turbans; Afro-Caribbean women wear plaited African hairstyles and African-style jewellery and clothes; young men wear red, gold and green Rasta tams and dreadlocks; Jewish men re-adopt the yamulka. Young British-born Afro-Caribbeans have evolved a dialect of their own that combines elements of the patois of the West Indies with local English dialects.

Sikh rally against turban rule

By Susan Tirbutt
Some of more than 1,000 Sikhs joined a rally in London yesterday to call on the Government to give them the statutory right to wear turbans in all British schools, institutions and places of work. They were also protesting at Lord Denning's controversial judgment last July that Sikhs are a religious, not a racial, group. The decision upheld a Birmingham headmaster's refusal to admit a Sikh pupil who wanted to wear a turban.

The Federation of Sikh Organisations of the United Kingdom has been lobbying the Home Office and MPs of all parties to amend the 1976 Race Relations Act, following the ruling.

The federation, which represents most of the estimated 250,000 Sikhs in Britain, wants the law changed to protect them from discrimination which they believe could result from Lord Denning's ruling.

When the act was being drawn up, it was proposed that it should ban religious discrimination, but this was dropped, and the Sikh community was assured that it would be protected.

Mr Indarjit Singh, a federation spokesman, said about 140 MPs of all parties had said they would support a bill to amend the act.

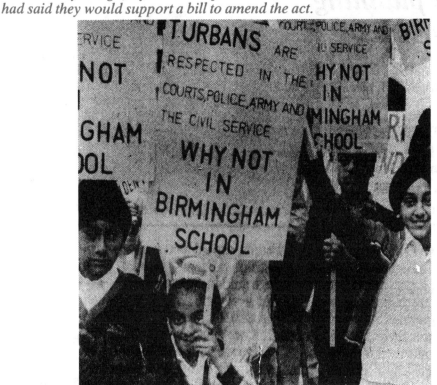

Young black people are asserting a right to their own identity.

The Guardian 27.9.82

Many black children have a strong sense of self-esteem and pride in themselves, their families, and their blackness. But some go through a period of rejection and dislike of themselves, their parents and anything that reminds them that they are not part of the dominant and 'superior' white group.

One thing is sure, that race and colour are never *not* issues for black children. As soon as children learn to distinguish colour and to identify themselves as part of a particular racial group, they begin to receive messages about the relative worth of their own and other groups. The messages conveyed, consciously or unconsciously, by authority figures such as health workers in their relationship with a child or its parents form a crucial part of the child's learning process and of his or her way of seeing and approaching the world.

Health workers need to be aware of the attitudes and values they communicate, consciously or unconsciously, towards black people and minority group cultures. No one is ever *not* communicating.

Race, and the experience of racism, should be acknowledged and discussed whenever appropriate. Racism is a central feature of the life of most black people in Britain. To ignore or choose to deny the existence of racism may give the impression of condoning it.

My experience is that workers rarely talk to the youngsters about race. Yet, when one listens to children and young people it is quickly apparent that colour and cultural differences are a constant issue for them and not something peripheral. When black people living in England experience constant attacks on their self-esteem, it is unwise for social workers, probation officers and teachers to assume that no positive intervention is needed to assist black children with their self-concept. Many social workers may acknowledge that the language of the playground is racially very abusive, but they often

93

argue that it does not mean anything at all. I suggest that this attitude merely reflects that social workers have yet to try and develop an understanding of what it is like to be black in a white society.

Asian social worker[14]

6.4 Family planning

Family size

There is no time for love in English families, no time for laughing. Even with children you just have one or two. Who can they play with? What will you do if those two get ill, or when they leave? That is not a family.

Punjabi grandmother in West London

Some factors that are likely to influence choice of family size:

- **family and social traditions and pressures;**
- **how women and men see their roles and personal priorities;**
- **who makes the decisions;**
- **the space and time available for children;**
- **income and economic circumstances;**
- **benefits or costs of children;**
- **availability of suitable contraceptive methods and ease of access to them;**
- **religious and moral beliefs.**

Economic factors

The choice of family size depends on many factors, not the least of which are economic.

Children in Britain, and in other industrialised consumer-orientated societies are expensive: a survey in *Parents* magazine in 1982 estimated the total cost to average parents of having a baby, including loss of income and taking in the period of pregnancy and the baby's first year of life, as £8,000.[15] The total cost to parents of raising a child to the age of 18 was reckoned by the Consumers' Association in 1980 to be £32,000.[16]

Children in Western Europe are major consumers. In a cold climate they take up a lot of space indoors; they increase lighting, heating and gas bills; they need warm clothes, shoes and protective wear. As a major consumer group they are the targets of high pressure advertising, and so are their parents. They need or want ever more prestigious and expensive toys, games, clothes, electric gadgets, holidays and so forth; they stay on at school until they are sixteen or more, dependent on their parents and under pressure to keep up with their friends in material terms. Once they become earners most young people leave home, often without ever having contributed to the household income. In an urban society they are unlikely to help their parents with the daily chores to the same extent that children can on a farm or in a rural village.

Whereas children may be both a source of family warmth and an economic asset in Third World countries, in industrialised countries they are expensive, an economic liability, and, to parents on a low income in inner-city areas with poor housing and few facilities, they may become more of a worry and a drain than a pleasure.

Economic factors and family size in Britain

A study of British couples, published in 1976, found that the question of how many children a couple felt they could *afford* was by far the most important determinant of family size. Four white British women gave these reasons for deciding to restrict the number of children they had:

Two's enough – for financial reasons. If I had any more I wouldn't be able to keep them.

Well they are too expensive for a kick off. I think it's far better to have one and do right

94

for it than have a few and scrimp and save all the time.

It's threefold. Financial, we don't have any relatives around so no help, both children have problems, and I want to get back to work.

We would like one of each. If I had a house I might have more, but if we stayed here I wouldn't have any more, there's not enough room.[17]

In Britain many people hold the view that couples who have more than three or four children, unless they are wealthy, are 'irresponsible' and 'feckless'. This view is likely to influence British health workers and the judgements they make about, for example, the size of ethnic minority families. But concepts such as 'responsible' and 'irresponsible' are culture-specific. Enormous variation in economic and social factors can mean that what is considered 'responsible' in one society is clearly 'irresponsible' in another.

Economic factors and family size in the Third World

Very different economic, political, climatic, religious and other factors may influence the norms of people now living in Britain who grew up in other countries.

In many areas of the Third World, for example, children represent security and wealth. A study of an unsuccessful population control programme in Punjab (India) concluded:

*The motivations of men and women originate in their social experience. Motivations do not exist in the abstract; their roots are to be found in a given social structure. . . . No programme would have succeeded, because birth control contradicted the vital interests of the majority of the villagers. **To practise contraception would have been wilfully to court economic disaster** [our emphasis].*[18]

Studies of family planning motivation and population control show repeatedly that for people in countries where there is no welfare state, no guarantee of support in old age, and where many hands are needed to run a home or a farm, children are vital economic assets. Population growth declines when communities and societies become richer, and industrial and agricultural processes become more mechanised.

Contraceptives increase people's control over their lives. But they only lower birth rates if people want less children. Experience suggests that people want smaller families only when they are sure that their children will survive, when incomes increase so that child labour is no longer essential, and when security improves so that children are not the only means of support in illness and old age.[19]

In many areas of the world large families are not just an economic necessity, they are a major part of what makes life worth living for ordinary women and men. Children may provide especial fulfilment and purpose for women, particularly if they do not consider it part of their role to work outside the home.

Research in Britain seems to show that second-generation ethnic minority families generally move towards current British norms of family size, apparently influenced largely by the different economic pressures in Britain. Couples who came to Britain as adults are more likely to have ideas about family size very much like those of couples of similar background in their country of origin.[20]

Providing family planning services in Britain

Certain factors may be important when working with or planning services for families from minority groups:

- **Unfamiliarity**: For people relatively new to Britain, or new to family planning services, the way in which they are offered may be confusing and frightening. Only the very bravest woman is likely to approach a family planning clinic where she knows nobody, particularly if her English is limited.

  In many cases domiciliary visits may be far more acceptable, since a relationship of mutual confidence between the woman and one particular health worker can be built up over time.

- **Responsibility**: In communities where a man is entirely responsible for protecting and providing for his wife and children, family planning decisions, like other important family decisions, may be made chiefly by the husband.

  If, for example, a woman's health might be harmed by another pregnancy it may be necessary to discuss this with her husband as well. In sexually conservative communities it is likely to be most acceptable for a male health worker to talk to the husband alone and discuss the issues. Mixed sex discussions of topics such as contraception may be excruciatingly embarrassing for all parties and if so are unlikely to achieve anything.

- **Religious factors**: members of certain communities may regard artificial contraceptive methods as contrary to the spirit or doctrine of their religion. The may apply, for example, to Jews, Muslims, Rastafarians and Roman Catholics.

Some **orthodox Jews** may be reluctant to use contraception. It is traditionally considered good to have a large family in obedience to God's command to be fruitful and multiply (Genesis 1:28). However, the health of the mother and of the whole family must also be considered and many orthodox Jews in Britain use contraception. Abortion is mandatory if there is a danger to the mother's life.

The Holy Quran, to which **Muslims** turn for guidance, contains no explicit ruling on contraception. However, it strongly forbids female infanticide, which was a serious social problem in Saudi Arabia at the time of the Prophet Muhammad. Many conservative Muslims feel that any interference with God's natural design is contrary to the spirit of Islam, and that God will provide for and bless any child whom He sends. However, the Holy Quran also urges Muslims to have no more children than they can look after and educate properly. This is taken by some Muslims to mean that artificial contraception is permissible provided both husband and wife agree and that it is responsibly used.

Governments of Muslim countries vary in the extent to which they encourage family planning programmes. In Bangladesh, for example, the attitude to family planning has changed considerably over the last ten years, and it is no longer a taboo subject.

*In Bangladesh the **mulavis** [the Islamic priests] have in recent years tended either to remain silent on the issue of contraception or to speak in favour of it, quoting the reference in the Quran to Muhammad's apparent sanction of the method of withdrawal or **coitus interruptus**. The government has been to great pains to distribute numerous leaflets putting forward a positive view of family planning based on Islamic teachings.*[4]

In Pakistan attitudes tend to be less favourable towards family planning.

Some **Rastafarians** may be reluctant to limit their families, basing their arguments on both religious and political grounds. The attempt to persuade black people to limit their families may be mistrusted as part of a clear historical pattern of white oppression and violence towards black people.

In the late 1960s when Jamaica and the West Indies were getting more politically and culturally aware, they started for the first time to show black people in advertisements there. It was also about this time that publicity about family planning began and, as it happens, the first time that black people ever appeared on advertisements in the West Indies the message of those advertisements was 'plan your family'. Rastas were then one of the most politically aware and active groups and they were the first to recognise and talk out against this. They became recognised as the group who are anti-contraception. In the 1960s a popular slogan in Jamaica was 'Family Planning – a plot to kill off the black race'.

Afro-Caribbean health worker

Like Jews, Rastafarians may also follow the Old Testament teaching: 'Be fruitful, and multiply, and replenish the earth' (Genesis 1:28).

The Vatican prohibition for **Roman Catholics** is very clear and uncompromising. Sex is for the production of children and no artificial measures must be taken to prevent conception, though 'natural' family planning methods are permissible. However, Roman Catholics in different countries often interpret this more liberally and many Catholics in Britain feel that they should follow the dictates of their own conscience rather than those of the Vatican.

For most people religion is likely to be only one of many factors affecting the choice of family size and of whether to use a contraceptive method.

For members of other religions not mentioned here there appear to be no clear prohibitions on contraception, though individuals may still feel that they do not wish to use a contraceptive method for personal religious or moral reasons.

- **The wider political context**: In introducing the topic of family planning to different communities it is important to be aware of the wider political context in which you and they live.

In many Third World countries foreign and national governments are funding high pressure population control programmes. Many of these are operated in such a way as to produce results of questionable benefit to the local population.

Good results appear to be defined as high numbers of sterilisation operations performed and cycles of oral contraceptives distributed rather than a higher quality of life for the Bangladeshi population. As one cynical USAID staff member put it 'The objective of the (US funded) Family Planning Programme is to eliminate the poor, not to eliminate poverty.'[21]

People from Third World countries now living in Britain may have had experience of coercive family planning programmes themselves and will certainly have heard stories about them. In some countries IUDs have been inserted in unsterile conditions and no thread attached; the heavier bleeding associated with IUDs has often led to severe anaemia; high dose oral contraceptives have been distributed to small often undernourished women; in India Sanjay Gandhi's sterilisation camps, during the 1970s, led to mass sterilisations in which men were brought in at random from their homes and from streets and markets and forcibly vasectomised. **For many people from Third World countries family planning programmes have therefore been seen as a clear attempt to force birth control on certain sections of the population, not as an attempt to increase the control that people have over their own lives or to liberate women from an endless cycle of pregnancy and birth.**

The concern of health workers in Britain that ethnic minorities should limit their families may also be interpreted in this light. Many black women with large families have reported hostile and insulting remarks from health workers and others.

Because I'm Asian too the other nurses get at me. When an Asian woman comes in to have her fifth or sixth baby they are so rude to her, especially if she doesn't speak English. They say terrible things right to her face, like, 'I'd do something to your husband if I could' or 'This one should be sterilised' and often she just smiles politely because she doesn't understand. And then they come and tell me to tell her that she mustn't have any more babies. They say, 'She's one of yours, tell her it's revolting to have so many children. Somebody should do something to her husband.'

Asian nurse in a maternity unit

Many black people are suspicious of the motives of the Health Service's evident concern to promote family planning for ethnic minority communities. They feel that there has been a single-minded concentration on getting ethnic minority women to use contraception but not the same concentration on other equally important health needs.

- **Depo-Provera**: Much of this concern has become focused on the injectable contraceptive Depo-Provera. Doubts over the long-term side effects have led to Depo-Provera being banned in its country of manufacture, the USA. In Britain the Committee on the Safety of Medicines has approved Depo-Provera for short-term use only, such as for three months after a rubella vaccination or until a negative sperm count following a vasectomy.

The Campaign Against Depo-Provera claims that Depo-Provera is being used in Britain to force birth control on those whom society considers feckless and unfit to breed, particularly on black and working-class women and on the mentally handicapped. There is concern that the unpleasant side-effects are not explained to women. These are irreversible for the full term of the injection: once the injection has been given nothing can be done to prevent any side-effects which may appear. There are also fears that Depo-Provera may be carcinogenic and that in some women it may lead to permanent sterility.

The Campaign also claims that Depo-Provera is given particularly to black women who speak little or no English precisely because it is so easy to give, because no communication about the mechanics of it is necessary, and because it requires no cooperation or understanding from the woman herself, unlike the pill or other contraceptive methods. Once given, no pregnancy can occur for three months, however unpleasant a woman finds the side effects.

In New Zealand, Depo-Provera is given to a disproportionate number of Polynesian women who are provided with no interpretation of what the English-speaking doctors tell them. Are they exercising their Right to Choose? Similarly, in Britain, the records of two family planning clinics in the East End of London revealed that in Clinic 'A' two-thirds of the women on Depo-Provera were described as Asian, in Clinic 'B' a third were Asian. Many spoke little or no English and the author of the study, Dr Wendy Savage, doubted whether more than one out of five patients had been given proper information about Depo-Provera.[22].

Many ethnic minority individuals and communities question the enthusiasm with which some health workers attempt to persuade them to use contraception. Are we increasing women's control over their own lives or are we exerting our control over them, their families, and their communities?

Choosing a family planning method

A woman won't use a method she's not happy with. It's not like buying a pair of socks. You have to make sure that she's really confident and happy in her mind before you let her go.

Family planning doctor

Very often the decision to use contraception at all is a difficult one. **A health worker should never try to pressurise a woman on this issue**; but once a woman has decided to use some kind of contraception, the health worker's task is then to make sure that she is provided with a method that suits her. Some methods are likely to be more acceptable than others. For example:

- For some Roman Catholics, Muslims and Rastafarians **natural family planning methods** may be most acceptable because they do not involve the use of any artificial barrier.

- **Methods such as the coil, Depo-Provera and the pill**, which may cause spotting between periods, may be unacceptable to women who feel unclean and do not perform normal routines when they are menstruating. Women who are devout Muslims, for example, must traditionally not say formal prayers, touch the Holy Quran or have sexual intercourse during a period. Many are distressed by bleeding between periods and do not know what they should do.

- For several reasons **the sheath** may be a popular method:

  In families where men take full responsibility for providing for children they may also make decisions on family size.

  No medical examination is required. Women who find internal examinations humiliating and shocking, or who disapprove of them for religious reasons, may find the sheath the most acceptable method.

  The husband can get the sheaths himself and his wife is not forced to attend a clinic or to brave nurses, doctors and chemists.

  When you talk about contraception, you are really discussing sex. For people for whom sex is a private or, perhaps, shameful topic, premeditation and planning are not required if a sheath is used.

- There is a belief among some health workers involved in family planning that **the diaphragm** is not appropriate for or acceptable to many women from ethnic minority communities, especially Muslim and/or non-English-speaking women. It is true that the principle on which it works is likely to be unfamiliar to many women, and some are initially embarrassed at inserting and removing a diaphragm.

This reluctance, coupled with a language barrier, sometimes discourages the health worker from suggesting it as a possible alternative. But individual family planning nurses and health visitors have found that it is a method which has a strong appeal to some women, since of all the methods available it gives the greatest degree of control over their own fertility. Experience has shown that if this factor is carefully explained, it may provide the motivation for some women to overcome lack of confidence or embarrassment about using it.

Explanation of the diaphragm may take some time and probably the help of an interpreter. But this choice of method should not be denied to non-English-speaking or Muslim women, as is sometimes the case, simply because the health worker has preconceived ideas about its acceptability or because it takes longer to explain.

Every contraceptive method has disadvantages. Full discussion is necessary so that all the positive and negative points of each method are understood. This is clearly impossible through a language barrier. If the client speaks little or no English it is essential to have either a health worker who speaks the client's language or an interpreter. Even clients with a working knowledge of everyday English may not be able to participate in a proper discussion about menstruation, contraception, side-effects, etc. and may need an intepreter.

Questions to think about[23]

- What are the attitudes of most people within a particular community towards family planning? Why?

- Do you know what *women* within the community think about how many children they want?
  What is the range of views among women within one community about family planning?

- Which methods are preferred and why?

- What doubts or anxieties exist about different methods and their effect on natural fertility?

- Do men often have different attitudes from women? Why?

- In what ways do family planning services meet people's needs? Are there ways in which they might abuse people?

- Should the health worker encourage parents to plan their families? All parents? Only some parents? Which? Should a health worker bring up the subject of family planning when a mother comes for other medical care, or when she brings her children? Should it only be discussed when a mother expresses interest? Should this depend on the needs of the individual family?

- Whose needs does family planning presently meet in your area?
  How could it better meet the needs of ethnic minority families?

Notes

1. Amin, Geeta, *Some Aspects of Social Policy Affecting Asian Women in Britain,* unpublished paper, 1977.
2. Ballard, Catherine, 'Conflict, Continuity and Change', in Khan (ed.), *Minority and Families in Britain*, Macmillan, 1979.
3. Cheetham, Juliet, *Social Work Services for Ethnic Minorities in Britain and the USA*, Dept. of Social and Admin. Studies, University of Oxford, 1981.
4. Ellis, June, (ed.), *West African Families in Britain*, Routledge, 1978.
5. Ellis, June, 'Foster Kids in the Culture Gap', in Cheetham *et al.* (eds) *Social and Community Work in a Multi-Racial Society*, Harper and Row, 1981.
6. Cooper, J. M., *Elderly West Indians in Leicester*, unpublished dissertation for M.A. in Social Service Planning, Dept. of Sociology, University of Essex, 1977.
7. Asian Community Action Group, 'Asians Sheltered Residential Accommodation', 1980, quoted in Glendinning, Frank, (ed.), 'The Ethnic Elderly: Cause for Concern' Unit *16:3 Ethnic Minorities and Social Community Work,* E354, Open University, 1982.
8. Ladbury, Sarah, *Cypriots in Britain*, NCILT, 1979.

9. Hiro, Dilip, *Black British, White British*, Penguin, 1973.
10. Haley, Alex, *Roots*, Picador, 1979.
11. Pringle, M. K. and Naidoo, S., *Early Child Care in Britain*, Gordon & Breach, 1979.
12. Crossfield family, *Seven of Us*, A & C Black, 1978.
13. Milner, David, *Children and Race*, Penguin, 1975.
14. Ahmed, Shama, 'Children in Care: The Racial Dimension in Social Work Assessment', in Cheetham *et al.*, *(eds)*, *Social & Community Work in a Multi-Racial Society*, Harper & Row, 1981.
15. *Parents Magazine*, June 1982.
16. *Guardian*, 23 Dec. 1981.
17. Cartwright, Anne, *How Many Children*, Routledge, 1976.
18. Mamdani, Mahmood, *The Myth of Population Control*, Monthly Review Press, 1972.
19. *New Internationalist*, No. 109, January 1982.
20. Iliffe, L., *New Society*, 6 April 1978.
21. Schweiger, Martin, *Family Planning in the Bangladeshi Community of Keighley*, unpublished dissertation for Master in Public Health, University of Leeds, 1982.
22. *Depo Provera*, The Campaign Against Depo-Provera, 1981.
23. Adapted from Werner, D. and Bower, B., *Helping Health Workers Learn*, Hesperian Foundation, 1982.

More information

If you want to find out more about family systems and family life in local communities in your area, a useful starting point is:

14 **Local needs: guidelines for doing your own research**
See particularly the questions on family life in
14.4 **Things you need to know**

The effects of migration on family life are considered in
3 **Migration and health**, especially
3.3 **Social and psychological pressures**

The problems of misleading generalisations and cultural stereotypes are discussed in
4 **Culture: a misleading explanation of health inequalities**, especially
4.2 **Stereotypes**

Further reading

See reading list in Chapter 16:
16.6 **Working with families and individuals**

See also relevant titles in the reading lists for other chapters: e.g.
16.3 **Migration and health**
16.4 **Culture: a misleading explanation of health inequalities**
16.7 **Health beliefs and practices**

7 Health beliefs and practices

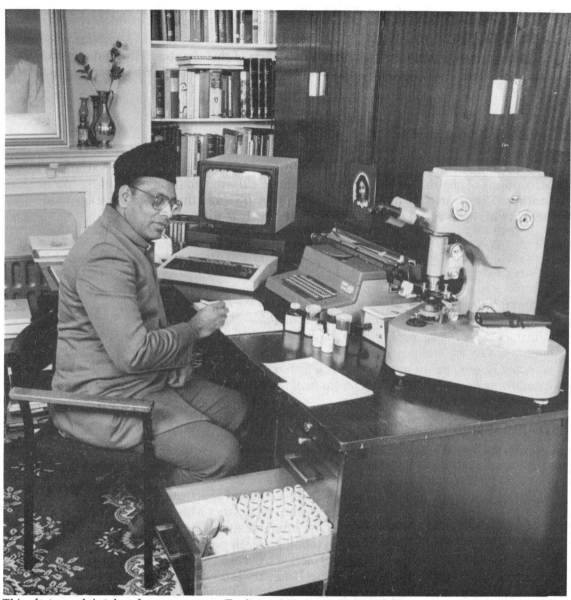

This photograph is taken from a paper on *Traditional Medicine* by Hakim, M. R. Qureshi, MA, MRUP.

7.1 Concepts of health

7.2 Expectations and experience of the health services

7.3 Use of traditional or alternative forms of health care

7.4 Working with different health beliefs and practices

Introduction

Beliefs about health and illness, ways of maintaining or improving health, and practices in caring for and curing the sick, vary widely. They differ between professional health workers and lay people, between middle-class and working-class people, between individual families, and between cultures. In the context of working with ethnic minority communities three aspects of health beliefs and practices are likely to be important:

- concepts of health
- expectations and experience of the health services
- use of traditional or alternative forms of health care.

These topics are explored in the first three parts of this chapter. The final section sets out some useful principles and practical suggestions for health workers wanting to find out more about traditional or alternative health systems.

7.1 Concepts of health

Ideas about health and illness are socially determined. There are wide variations in perceptions of health and illness both in a single culture and from one culture to another. **The greater the difference between your own and the patient's background, the more his ideas about health and illness are likely to differ from yours.**

Beliefs about health and illness, the causes of disease, the appropriate reactions to ill-health, where to seek treatment, and how to prevent disease, are as much part of a culture as language, religion or family patterns, and as distinct as the patterns of behaviour in other cultures. If people from different cultures hold different views on health, it is likely that they will react differently to the health services. The health services in Britain are based on a model of health and disease causation that is part of British culture. Because it is part of the culture it is 'taken for granted' and hence not questioned by the majority of the population; prescribed behaviour is logical within the accepted system, but to someone from a different culture the 'normal behaviour' may seem strange or illogical. Beliefs about health and illness are part of a 'world-view', and cannot be evaluated in isolation.[1]

'Superstition' or a different kind of logic?

Different health beliefs and practices do not come about by accident; they are not arbitrary. **Because it is sometimes not easy to understand the logical basis of a particular belief or practice, it doesn't mean there isn't one. It need not be logic based on the laws of Western medical science to be valid and practical.** The value of a belief or practice may lie in its religious significance (e.g. strict Muslims, Jews and Rastafarians regard pork as unclean); its ritual meaning (e.g. nurses changing their aprons when a patient dies); or the psychological support it provides (e.g. GPs prescribing tablets for their placebo effect). Physical and biological phenomena may be explained in symbolic or metaphorical imagery rather than in literal terms. The value of a particular therapy may lie in its power to stimulate the body's self-healing mechanisms.

Differences between the health worker's and patient's view of illness

If you are working with people from different communities you will need to discuss some of the points below to ensure that the preventive health care, advice and treatment you suggest is appropriate and acceptable in the eyes of the patient – otherwise it may be useless.

- Is good luck or good management seen as the main explanation of good health?
- What measures do people expect to take to prevent illness?
- Who defines illness? How is it defined?
- Is a distinction made between mental and physical illness?
- What are the causes of illness?
- What conditions are considered normal or abnormal?
- What can or can't people expect to have treated?

- What is regarded as adequate or normal functioning for the individual's age or sex?
- What is a normal level of energy or activity? Of pain? Of restrictions on mobility?
- What are the relevant factors in diagnosing illness?
- How is illness cured or treated?
- What kind of treatment do people expect?
- What can a person reasonably be expected to go through to be cured?
- What support and help does a person expect to draw on during illness?
- What is the expected role of health professionals, family and friends?
- How much is the individual expected to do for himself?

Some of these questions are discussed in more detail below, along with a few practical suggestions.

Good luck, good management and preventive health care

Most preventive health programmes are based on the principle that health is the result of good management; the message of most health education campaigns is that health is the responsibility of the individual and ill health can be avoided through the individual's efforts to alter his personal behaviour.

But for people who are on low incomes, who lack the basic necessities of life and who feel socially isolated, health is largely determined by factors over which they may have little control – low quality housing, inadequate diet, poor working conditions, etc. The choices they can make about their own health and that of their children, and the extent to which they can follow advice about health are limited by these wider constraints.

The individual who feels that health and illness are outside his personal control will see little value in preventive health advice that advocates changes in personal behaviour, but ignores the impact of social, environmental and economic conditions on health. **This is why an increasing number of health educators argue that health education must take on a broader role, recognising a collective responsibility for health, and helping to increase people's ability to change their home and work environment through collective action.**

Defining illness

Once a sick person decides to consult the GP about his symptoms, it is the GP who then defines the illness: she decides whether the symptoms warrant a prescription, sick note, blood test, X-ray, referral to a specialist, or no action but simply reassurance.

The majority of a GP's patients present with fairly common and familiar symptoms. But patients from different backgrounds may present with symptoms in an unexpected way:

- **Symptoms regarded as minor by the GP may mean something far more serious in the patient's country of origin.** For example, coughs and colds, regarded as minor seasonal illnesses in Britain, often reach epidemic proportions in the Punjab where most people have little immunity and low resistance to them. In Britain diarrhoea in infants can be serious but is not usually a killer. In hot climates dehydration from diarrhoea kills thousands of infants every year.

- **Patients may present with symptoms common in their country of origin but unfamiliar to the doctor.** 'A GP colleague told me about a Bengali woman who complained constantly of "burning hands" which completely baffled him. . . . In fact, she could well be trying to describe the kind of sensation produced by Vitamin B deficiency, which causes pellagra . . . which is common in Bangladesh, . . . I treated several patients suffering from "burning hands" while I was out there.'

- **There is always a danger of under-diagnosis with ethnic minority patients, if doctors are not alert to the different patterns of illness in different ethnic groups.** For example, a GP may not realise that 'aching bones' in a pregnant Asian woman could be an indication of osteomalacia; she may not recognise the characteristic symptoms of a sickle cell crisis in a West Indian child.

Mental and physical illness

The distinction made by Western psychiatric medicine between 'mental' and 'physical' illness may not correspond at all with the way illness is perceived in other societies.

The dichotomy between 'physical' and 'mental' illness (tempered by the somewhat lame qualification that the mind and emotions can have some effect on the body and its physical ills) is a notion springing out of Western medical tradition. Healers in other cultures may have a very different way of looking at the 'body' and the 'mind', often more wisely not differentiating at all between 'physical' and 'mental' because they understand the essential unity of the two.[2]

Some psychiatrists have questioned whether 'mental illness' is not itself a cultural concept shaped by Western medicine.

Different societies have their own way of describing what we usually call mental illness. It may be thought of, as it is by most psychiatrists, as analogous to physical illness, or it may be perceived as a religious phenomenon – spirit possession or the consequence of witchcraft – or even in terms of abnormal or anti-social behaviour. . . .

Why do different societies have different concepts of mental illness? Is it that non-Europeans fail to recognise something that is quite obviously there? Or is 'mental illness' really a cultural idea, like spirit possession or witchcraft?[3]

A growing number of professionals now recognise the need for trained bilingual workers and counsellors who can bridge the cultural gap between the practitioner's and the patient's view of the world, especially in the field of mental health and psychiatry.

Causes of illness

Western medicine tends to view illness as something which affects only specific organs or bodily functions, rather than the whole person. In some societies illness is seen much more in terms of the whole body, the individual's state of mind, and social relationships. Western medicine is concerned with *how* a person becomes ill (the specific causes of a particular disease), but Western medical science is less concerned with *why* a particular individual should happen to succumb to that particular disease at that particular time, even though the patient is often preoccupied with finding an explanation. In some cultures there is greater concern by the healer to explain *why* a particular person becomes ill. Illness may be attributed to bad luck, bad management, spiritual affliction, poor diet, emotional or psychological stress, punishment for shameful behaviour, the ill-will of another person, or malignant spiritual powers. This will directly influence the kind of treatment that is seen as appropriate.

Normal and abnormal conditions

Whether a condition is regarded as normal or abnormal depends on the individual's lifestyle, environment, and the consequent priority attached to particular needs and tasks. In Britain, for example, the elderly are often expected to be less mobile and alert: arthritis and senile dementia are regarded by some people as 'normal' or 'inevitable' in old age. Similarly, back pain is so common in people over 40, that sufferers are often told they have to learn to live with it.

People from other backgrounds may use different criteria from a Western doctor in deciding whether a condition is normal or not. For example, certain endemic diseases (such as the eye disease, trachoma, which is common in Vietnam) may be regarded by some people as an everyday affliction that has to be put up with.

Diagnosis

Factors other than those used in orthodox Western medicine may be significant in the process of diagnosing an illness. For example, in traditional Chinese and Ayurvedic (Indian) medicine a complex system of pulse-taking is a major diagnostic tool.[4] In homeopathic diagnosis, the patient's complexion, colouring, personality, likes and dislikes, and dreams may all be significant in determining appropriate treatment.

Treatment

As far as possible, the therapy prescribed should match the patient's views of appropriate treatment. Depending on what the individual believes to be the cause of his illness, he may expect the practitioner to prescribe one or several of the following: medication, rest, exercise, prayer, massage, diet, and change of routine.

Preferred forms of medication vary from one country to another. The English take tablets; the Italians prefer suppositories; in some Third World countries (for example, Vietnam, Bangladesh) injections are seen as the most effective medicine.

Some people may have very high expectations of the effectiveness of Western drugs and hope for an immediate cure when this is simply not possible. **Find out what a person's expectations are and explain carefully what a particular medication can or cannot do. It may be important to emphasise that a particular drug is only suitable for the condition it is prescribed for, and should not be used for other conditions or by anybody else.**

The desirability of treatment

The health worker's job is to help people get well, or at least to improve their quality of life during illness as far as possible. But sometimes a patient simply does not want to go through the protracted effort and discomfort involved in treatment.

My uncle had cancer and he refused to have chemotherapy. He'd reached a point where he decided he didn't want to go on. 'I'm going to die sooner or later anyway', was his attitude. He said, 'I just don't want to go through all that rigmarole and messing about – it's not worth it any more.'

English nurse

It is important to respect the fact that in the patient's view, some treatments can represent a reduction rather than an improvement in the quality of life.

On the other hand, there have been cases where patients initially refused treatment because they mistrusted Western medicine or because treatment was complicated or protracted and the details were not properly explained to them. In these circumstances it is essential to use a bilingual worker with counselling skills who can both convey the patient's fears and anxieties to the health care team and explain the treatment fully to the patient.

Support during illness

In some communities, care during illness is regarded very much as a family responsibility, while in others the individual may be expected to brave it out on his own. **Try to find out what part other family members expect to play, who expects to be involved in decisions about care and treatment. It may be important to discuss instructions and advice with other family members as well as the patient.**

7.2 *Expectations and experience of the health services*

People's own ideas about health and illness will affect what they expect of the health services and how they use them but this also depends on several other factors:

- **What kind of health care system are people used to?**
- **Where do people expect to go for help or treatment?**
- **How easy is it to find out about and get access to the services currently available?**
- **Are existing services appropriate to needs?**
- **Do individual health staff have a positive or negative attitude towards patients from different backgrounds?**

What kind of health care system are people used to?

People who have not grown up in Britain may be used to a system of health care that is completely different from the NHS. In some Third World countries Western medical facilities are extremely scarce. They may be confined to the more developed or urban areas; they may only be available to those with enough money to pay expensive consultation and treatment fees.

Alternatively there is sometimes an uncoordinated range of Western medical facilities available in one area. There might be, for example, a private clinic for European expatriates, a free government health clinic, a public health department running immunisation programmes, a group of missionaries running a small hospital and an aid team operating a mobile dispensary, all functioning independently of each other.

People on low incomes in rural areas may have relied far more on traditional or informal systems of health care (see below).

In some Third World countries Western and traditional health care systems are not mutually exclusive, as they tend to be in Britain. For example, the governments of India, China and Vietnam among others have actively encouraged the research and development of traditional medicine as an integral part of the state health care system[5].

Where do people expect to go for help or treatment?

In every community there is a chain of referral used when a person becomes ill, injured, pregnant, etc. For example, an English mother in a Yorkshire town worried about eczema in her six-year-old daughter sought advice in the following order:

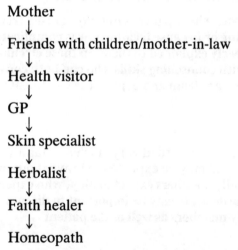

Mother
↓
Friends with children/mother-in-law
↓
Health visitor
↓
GP
↓
Skin specialist
↓
Herbalist
↓
Faith healer
↓
Homeopath

Patients from a different background are likely to use different chains of referral. For example, an Indian mother living in a Punjabi village might seek help for the same problem in this order:

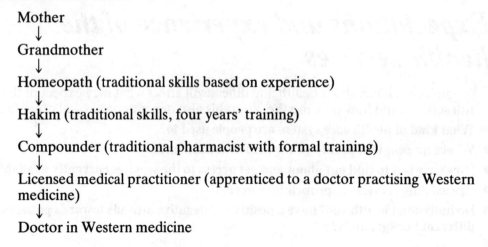

Mother
↓
Grandmother
↓
Homeopath (traditional skills based on experience)
↓
Hakim (traditional skills, four years' training)
↓
Compounder (traditional pharmacist with formal training)
↓
Licensed medical practitioner (apprenticed to a doctor practising Western medicine)
↓
Doctor in Western medicine

Some members of ethnic minority communities are likely to need specific information about the expected chains of referral for different health needs in Britain. In some communities, men may prefer to seek help from other men, and women from other women. Wherever possible, health workers should be sensitive to the fact that some people are acutely embarrassed at having to see a practitioner of the opposite sex.

The role and status of health workers

People who come from a background where the role and status of health workers is different may not know what to expect of a GP or hospital nurse, etc.

The family doctor: In this country a person is expected to register with a GP who is then consulted for all health problems. NHS patients are not expected to shop around for a doctor: most people seem to choose their GP by geographical accessibility and then stay with him for good, unless they move elsewhere.[6] But in some countries there is no system of registering with a doctor and it is quite normal to refer to different doctors for different problems, or to several doctors for the same problem.

In Hong Kong it's common to try out two or three doctors for the same problem, if you don't seem to be getting anywhere, and a lot of Chinese in Britain prefer to get two or three opinions when we're ill. I must admit I find it odd that people see their GP as the only option. I mean, you wouldn't go on taking your car to a garage that couldn't fix it, would you?

Chinese health education worker

Nurses: Nursing may be disapproved of as a female profession by older or more conservative members of some communities.

Older male Muslim patients are often unaccustomed to dealing with women in positions of authority or with professional status and may sometimes be embarrassed and difficult with female health workers. This is particularly likely with nurses, who generally have a low status in traditional Muslim and Asian societies since they have physical contact with strange men.[7]

How easy is it to find out about and get access to the services currently available?

When a particular community or patient group doesn't make use of the health services as expected, attention is often focused on what's wrong with *them*, rather than on asking what's wrong with the delivery of the services.

*I heard a community doctor describing the **particularly terrible** problem they had in their urban area because the Asian immigrants there were from a rural background. In other words, the more different the clients are from the health worker and the British environment, the more of a problem they are. Another view that is often voiced is that advice given to Asians is not listened to and the communication problem or ignorance that is causing this is therefore a great problem. Then there is the difficulty that Asian patients may not attend for appointments, seem to change their surnames, keep changing their family doctor and generally not follow instructions – they are therefore seen as un-cooperative.*

All this is based on three assumptions – that immigrants should know as much about the NHS as someone born in Britain, that there should be one-way communication only – i.e. from the professionals to the patients – and that medical care is the most important factor affecting health. All these assumptions are false, I believe, and are leading to this 'problematic' view of immigrant patients.[8]

If services are not reaching a particular community, or if the community is making use of services in an unexpected way, these are some of the factors for consideration:

- What information is available about the way the services work? In plain English? In the community's own language, if relevant?
- If a significant proportion of people are not literate in English or their own language, are there bilingual workers available to explain how hospital and community health services work? And to provide professional care?

- Are surgeries and clinics physically and geographically accessible?
- Are the times of surgeries, child health clinics, ante-natal clinics, etc. suitable for the population they serve?
- Do community health staff such as GPs, Health Visitors, community midwives and nurses always explain their role to patients?

Some members of ethnic minority communities may face real problems in making use of the health services available to them because NHS practices conflict with their own values or beliefs. For example, services may be inappropriate because of:

- religious or cultural conventions about contact between men and women;
- religious or cultural differences in food habits;
- language and communication difficulties.

Suggestions for coping with these and other aspects of service provision are discussed in Chapter 10.

Do health staff have a positive or negative attitude towards patients from different backgrounds?

The support and understanding of health staff can go a long way towards smoothing out some of the difficulties that ethnic minority patients can experience in using the health services. On the other hand, the health worker who has negative expectations of ethnic minority patients may be making her own job more difficult than it need be. Patients who sense a negative attitude may in turn react negatively to the health worker. The benefit that the patient should derive from health care may be reduced in various ways:

- If patients think that health workers will disapprove of their traditional health beliefs, they may be reluctant to disclose relevant information about, for example, traditional treatments being applied.
- If health workers respond with impatience and irritation to patients who do not speak English very well, they are likely to become increasingly withdrawn, isolated and unhappy. Some patients may try to avoid contact with unsympathetic health workers altogether by pretending to understand no English at all.
- If patients feel they will be pressurised by health workers to eat food they consider unsuitable, they may refuse hospital treatment or discharge themselves.
- Women who have large families will be reluctant to use the health services if they are continually told that they have too many children and must not have any more.
- Ethnic minority women may drop out of ante-natal classes if they feel that class teachers are not sympathetic to their particular needs and anxieties:

I felt very left out. They made me feel very self-conscious. My English is not good you see. I was left alone so I stopped going. We were two Asian mothers and we both stopped going. If there were a group of Asian mothers – yes, I'd go – I'd feel better.

Asian woman[9]

Professional expectations are also discussed in 2.6 and 12.3.

7.3 Use of traditional or alternative forms of health care

As the examples at the beginning of the previous section show, most people, whatever their background, make use of various sources of help for different problems, ranging from the informal but often experienced advice of members of their own community, through various kinds of alternative or traditional healers (who may or may not charge for treatment), to the formalised services of orthodox Western medicine. People thus seek help from some point on a spectrum which looks like this:

INFORMAL	TRADITIONAL/ ALTERNATIVE	FORMALISED
e.g.	e.g.	e.g.
Mother	Acupuncturist	General Practitioner
Aunt	Herbalist	Health Visitor
Sister-in-law	Homeopath	Casualty department
Respected older member of community		
Friend		

The point they choose depends on their background, culture, income, the terms in which they see their illness, and what they believe different practitioners can or cannot do for them. For example, many people who have grown up with the NHS would try alternative medicine only as a last resort. They share the view of many members of the medical establishment in Britain that traditional or alternative medicine is the domain largely of quacks and charlatans.

On the other hand, for people from Third World countries, alternatives to orthodox Western medicine may be a much more potent option, for the reasons discussed above.

Many people settled in Britain have grown up in communities where there are one or several alternatives to Western medicine. They are likely to go on making use of traditional healers in this country when they feel it is appropriate.

For example, people from the Indian subcontinent (India, Pakistan and Bangladesh) may go to a *vaid* or *hakim* for treatment. The Chinese and Vietnamese may consult an acupuncturist or herbalist from their own community.

The extent to which members of a community make use of their own traditional medicine varies widely. Families and individuals will seek help from the source they feel to be most appropriate for a particular illness. People who have grown up in a country where traditional medicine is an integral part of the state health care system (see above) may see no sharp distinction between traditional and Western medicine.

Why are traditional beliefs important in health care?

Belief in the value of traditional medicine, whether it has a proven scientific basis or not, is likely to be very important to a sick person, possibly as important as his religious beliefs. Traditional health beliefs may even be based on or closely bound up with the patient's religious philosophy.

If you are working with members of a community that has a strong tradition of alternative health care, it is useful to find out as much as you can about the system, for the simple reason that it is more effective to work with people's beliefs than against them. If your advice or treatment contradicts an individual's own health beliefs, it may be discounted; if you discount the patient's beliefs, he may be deterred from disclosing relevant information. The patient may even lose confidence in you and the health service, and delay seeking treatment when it is important.

At the immediately practical level, the more the health worker can find out about the patient's own beliefs, the less misunderstanding there is likely to be. Knowledge of a community's traditional health system means that the health worker can provide suitable advice or treatment in the confidence that the patient sees it as appropriate and will act on it.

An Asian woman came to talk to us about how Asian mothers look after themselves during pregnancy. She was talking about religious beliefs and how they affect diet, and also about this idea that pregnancy is a hot condition so women eat cold foods. Well suddenly things fell into place because we'd had an Indian woman in the week before on the antenatal ward and she kept saying she couldn't eat this and that, she wanted cold food. . . . Well, we kept offering her ice cream, and we couldn't understand why she wouldn't touch it. . . . The difficulty is that it seems to vary a lot . . . what one person counts as hot, another counts as cold . . . and some don't bother . . . so the menu takes a bit of negotiating, but at least I've stopped offering people ice cream!

Staff midwife

It is not simply that a negative approach to traditional medicine may have a negative effect on the practitioner–patient relationship. Some of the therapies of alternative and traditional medicine are positively beneficial in themselves, used either as an alternative or complementary to conventional medical treatment. This is one reason why, in some countries, traditional medicine receives financial support from the state.

It is argued that the health care system in Britain is itself beginning to move in this direction, as an increasing number of NHS doctors are prepared to consider the potential value of treatments such as acupuncture for the relief of chronic pain, osteopathy for non-specific back pain, homeopathy for allergies and possibly rheumatoid arthritis, etc.

I think it's rather difficult nowadays to know what to call conventional and what to call unconventional medicine. This is probably a good thing because the distinction is becoming blurred. I think that any treatment at all which claims to have any effect should be looked at dispassionately and objectively by people who know what it is doing. The only way you can test things is by looking at them. It's no use refusing to have any truck with something just because it has been done by someone who is a bit way out.

Medical researcher[10]

There has certainly been a growth of interest in alternative medicine among ordinary peoople in Britain in the last few years. People are attracted to it for the same reasons[11] that unorthodox medical systems remain and will continue to remain a strong tradition in some ethnic minority communities:

- **The traditional practitioner can often spend more time with the patient than a busy NHS doctor.** The average length of consultation in a GP's surgery is six minutes. The traditional practitioner may spend anything from 15 minutes to an hour with the patient. If nothing else, the patient is likely to get psychological benefit from the attention the traditional practitioner can give to his problem.

- **Some people may prefer traditional medicine because they are afraid of, or unable to tolerate, unpleasant side effects from drugs.** The attraction of homeopathic remedies, for example, is that doses come in minute quantities so that even if they do not achieve a cure, they cannot harm the patient.

- Traditional medicine may be able to provide **relief for problems that conventional Western medicine sometimes cannot help**, such as backache, migraine, allergies, rheumatism and arthritis.

- Patients may prefer to go to an alternative practitioner because they can retain **a greater degree of control over what happens to them.** Some people feel that conventional medicine is organised in a way that removes control from patients and expects them to be passive and accepting. Paying an alternative practitioner for treatment gives the individual a greater say in what happens to him during illness. This is not a justification for the privatisation of the NHS but rather it is an argument for giving patients more control over what happens to them when they seek NHS treatment.

- The patient's loss of control is in part related to the fact that **conventional Western medicine is based on an engineering approach to the human body and the diseases that affect it.**[12] The individual is fragmented into functioning or non-functioning parts. Health care tends to be correspondingly fragmented into different departments that specialise in the workings of those particular parts (e.g. gynaecology, haematology, nephrology, etc.), often, it is argued, to the exclusion of the rest of the patient and his social needs. **In contrast many traditional and alternative medical systems are based on a holistic philosophy:** illness is looked at in terms of the whole body, the individual's state of mind and social relationships.

Holistic health systems

Some of the information below is adapted from an article in *Community Nursing*, December 1981, by Hilary Homans and Antoinette Satow.

To illustrate what is meant by a holistic approach, three traditional medical systems are described below. Most people settled in Britain who originate from West Africa, South East Asia and the Indian sub-continent are probably familiar with one of these systems of traditional medicine, but bear in mind that families and individuals vary widely in the extent to which they make use of them.

- **Today theories of traditional medicine are not necessarily interpreted literally, even though regarded as effective in practice.**

- **There are many local variations and popular interpretations of traditional therapies.**

- **Younger and more Westernised members of the community may disregard traditional beliefs and practices altogether.**

Nigerian medicine

Our first example of a traditional medical system is from West Africa. The basis of traditional medical practice in Nigeria is similar to that found in many other parts of Africa. African medicine can only properly be understood in its wider context as part of a broad religious and philosophical framework through which the individual interprets his existence.

The people of Nigeria's western region, the Yoruba, have developed a complex philosophical system in which man is seen as being at the centre of a web of personal and spiritual relationships. The individual's ancestors, the gods and spirits, and the plants and animals of his environment, all have an influence on his present existence, and consequently influence his state of health.

The traditional healer is likely to focus far more attention than a Western doctor on the individual's personal life in diagnosing an illness. In identifying the causes of the illness, healer and patient may consider possibilities such as the influence of ill-disposed persons or malignant spiritual powers, or some disturbance or imbalance in the individual's private life or social relationships. Minor illnesses are often treated by a herbalist, but for more serious and for mental illness a person may go to a healer who makes his diagnosis by divination. The healer, or diviner, often provides a valuable form of psychotherapy, by prescribing ritual and practical measures aimed at a fundamental reorganisation of the patient's personal relationships.

Chinese medicine

The philosophical principles underlying Chinese traditional medicine also take into account the relationship between the whole person, his environment and his culture. The normal functioning of the body is seen as depending on an equilibrium between two opposite energies, *yin* and *yang*. According to Chinese medical theory there are also five elements (wood, fire, earth, metal and water) which influence health and illness and the functioning of the major organs in the body. Disease occurs when the balance of *yin* and *yang*, or of the five elements, is disturbed. For health to be restored the imbalance must be corrected. The aim of the traditional practitioner is to restore the equilibrium of these vital forces so that the patient himself is then able to overcome his illness.

Illness is diagnosed by questioning the patient about his complaint and medical history, by observation of general appearance, colour, respiration, and by pulse-taking.

The traditional practitioner uses a variety of methods to restore equilibrium in the body's energies. He may, for example, prescribe exercise, herbal treatment, acupuncture, or a therapeutic diet. A balance of *yin* and *yang* can be restored by prescribing 'hot' or 'cold' foods as appropriate and correct diet is regarded as important in maintaining health and preventing illness.

Ayurvedic medicine

The traditional Hindu system of medicine, Ayurveda, is based on a similar philosophy. Ayurvedic medicine also views health as a state of equilibrium and disease as a state of disharmony in the body as a whole. Treatment is aimed at finding appropriate internal remedies, using all available means to restore the normal balance or equilibrium.

According to Ayurvedic medicine a person's constitution is made up of three humours: *vata* (wind), *pitta* (bile) and *kapha* (phlegm). When these three humours are in a state of balance the body is healthy. To maintain a balance of humours the individual pays specific attention to what he eats. Health is measured in terms of good appetite, healthy diet and defaecation. Common illnesses are often attributed to poor food digestion.

In Ayurveda, as in Chinese medicine, foods are believed to have hot and cold qualities, according to the effect they have on the body. Foods are seen as particularly important when a person is sick or when the body is in a state of imbalance – for example, during pregnancy.

Preventive care

In each of these traditional systems, health maintenance is of prime importance. Detailed instructions and prophylactic measures are observed to prevent illness. If illness does occur, the whole person is treated by an adjustment of diet and/or the prescription of traditional remedies. The illness is often attributed to a digression from the rules governing health behaviour – for example, eating certain foods at the wrong time of day. Or the illness may be seen as a disturbance in the social order or environment.

Social relationships

The importance given to the environment and social relationships as causes of illness contrasts sharply with the Western medical system, which views specific pathologies as the cause of illness. Because of the emphasis on treatment of specific disease there is a tendency for orthodox Western medicine to underestimate social and environmental factors.

The difference in philosophies between Western and traditional medical systems leads their respective practitioners to adopt fundamentally different approaches. The traditional practitioner is likely to spend more time looking at the individual's circumstances and social relationships, and establishing a personal rapport with the patient. Because Western medicine is based on the medication and treatment of specific diseases, health services are organised in such a way that factors like the patient's material circumstances and the relationship between practitioner and patient come to be seen as secondary considerations in medical practice.

This is one reason why some members of ethnic minority communities in Britain prefer to seek treatment from a traditional practitioner. **The traditional practitioner is likely to share their background and beliefs, and often provides a service which is more flexible and, in some circumstances, more appropriate than that provided by NHS practitioners.**

Traditional and Western medicine: a patient's view of the differences[13]

Traditional healer	NHS health worker
• Shares same language and culture – sees illness in same terms as her patient.	• Different language and cultural background – sees illness in terms patient may not understand.
• Easily accessible, can be contacted without going through formal procedure. Patient can refer himself.	• Is part of a complex system of services. Patient cannot refer himself to some professionals but has to go through complicated procedure.

- Often gets to know her client over a course of treatment

- Will use medicines and treatment familiar to the patient. This increases the patient's level of understanding about treatment.

- Patient feels he has control over what is happening to him.

- May be one of several professionals involved in care of the patient – represents just one face in a chain of contact with strangers.

- Care may involve the use of sophisticated drugs and equipment, and complicated procedures. Patient has a greater need for information but often gets less explanation because of difficulties anticipated with the language barrier.

- Patient feels loss of control over what happens to him.

7.4 *Working with different health beliefs and practices*

Below are some suggestions about practical ways of finding out more about the health beliefs and practices of different communities. There are also suggestions for practical action to ensure that the community and health staff are aware of differences in their own beliefs, practices and expectations of each other.

In deciding what practical steps to take, it will be helpful to bear in mind four principles:

- **Professional practice, if it is to be effective, should aim to provide health care resources and services that fit in the lifestyle, needs and priorities of the community.**

- **Trying to change the traditional beliefs and practices of a community because they don't fit in with the expectations of health service institutions is not likely to be productive.**

- **Proposals for practical action should be made as far as possible in consultation with representatives of the community. Find out what changes, if any, members of the community would like to see.**

- **It is easier and more useful to explore in detail health beliefs and practices that relate to your particular discipline. By exploring one area in depth and asking questions based on your own observation and experience, you are more likely to discover information that would be missed by more general research and that people might not think to offer unless specifically asked.**

Checklist: practical action

- Find out about the health beliefs and practices of the community you are working with by reading any available information and comparing it with what people from the local community say. Check the accuracy and relevance of written information by talking to families you work with and asking friends and colleagues from the community.

- Find out how many people go to traditional healers and for what kind of problems. If possible, try to meet and talk to any traditional healers living in the area. Bear in mind that unless they know you well and trust you, people may only tell you what they think you want to hear.

- Find out what illnesses are regarded as serious within the community. Talk to people about their views of the causes of illness, and effective preventive measures, diagnosis and treatment.

- Find out what symptoms are regarded as serious. If they are very different, find out why and draw these differences to the attention of the families you are working with. Make sure that colleagues are aware of the differences, and understand that patients may need particular reassurance over symptoms that health staff do not regard as serious.

- Give guidelines about symptoms that should be seen by a doctor.

- Try to build up a picture of the normal chain of referral within the community, by asking people who they go to for a particular illness, and through your own observations. If a significant number of people in a particular community are referring in an unusual way, or using the health services in an unexpected way, find out whether they are aware that health staff expect a different pattern.

- Give clear guidelines and explanations to patients who don't know how the health services work.

- Explain carefully your role, and your relationship to other health staff who may be involved, in terms that patients can understand.

- Where possible, try to develop positive ways of working with, rather than against, the community's own referral network. Health education initiatives, for example, are likely to be more effective if they use these networks. It may be possible to involve members of the community, such as traditional healers and respected older women, in health education programmes, and in disseminating health education information.

- Don't discourage traditional therapies unless they have been proved to be positively harmful. Respect the fact that traditional remedies provide, at least, valuable psychological support, and often, effective relief of symptoms.

Notes

1. Abbas, Valerie, *A Theoretical Examination of the factors involved in health education with ethnic minority groups*, Dissertation submitted for the requirements of Diploma in Health Education, University of Leeds/Leeds Polytechnic, 1981, p. 9.
2. Brownlee, Ann Templeton, *Community, Culture and Care: a cross cultural guide for health workers*, C. V. Mosby, 1978, p. 183.
3. Littlewood, R. and Lipsedge, M., *Aliens and Alienists: ethnic minorities and psychiatry*, Penguin, 1982, p. 33.
4. Diagnosis by pulse-taking is discussed in Leslie, Charles, *Asian Medical Systems*, University of California Press, 1976 (Ayurvedic System) and
Crozier, R. C., *Traditional Medicine in Modern China*, Harvard University Press, 1968.
5. For an account of the Vietnamese health care system see McMichael, Joan K. (ed.), *Health in the Third World: Studies from Vietnam*, Spokesman Books, 1976.
6. Cartwright, A., and O'Brien, M., 'Social class variations in health care and in the nature of general practice consultations' in Stacey, M. (ed.), *The Sociology of the National Health Service*, Sociological Review Monograph no. 22, 1972.
7. Henley, Alix, *Caring for Muslims and their Families: religious aspects of care*, National Extension College, 1982, p. 43.
8. Ruck, Nicola, 'The Health needs of an Asian community', *Health Link*, no. 1, Journal of the Community Health Group for Ethnic Minorities, (London), 1981.
9. Amin, Geeta, *Some aspects of social policy affecting Asian women in Britain*, paper presented to Asian Women's conference on Our Role in Great Britain Today, 16 July, 1977, p. 2.
10. Dr David Bowsher quoted in Eagle, Robert, *A guide to alternative medicine*, BBC, 1980, p. 7.
11. Eagle, Robert, *A guide to alternative medicine*, BBC, 1980, p. 9.
12. Stacey, M., *Concepts of health and illness: a working paper on the concepts and their relevance for research*, (unpublished paper), 1976.
13. Mares, Penny, *The Vietnamese in Britain: a handbook for health workers*, Health Education Council/National Extension College, 1982, p. 60.

More information

Different family systems and the role of family members in health and health care, see
6 Working with families and individuals

Different dietary traditions, see
8 Foods and diets

Training to enable health workers to work effectively with patients' beliefs and practices, see
12 Health worker training and professional values

The risk of cultural stereotyping, see
4 Culture: a misleading explanation of health inequalities

Practical action, see
14 Local needs: guidelines for doing your own research

Further reading

See the reading list in Chapter 16
16.7 **Health beliefs and practices** and relevant publications in the reading lists for other chapters, e.g.
16.6 **Working with families and individuals**
16.8 **Foods and diets**

8 Foods and diets

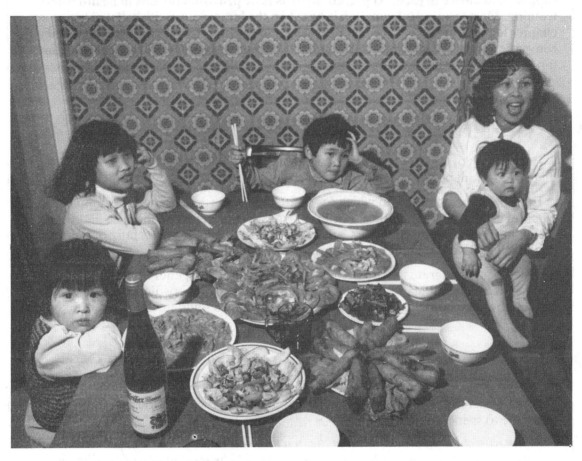

Introduction

Diets can be crucial in both preventive and curative health care, and dietary advice is becoming an increasingly important part of many health workers' roles. But to be effective, this advice must be closely related to what people normally eat and like.

In a multiracial society health workers may need to be informed about the traditional diets of families or individuals from different communities in order to give effective support and advice to each. At present there is little provision for this in health worker training. Most training information is based on the indigenous British diet. This chapter looks at some of the economic, social and religious factors influencing dietary conventions in different communities in Britain, and sets out some practical guidelines for health workers concerned with the nutrition and dietary needs of patients.

8.1 Diets of different groups

Each region or country has developed its own local diet over many centuries. Local diets in different parts of the world differ a good deal.

Each has evolved based on which foods are available (depending for example on climate, geography, agricultural patterns, transport systems, economics and food technology), and on social factors, such as religion, culture, class, family organisation and lifestyle. Each contains a balance of essential nutrients.

When people migrate they take their diet with them, and generally attempt to recreate it as one familiar feature in an unfamiliar and often hostile world. The tremendous psychological importance of familiar food should never be overlooked.

8.2 Socio-economic factors affecting diet

A major determinant of a family's diet and health is obviously the amount of money available to spend on food.

Families with children ate less food in the first three months of 1982 compared to 1981, according to figures from the National Food Survey. The food intake of families with three children was only 83 per cent of the recommended levels for energy and iron consumption. These figures must give rise to fears about the welfare of children in low-income families as unemployment continues to rise and the value of benefits to fall.[1]

Black people in Britain tend to be mainly in lower-paid jobs and to suffer disproportionately from unemployment. Their diets are therefore likely to be affected by poverty, and where there are nutritional problems, these are as likely to be due to lack of cash as to any other factor. People unfamiliar with the cheaper foods available locally may require some help and advice in buying foods that fit in with their family's normal diet.

8.3 Religious aspects of food

For some members of minority groups food has a spiritual significance that it has almost entirely lost in the West. Certain foods are prohibited and these prohibitions form an unquestioned part of many people's daily lives. Listed below are religious restrictions that may affect the diets of Hindus, Sikhs, Muslims, Jews, Rastafarians and Seventh Day Adventists. Members of other groups may also follow religious dietary restrictions.

How far individuals follow such restrictions will depend on their own religious views. **Most devout or conservative members of these groups will follow dietary restrictions carefully, but some people may decide to ignore them or only to adhere to** those they consider most important. **Individual decisions will vary widely, and for each individual the decision is a question of personal conscience.** It is important to find out whether clients follow any religious dietary restrictions, and neither to assume that they do, nor that they don't.

Adhering to religious food restrictions is not a matter of people being faddy about their food. Respecting an individual's culture and religious choices is part of respecting that individual.

Hindu dietary restrictions

In Hindu belief all living things are sacred and interdependent and it is considered wrong to take another creature's life to sustain one's own. As a result **many devout Hindus are vegetarian** and do not eat meat, fish, eggs or anything made with them. The cow is particularly sacred to Hindus, representing the gentle, giving, loving qualities of a mother, and the eating of beef is strictly forbidden.

Alcohol is also forbidden since it reduces one's control over oneself.

Hinduism however does not have a central authoritative set of regulations and so, within a general ideal of vegetarianism, different sects, families and individuals may make their own decisions about what they can and cannot eat. Such decisions carry a strong moral commitment which should be respected by health professionals.

Some Hindus, mainly women, may fast on one or two days a week. Fasting usually involves restricting food intake rather than eating nothing. For example, some women may eat only one meal in the day, or may eat only dairy products or only fruit or nuts all day. Some people may fast for special intentions, such as a successful pregnancy or recovery from an illness. Some people may eat nothing all day when they fast. Fasting is considered both physically and spiritually beneficial.

In general, those people likely to follow religious dietary restrictions most strictly are women, who are often regarded as the custodians of a family's moral and religious values; people who worship regularly and are devout practitioners of their faith; and older people.

Sikh dietary restrictions

Sikhism began as an offshoot of Hinduism in the sixteenth century. It has retained many features of Hinduism, and some Sikhs, particularly women, follow similar dietary restrictions to Hindus. **Few Sikhs eat beef.** Drinking **alcohol** is strongly disapproved of by conservative Sikhs.

Muslim dietary restrictions

Muslim dietary restrictions are laid down in the Holy Quran and are regarded as the direct command of God. They are part of a set of rules designed to create a disciplined life.

Muslims may not eat pork or pork products or anything that contains or is made with them. They may eat all other meat provided that it is *halal* (Arabic, meaning permitted): to be *halal* the name of Allah must be pronounced over the animal, its throat must be quickly cut and the blood must be allowed to drain.

Alcohol is strictly prohibited.

All healthy adult Muslims must **fast** during the 30 days of the month of Ramadan (pronounced Ramzan in Urdu). For Muslims **fasting involves eating and drinking nothing between dawn and sunset.** Since the Islamic year is lunar and contains only 355 days, Ramadan falls 10 days earlier in the Western calendar each year. In 1984 Ramadan began on 2 June and ended on 3 July.

Estimated dates of Ramadan (check with your local mosque for precise dates)

1985	22 May	20/21 June
1986	12 May	10/11 June
1987	2 May	31 May/1 June
1988	22 April	21/22 May
1989	12 April	11/12 May

Certain people are exempt from fasting during Ramadan: the elderly and infirm, women who are menstruating, pregnant or breast-feeding, people on a journey, and anyone who is too ill to fast. Everyone except the elderly and infirm must make up the number of days fasting they have missed as soon as possible after the end of Ramadan. People who are not fasting may not cook or eat in front of anyone who is fasting in case they should tempt them to break their fast. Fasting is highly valued among Muslims, both for its spiritual benefits and because it enables people to share in and understand the suffering of those people who never have enough to eat.

Jewish dietary restrictions

Most devout Jews adhere to Jewish *kashrut* or dietary laws. As in Islam, Jewish dietary laws are part of a code of discipline.

Jews may not eat pork or pork products or anything that contains or is made with them. **Shellfish and any fish without fins** or scales are also proscribed. Jews may eat meat from an animal that has a cloven hoof and chews the cud, and from any herbivorous bird, but all meat must have been killed in a special way so as to be *kosher* (Yiddish, meaning fit). To be *kosher* the throat of the animal or bird must be cut quickly and the blood allowed to drain. The meat is then salted and steeped in water to remove all remaining blood. Only perfectly healthy animals and birds may be used for food.

Milk and meat may not be used together in cooking. When preparing and serving food, meat and milk foods must be kept apart and separate utensils must be used. **This latter rule is generally only observed by more orthodox Jews.**

Devout Jews may **fast**, taking no food or liquid, for 25 hours at the feast of Yom Kippur – the Day of Atonement – in September or October. People who are ill are exempt from fasting.

During Pesach (Passover) in March or April, all foods that contain **yeast** are prohibited. These include leavened bread, cakes and biscuits, beer and vinegar.

Rastafarian dietary restrictions

Most Rastafarians are **vegetarian**, but some eat any meat **except pork**. All products of the vine, such as wine, currants, raisins, or grapes, are forbidden. Some very strict Rastafarians eat only food cooked in vegetable oil. They may wish to eat in privacy.

For strict Rastafarians, the importance of diet cannot be overemphasised. The techniques of Western medicine are themselves viewed with suspicion as the movement advocates the use of natural and herbal remedies. If Rastafarians believe they will be pressurised to eat food they consider unsuitable they may refuse hospital treatment or discharge themselves.

Rastafarians regard the kind of food eaten as a reflection of the health of body and soul, and eat only 'pure' foods. By and large, what is eaten and what is not eaten is an individual decision, but in general Rastafarians are vegetarian. Some are vegan, others will eat eggs, cheese and other milk products, and some will take fish. Food additives and preservatives are avoided, as they are believed to pollute food. Canning is regarded as reducing the goodness of food, so tinned foods are not eaten, although frozen food is acceptable.

Rastafarians regard unprocessed foods as particularly beneficial, so wholemeal flour and brown rice would be taken in preference to white flour and rice.[2]

Seventh Day Adventist dietary restrictions

Many West Indian Christians are Seventh Day Adventists. They do not eat any **pork or pork products**.

Members of some other groups may also follow certain dietary restrictions or may fast at certain times. For example, some Christians give up sweet and rich foods during Lent, some Hindu women may avoid salty foods during particular periods of the year, some Buddhists may refrain from eating meat on the days of the full and new moon. Many groups avoid drinks that are considered to be stimulants, such as alcohol, tea or coffee. **If possible, check in advance whether there are certain foods that a person does not wish to eat, or certain times when they will fast.**

8.4 Eating a balanced diet

Every culture contains the concept of a balanced healthy diet, though this may be organised in different ways. **In most cultures except the European there are age-old traditions which divide almost all foods into two groups, defined as 'hot' and 'cold' in,** for example, most of Asia, South America, and parts of Africa, and as '*yin*' and '*yang*' among Chinese people.

To sum up, what any of us eats is largely a question of the culture to which we belong and the foods with which we are familiar.

In general, we eat: what we know
what we like, in terms of taste, texture and idea
and what we believe is good for us.

We don't eat: what we don't know
what we don't like, in terms of taste, texture and idea
or what we believe is bad for us.

The diets of most minority group families in Britain are a synthesis of their traditional diet and a British diet. Those people most newly arrived in Britain will tend to eat fewest British foods; young people born and brought up in this country may eat a mainly British diet. It is not possible to make blanket statements about the diets of different groups, only to suggest possibilities and factors which may be important, and which health workers may find useful when discussing food and diets with members of minority groups.

Some factors which may increase rate of change	Some factors which may decrease rate of change
– many years in U.K.	– newly arrived in U.K.
– fluent, confident English	– lack of English and confidence
– few traditional foods available	– traditional foods easily and cheaply available
– positive contact with British families	– little contact with British families
– contact with other women who buy local foods	– religiously and culturally conservative
– food advertising	– religious restrictions on permissible foods
– women going out to work	– women staying at home
– school-age children	– older women in charge of shopping and cooking.
– British convenience foods easily and cheaply available	

Dietary change

Every family in Britain makes some inevitable adjustments to its diet over time, but, like anybody else, minority group families will not generally make major changes in their eating habits unless they can perceive a good reason for doing so; any new foodstuffs that they adopt will usually be prepared in ways with which they are already familiar. Inessential or peripheral items in the diet are more likely to be changed than the most essential central items.

The effects of conscious adaptation by minority groups to British foods and dietary habits are not necessarily beneficial in nutritional terms. Health workers may need to stress more the value of the family's traditional diet and to point out that many features of British diets are undesirable and should not be adopted.

Many Western governments have set up committees to formulate dietary goals for their countries, and all of them have independently come to very much the same conclusions. Without exception they have recommended that we should decrease our consumption of fats and sugar and increase our consumption of starch foods, preferably not highly refined; we should increase our fibre intake, eat more fresh fruit and vegetables and perhaps eat less meat and more foods like pulses and lentils.

One striking feature of these recommendations is that they would shift Western diets very much closer to the traditional diets typical of Third World countries. By the standards of these generally agreed goals, the overall dietary patterns typical of these countries are nutritionally superior to those of the West. The nutrition-related problems of the Third World usually stem from lack of food, rather than bad dietary patterns. By contrast, most of the major health problems more typical of the West – the so-called diseases of Western civilisation such as coronary heart disease, diabetes, stomach ulcers and diverticular disease – are, to a considerable extent, the product of the Western diet.[3]

Main features of some local and national diets

	traditional British diet	diet of northern Indian subconti- nent	Chinese/ Vietnamese diet	Caribbean diet	West African diet
staples	potatoes bread (wheat)	rice or *chapatis* (wheat)	rice or noodles (rice or wheat)	rice, yams, plantain	yams and cassava (gari) plantain
main sources of protein	meat fish dairy pro- ducts	meat, fish (non-vegeta- rians only) dairy pro- ducts cereals pulses	cereals pulses meat fish	fish chicken goat other meat pulses	meat stews chicken goat fish
main fats	butter margarine vegetable oils lard	*ghee* (clar- ified butter) vegetable oils	vegetable oils lard	vegetable oils especially coconut oil	vegetable oils especially palm oil

Traditional methods of preparation

Although basic diets all over the world contain similar ingredients, methods of preparation may differ.

For example, most **northern Indian cooking** involves a kind of dry stewing in which ingredients are initially fried fairly fast and then covered and left to cook, sometimes with a little water added. Pulses are boiled and then quickly added to other fried ingredients. Vegetables are rarely if ever boiled. Different spices are added to each dish.

Some northern Indian vegetables[4]

aloo	– potato	*palak*	– spinach
baingan	– eggplant, aubergine	*papdi*	– double beans
band gobi	– cabbage	*peta*	– ash gourd
bindi	– lady fingers	*pyaz*	– onions
fali	– green beans	*saijan*	– drumstick
ful gobi	– cauliflower	*salad*	– lettuce
gajar	– carrot	*sarson-ka-saag*	– mustard leaves
gooar	– cluster beans	*shakarkundi*	– sweet potato
hara dania	– coriander leaves	*tamater*	– tomato
kadoo	– pumpkin	*tar*	– cucumber
karela	– bitter gourd	*tindoora*	– round gourd
matar	– peas	*torai*	– ridge gourd
mooli	– white radish		

Note that potatoes, which in Britain are used as a staple, are used as a vegetable in Asian cooking.

The main **English methods of cooking** are boiling (particularly vegetables), frying, and baking or roasting. Few spices are used. Thick soups and stews are often eaten in the winter.

Caribbean cookery has been influenced by the diets of many countries, including Africa, Spain, China, France, Britain, Portugal, Holland and the Indian subcontinent. Different flavours and methods of cooking predominate in each island. Fish is the main source of animal protein and generally the most important food, as in many island diets. The main pulses used are kidney beans, black-eyed peas and *gunga* peas. Many West Indian dishes are baked or stewed.

Varieties of fish eaten in the West Indies, many of which can now be bought in Britain

Barracuda	Dolphin	Mullet
Bonito (tuna)	Flounder	Oyster
Bluefish	Flying fish	Sailfish
Butter fish	Grouper	Salmon
Calepeave	Hassar	Shark
Cavilli	Herring	Shrimps
Clam	Jack	Snapper or Redfish
Cod (salted)	Jonga	Tarpon
Conch	Kingfish	Titiri
Crab	Lobster	Tuna
Crayfish	Mackerel	Turtle
Cutlass	Marlin	Whelk

Some common West Indian vegetables

Ackee	Cristophene (Chocho)	Pumpkin
Arrowroot	Cush Cush	Potato
Avocado	Dasheen	Spinach
Eggplant	Eddo	String beans
(Melongene)	Green banana	Sweet peppers
Breadfruit	Lettuce	Sweet potato
Cabbage	Okra	Sorrel
Callalloo	Peas	Tannia
Carrot	Pigeon peas	Tomatoes
Cassava	Plaintain	Yam
Corm		

Much **Chinese cooking** uses the stir-fry technique, in which meat, vegetables and other ingredients are chopped small and then fried very quickly until cooked. Vegetable or meat broths may also be eaten, with noodles or rice.

Methods of preparing food are usually handed down from mother to daughter and often learnt at an early age. They are unlikely to change radically when people migrate. The new local foods most likely to be adopted are those that can be prepared in a familiar way.

Sources of protein

Most diets rely on a combination of vegetable and animal sources of protein, though in wealthier industrialised societies there has been, at least until recently, a greater emphasis on animal protein.

In less affluent societies even non-vegetarians may eat little animal protein, possibly giving what meat or fish there is to those, usually the men, who do heavy manual work. Many non-vegetarians therefore rely a good deal on vegetable protein, and **in many diets pulses and cereals are regularly eaten together to ensure complete protein intake.** Examples are *chapatis* or rice with *dal* in the Indian subcontinent, *tacos* or *tortillas* with beans in Central America, sweet lentils with rice, and peanuts with noodles in South-East Asia, baked beans on toast in Britain.

Combinations like these are often a very important part of people's diets. They are handed down through the generations and have always played a key role in keeping people well nourished, even though nobody has in a sense been aware of their importance nutritionally. But once you start playing around with diets, leaving out some of those foods that may be low status or whatever, and adding other new foods, you risk creating all sorts of imbalances and deficiencies in the diet. You can see this in the British diet now, we went off bread and potatoes and things and went for more exciting and higher status and richer or more refined foods. And now we've got a high incidence of diet-related diseases. Changing diets can be a dangerous game.

Nutritionist

Asians often lose confidence in their eating habits when they arrive here and tend to break their pattern in a way that is bad for their health. Some Hindus turn over to a western diet in the end and eat chips and pies, but abandon their vegetable curries and beans, and stick to their religious observance of not eating meat. The result is an unbalanced mixture of east and west.

Asian dietitian

A balanced diet

Certain foods, 'hot' or *yang* foods, are believed to raise the body temperature, excite the emotions and increase activity. Other foods, 'cold' or *yin*, have opposite qualities; they cool the body temperature, calm the emotions, and make a person cheerful and strong. These categories have nothing to do with physical temperature, but 'hot' or *yang* foods are often spicy or high in animal protein; 'cold' or *yin* foods are often bland and many are vegetable in origin. Too many of either type can unbalance the body and the emotions and cause problems. The precise foods defined as hot or cold, *yin* or *yang*, will vary from community to community and from family to family.

Eating a balanced and healthy diet will tend to be most important to people if they are ill or somehow under the weather, and at crucial times when it is important to be as healthy as possible, such as during pregnancy and while breast-feeding. At these times people may take care to eat more of one kind of food or another to ensure maximum health.

Some members of minority communities in Britain, particularly people from rural areas or families with older members, will hold to these beliefs and may control their diet carefully. Any discussion about a change of diet must take account of this, since some people may be unable to eat some of the foods that are advised. People in hospital may also reject certain foods which they believe would be bad for their condition. In most non-Western medical traditions a central part of the medical practitioner's advice involves dietary change: people are advised to eat more or less of certain foods to get well and ensure continued good health.

People will not necessarily articulate their beliefs in terms of 'hot' and 'cold' foods. They may simply feel convinced that there are certain foods which one should not eat, or which are particularly good for one, at certain times.

Hot and cold foods in the Vietnamese diet[5]
Below are some examples of heating and cooling foods, but remember that interpretations of this principle vary from region to region in Vietnam and even from family to family, so that individuals may have differing views about which foods fall into which categories.

Hot		*Cold*	*Neutral*
fried foods	sea food	boiled and steamed foods	rice*
butter	Chinese cabbage	green leafy vegetables	bread
ginger	chocolate	most fruits	
garlic	sugar	bean shoots	
onions	coffee	bean curd	
potatoes	cocoa	melon soup	
yams	Coca Cola	barley water	
nuts	duck	carrot water	
red meat	goose	chicken	
oily fish			

---

* Rice gruel is regarded as cooler than boiled rice because of the quantity of water used in cooking.

Acupuncture has been found to make sense. Why not hot and cold food? We don't know enough about it yet, but I wouldn't dismiss it.

Health worker

8.5 *Weaning*

The age at which mothers in different societies begin to wean their children onto solid foods varies a great deal, and may be anything from four months to two years. Decisions on when to begin weaning are influenced by such factors as local custom and tradition, advice from relatives, friends and professionals, class and economic circumstances. **In most Third World countries babies are weaned later than is current practice in Britain.** Late weaning in areas where undernutrition is common generally increases an infant's chance of survival.

In all societies, weaning involves a pureed, softened, mashed, or pre-chewed form of a local staple, for example, barley, corn, rice, wheat, flour, semolina, dal, potato, yam, banana or plantain. Small quantities of fruit, cooked vegetable, meat or fish, may be added. If soups, stews, or curries are part of the local diet, some of the liquid may be mixed in with the staple. Where babies are weaned relatively late, the weaning foods may be fairly firm in texture, and may be given with the hands, rather than, as is common in Britain, with a spoon. Some children are simply weaned onto bits of suitable food from the family meal, perhaps slightly mashed and without the stronger and hotter spices.

In Britain current practice is to encourage mothers to start supplementing a baby's milk diet between three and eight months. There is an established tradition of a British 'in-between' diet to bridge the gap between milk and an adult diet. Most babies are weaned onto the different stages of baby foods and packaged cereals, and then onto pureed versions of the family's everyday food.

The earlier weaning generally advocated in Britain can cause problems for some mothers who have not weaned children so early before and who may be unsure how to prepare food for such very young babies. Some mothers may need help and advice in feeding their babies at this stage. Older women in the family are unlikely to have had experience of weaning early and often cannot advise or help. They may also worry about the effects of introducing solids so early.

Health workers who are unsure about which of the family's foods are suitable as weaning foods, or who have difficulty in communicating with the family, often simply recommend a diet of proprietary baby foods. This can sometimes lead to problems.

Many proprietary baby foods are unsuitable for people who follow religious dietary restrictions, for example, vegetarian Hindus and Sikhs, Muslims and Jews. Some mothers avoid prohibited foods by buying only products that they know contain no meat at all, such as puddings or custards. A long-term diet of sweet dishes alone is not sufficiently nutritious and leads to tooth decay and a very sweet tooth. It is also an unnecessary expense. However the names of proprietary foods may be passed around women within the communities and some people may feel that they must be excellent and sufficiently nutritious simply because they are British.

Problems may also arise later when parents try to wean a child off proprietary foods onto the family's normal diet. Children who have accepted the flavours of British-style baby foods may refuse to be reweaned onto the different flavours of their own food. This can cause long-term problems. If a mother cannot rewean her child onto suitable family foods, it is likely to stay on a long-term diet of proprietary baby foods.

I have constantly stressed the benefits of breastfeeding. Many women who have breast-fed their babies in India assume they should start bottles once they get here. And it's often the fathers who favour switching to what they think is the Western way.

So I always try to make sure that fathers and perhaps even mothers- and fathers-in-law are there when I give dietary advice. Asian women are reluctant to introduce cooking or eating patterns which go against the ideas of their elders.

PART 2: HEALTH NEEDS AND EXPECTATIONS

Tinned baby foods are another of my recurring fights. I always try to encourage mothers to go on with the pattern they knew back home – putting babies straight onto the family foods as soon as they are off the breast.

Sometimes mothers even ask whether it is all right to give their children plain water. Faced with shelves of sweetened fruit drinks they begin to believe they must be necessary. And mothers don't always realise they are actually forming children's taste by what they buy for them.

Asian dietitian

Most ethnic minority mothers will have no problems with weaning their babies. Many will choose to use a convenient combination of proprietary British baby foods and traditional weaning foods. Nevertheless, it may sometimes be important to **stress the value of the family's traditional foods** and to advise mothers on how to prepare suitable locally available foods for young babies. An attitude which undermines a mother's confidence in her own foods is *not* helpful.

She's very good. She gives her children English food.

Health visitor about an Asian mother

8.6 *Nutritional problems*

Every traditional regional diet is naturally balanced. **No regional diet has nutritional deficiencies built into it, though where certain foods that are normally part of the diet become unavailable or are too expensive or are rejected, some people may become poorly nourished:** in Britain, for example, elderly people often suffer from nutritional deficiencies because of poverty or lack of interest in food. Increased affluence may cause people to substitute refined or richer (high fat, high sugar, high animal protein) foods for traditional whole foods.

Dietary deficiencies are proportionately no more of a problem among ethnic minority groups in Britain than among the majority population. When, however, individuals or families from minority groups do suffer from nutritional deficiencies, the advice that they receive from health workers may not always be useful or well informed.

They used to complain about some of the Asian vegetarian mums here being undernourished. Well, I'm a vegetarian, and I know my diet's adequate. You can have just as good a diet if you're vegetarian. Better, I think. It's much healthier. But in the early days, the nurses didn't know what to say to the vegetarian mums. A mum would come in and they didn't know how to help her, how to give her advice that she could follow. It's getting a lot better now.

Asian nurse

A few dietary problems may be caused when people migrate to a different climate where certain nutritionally important traditional foodstuffs are no longer available. For example, the lack of sunlight in Britain may lead to additional requirements for dietary Vitamin D among Asians, Vietnamese and other groups; factors such as a less abundant and varied supply of green leafy vegetables may lead to iron deficiency anaemia among some vegetarian women in Britain; it has been suggested that methods of cleaning and packaging in Britain wash off the residual Vitamin B12 on vegetable produce, and that some Indian vegetarians in Britain (though not in India) may lack Vitamin B12.[6,7]

Vietnamese rice contains six times as much calcium and nearly four times as much iron as rice imported to Britain. Tropical fruit and vegetables also have a higher content of calcium, iron and certain vitamins than vegetables grown in Britain. A major source of calcium in the British diet is milk, but milk and milk products are used in small quantities by the Vietnamese. A combination of these factors may lead to calcium and iron deficiency.[5]

It is essential to have a basic idea of the normal everyday diets and nutritional patterns of all the families with whom you work, in order to be able to give appropriate advice when it is needed.

8.7 Practical action: giving nutritional advice

The same basic rules about giving nutritional advice apply to minority group clients as to everybody else. There may, however, be some additional factors to take into account.

- **Find out about the client's normal diet**
  Find out which religious and regional group and social class the family comes from. Find out what you can about the general dietary norms and traditions of this group so that you have some basic ideas to start from. Questions based on some existing knowledge indicate your interest and professional competence and will increase people's confidence in you.

  Give advice that is based as far as possible on what your clients already choose to eat, and indicate clearly that this is what you want to do. Be aware of individual and family differences and preferences. **It is almost always possible for you to give nutritional advice that builds on and does not clash with people's existing dietary practices.**

- **Find out about any dietary restrictions the client follows**
  Some minority group families are afraid that British health workers will laugh at or despise their customs. They may tell you what they think you would like to hear or will approve of rather than expose themselves to ridicule. Expect many people to follow religious or cultural restrictions on food, and accept without question the restrictions that they do follow. **Indicate clearly your respect for and understanding of your client's dietary choices.**

  But do not assume that every client follows all the traditional customs and practices.

- **Work with all those people who are responsible for decisions about diet**
  In most English families a young mother is responsible for decisions about what she cooks for her family and what she and they eat. In minority group families there may be several people responsible for such decisions. It may, for example, not be the young mother alone who needs explanation and support, but her mother-in-law, older sisters-in-law or her husband. Their support is crucial and their opposition unbeatable. **Work within the decision-making structure of the family to avoid embarrassment and frustration**. The person who cooks may not be the one who does the shopping. In some families, for example, the men do the shopping and will need to be informed.

  Find out who are the key people to work with in each family.

- **Look critically at any radical dietary changes you might advise. Are they really necessary for the client's health?**
  Advice that is standard and easy to follow for most people on a traditional English diet may require major changes for people who have a different traditional diet. As far as you can, give your advice in terms of the foods the family already eats. Advise as little radical change as possible. If change is really necessary, concentrate on the one or two most important items. **Explain why you are recommending changes.**

- **Try suggesting some new foods that are cheap and easily available**
  Many people fairly new to this country would like to use, for example, some of the cheaper British vegetables but do not know how to prepare them. If it seems appropriate, tell people the names of suitable foods that you think they might be able to use in their cooking. Explain what they are like and why they are useful. If possible, demonstrate how to prepare them.

  Bear in mind that the foods most likely to be accepted are those which can be cooked according to the family's normal methods.

- **Make sure that your client understands your advice**
  Make sure your advice is clear and simple to follow. **Use an interpreter** if you cannot communicate effectively in English.

- **Build up a relationship of mutual trust, liking and honesty**
  Most cultures stress the importance of personal relationships in any interaction.

Some people may be more likely to follow your advice because they like you and feel that they have a personal relationship with you as a friend, rather than because of your professional status, training or knowledge.

To build up an effective relationship requires extra time and effort, especially across cultural and language barriers, but without it, very little is likely to be achieved.

8.8 *Food in hospitals and institutions*

Although the situation is beginning to improve, some ethnic minority hospital patients have suffered from a surprising lack of sensitivity among medical nursing and catering staff who have not considered the importance of familiar food in hospital.

Aslam no longer throws his dinner at us, now we've discovered what he eats.
Nurse in a centre for the adult mentally handicapped.

Problems with food are frequently mentioned when Asian and other minority group patients are asked about their experience in hospitals.

At a well known hospital in South London the maternity ward has a high number of expectant Asian mothers. On questioning one of the medical social workers about the dietary needs of Asian mothers I received the following reply:
'Oh yes they all like the food – I think so anyway. They never complain so I suppose it's all right. It must be difficult for them but we've never really discussed it at this hospital. Yes, we have nearly 40 per cent of our beds in the maternity department taken up by Asian mothers.'

Asian mother in the maternity ward of the same hospital:
'They think I like the food. We people never like this food really, do we? I don't eat much of it. My husband sometimes brings food in for me. He knows I don't eat this English food. Sometimes the nurses make sarcastic comments when he brings food for me – but I have to eat, don't I? They tell us we must have a balanced diet but they don't care whether we eat or not.'

Worker at a London hospital:
'We have 50 per cent Asian women in maternity. We know most of them are vegetarian, we asked them if they would like to have some boiled rice and maize [which for a European would be like having mashed potato on its own!!]. They unanimously refused.'[8]

The food provided on the normal hospital menu is often unfamiliar and may be forbidden and many patients will refuse it. The name of a dish often gives no clue to its ingredients: shepherd's pie, hot pot, jam roly poly, toad in the hole, and spotted dick. If people do not know what is in the dish and what cooking fat was used they may not be able to eat it.

For people who follow religious dietary restrictions there are certain rules:

• **Food which contains any proscribed ingredients at all cannot be eaten:** eggs fried in bacon fat, puddings cooked in tins greased with lard, are forbidden to Jews, Muslims, Rastafarians and vegetarians. Cakes containing eggs are forbidden to strict Asian vegetarians and all vegans.

• **Food which has been in contact with proscribed foods cannot be eaten:** a salad from which a slice of roast beef has been removed has already been contaminated to most vegetarians. A Muslim or Jew cannot eat from a dish that has contained non-*halal* or non-*kosher* meat or gravy. Potatoes or vegetables with meat gravy on them may be unacceptable to Jews, Muslims and many vegetarians.

• **Utensils that have not been washed since they were last used for proscribed food, contaminate any other food that comes into contact with them.** The same spoon cannot be used to serve stew for other patients and potato for Muslims or vegetarians.

Some very conservative Asian vegetarians and Muslims consider that if a utensil has ever been used for proscribed food it contaminates all other foods. They will refuse all food that has been prepared outside their own homes. However, in hospital and other institutions it may be impossible to keep utensils and cooking pots completely separate. Most devout people feel able to accept this so long as they are sure that all utensils and cooking pots have been well washed since they last touched prohibited food.

Providing familiar food

Someone ill in hospital or having a baby is least likely to be able to cope with new foods; they need the comfort of food that is familiar and soothing. A good diet is also necessary to speed up healing and recovery processes.

I gave the cooks recipes and showed them how to cook them but they didn't always do them and there were complaints earlier this year. The doctors said the vegetarians were not getting enough to eat.

Asian dietitian

For many ethnic minority patients a spell in hospital may be their first encounter with British food. Being presented with strange, possibly distasteful, and in some cases religiously or culturally unacceptable food is likely to be particularly upsetting for a sick person.[2]

The dietary needs of minority groups can pose new questions for caterers in hospitals and other instititions, since the choices on a standard English menu may not provide an adequate or acceptable diet.

A recent DHSS publication, *Catering for Minority Groups*, begins:

Catering managers in the National Health Service have a responsibility to provide suitable food for all patients but the needs of some groups are not easily identified. It is important that patients are provided with food which is suitable, familiar and acceptable.[9]

How different NHS institutions respond to this situation will depend very much on the size of local ethnic minority populations, their cultural and religious backgrounds, and the differences between their normal diet and the standard British diet on which hospital menus are based. An increasing number of hospitals in multiracial areas are providing meals for Asian patients, but few are yet catering for other groups, whose standard diets may be equally different.

A recent survey of local hospital dietary provision by Haringey Community Health Council recommended, among other things:

- *halal, kosher,* **vegetarian and other meals to be offered to all patients as alternative menu choices.** (Strict Asian vegetarians do not eat eggs or cheese, so the standard British vegetarian alternative of omelette or cheese salad is not adequate.)

- **the use of frozen meals** suitable for ethnic minority groups where the hospital kitchens did not provide them.

- the **inclusion of some foods that would appeal to the West Indian and Cypriot members of the community**, based on suggestions from West Indian and Cypriot catering staff.

- **increased milk and yoghurt consumption to supplement vegetarian diets.** These should be made freely available to patients on request.

- the provision of **spicy sauces**, such as tabasco and hot pepper sauce, **pickles and chutney**, to render some of the blander food on the menu more acceptable to groups who prefer spicy food.

- where patients find the hospital food unacceptable, **encouraging relatives to bring food in, and the provision of facilities for storing and reheating foods.**

- **leaflets** for patients in all relevant languages, including English, explaining all the available options and choices of food available to them.

- where special food is provided, **leaflets** for patients in English and appropriate languages **to explain that the food is prepared in accordance with religious requirements.**

– **training and information for all catering and ward staff** on cultural and religious aspects of diet.

The survey also stated:

Our overall impression in talking to ethnic minority group patients was that most were slow to criticise and quick to praise. Some had spent days stoically and uncomplainingly eating potato, and vegetables, or munching through plates of salad, until nursing staff or relatives came to the rescue with more suitable and appetising food. Ethnic minorities in this country do not find the experience of being outsiders unusual. Many have difficulty with English and are unable to communicate their needs and problems; and of those who can communicate most have repeated experiences of rejection and dismissal from the institutional level right down to the individual level. One West Indian man's comment illustrates the reticence of other patients:
'I don't eat much, but I don't want you to take this, because this hospital is not just for me. Most people in this ward eat the meals, they are good for most people. I don't need special arrangements just for me.'

Although this man had been in England for twenty years, he still expected little from the society which he had no doubt worked for and contributed to consistently over this period. His attitude is by no means unique.[2]

Questions to think about: providing a suitable meals service for ethnic minority groups

Here are some questions you may like to consider:

● How will you identify the needs of local groups?

● Whom will you involve or consult? Inside the hospital? outside it?

● What factors will you take into account when planning the menus?

● How will you ensure nutritionally adequate meals?

● How will meals be served?

● Which staff will be involved in preparing the meals? Serving them? What will you do to ensure their cooperation?

● What special arrangements, if any, will you make in the kitchens?

● How will you ensure that the food you provide is acceptable to the people for whom it is intended?

● How will you ensure that they know about it?

● How will you cater for patients from minority groups with a small local population, for whom it may not be feasible to provide a regular meals service?

Notes

1 *London Voluntary News*, Oct. 1982.
2. O'Brien, Maureen, *Hospital Food for Ethnic Minority Patients*, Haringey Community Health Council, 1981.
3. Sheiham, Helena and Quick, Alison, *The Rickets Report,* Haringey Community Health Council, 1982.
4. Henley, Alix, *Asian Foods and Diets: A Training Pack*, National Extension College, 1982.
5. Mares, Penny, *The Vietnamese in Britain: a handbook for health workers*, Health Education Council/National Extension College, 1982.
6. Britt, R. P. and Harper, Christine, M., letter in *The Lancet,* 9 Oct. 1976.
7. Rose, Michael, letter in *The Lancet,* 25 Sept. 1976.
8. Amin, Geeta, *Some Aspects of Social Policy Affecting Asian Women in Britain*, unpublished paper, 1977.
9. Department of Health and Social Security, 'Catering for Minority Groups' *Catering and Dietetics Branch Manual,* Vol. 6, 1982.

More information

Communication skills and giving dietary advice, see
5   **Communication**, especially
5.6 **Practical action: improving communication across a language barrier**

Health education, see
13 **Health education**

Rickets and Vitamin D deficiency, see
9.5 **Rickets and osteomalacia**

The risks of imposing dietary change, see
4.1 **Cultural differences**

Finding out more about foods and diets, see
14.4 **Things you need to know**, especially **Foods and diets**
14.7 **How to ask questions**

Further reading

See the reading list in Chapter 16
16.8 **Foods and diets**

9 Patterns of illness

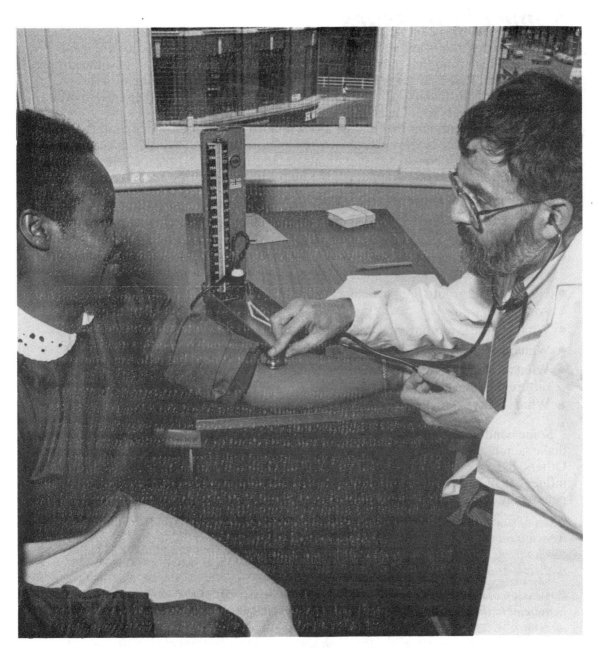

Introduction

There are important variations in patterns of illness among the different ethnic groups living in Britain. A knowledge of these variations is essential if health workers are to be effective in the care they provide. This chapter examines some of the factors contributing to different patterns of illness; it sets out some introductory information about four specific diseases and the key issues surrounding their management.

9.1 Some of the issues

Most health workers are aware that different ethnic groups experience different patterns of illness and that the incidence of certain conditions is higher in some groups than in others. **Research suggests that most health workers are familiar with those conditions that particularly affect the majority population, but that they receive little and often inadequate training about the nature, symptoms, prevalence and management of conditions that mainly affect minority communities in Britain.** As a result these diseases, however serious, often go unrecognised; health workers do not know what to do, or how to advise patients or their families; British people suffering from these conditions often do not get the help and support they need.

Do you know the answers to these questions?

- What is the incidence of cystic fibrosis in the white population? And in other ethnic groups?
- What is the difference between sickle cell disease and sickle trait? What would you do to avert a sickle cell crisis?
- Which ethnic groups are particularly affected by thalassaemia? What are the symptoms?
- What are the symptoms of Tay-Sachs disease?
- Which groups are particularly at risk from osteomalacia?
- What are the differences in the prevalence of hypertensive disease among the different ethnic groups in Britain?
- Which cancers are particularly likely in different ethnic groups?

Some conditions that affect particular ethnic groups in Britain, such as thalassaemia, cystic fibrosis and sickle cell disease, are caused by **genetic mechanisms.** Others, like rickets, osteomalacia, skin cancer and hypertensive disease, are chiefly influenced by **social, economic and environmental factors**, though they may also be genetically influenced to some extent.

Each of us carries a number of harmful genes and may develop a genetic disorder or transmit one to our children. Every disease is either caused or influenced by genetic mechanisms. Common examples include heart disease, high blood pressure, cancer, diabetes, and allergies. Even longevity is genetically influenced.

Possession of certain genes by people living in defined areas of the world has proved to be beneficial to their health. This advantage has best been shown for sickle cell anaemia. . . . Many years ago it was noticed that in areas where malaria was rife, there was also a high frequency of sickle cell anaemia. Ultimately it was clearly shown that those individuals carrying the gene for sickle cell anaemia were much more resistant to malaria. You will recall that sickle cell anaemia is a recessive disorder, and the gene is carried equally by both parents. While the individual affected by this anaemia is ill, the carriers are not. Indeed carriers turn out to have an advantage or be 'fitter', in that they are able to resist malaria much better than those of us without the sickle cell gene.

Other genetic adaptations to disease are known that also confer advantages on the bearer of the specific gene. Thalassaemia, for example, is a fatal, hereditary anaemia similar to sickle cell anaemia (involving changes in bones and skin and spleen enlargement) found mainly in people who live in or originate from the Mediterranean region: especially Italians and Greeks, as well as Africans and Indians. Again carriers are more resistant to malaria. Female carriers of the sex-linked enzyme disorder called glucose-6-phosphate dehydrogenase are more resistant to malaria; this disorder also occurs in those who live in the malarial belts of the world.[1] [our emphasis]

Ethnic group(s) in Britain particularly affected by particular conditions

Cystic fibrosis	people of northern and central European origin
Tay-Sachs disease	people of European Jewish origin
Thalassaemia	people of Mediterranean, North African and Asian origin
Rickets and osteomalacia	people of Asian origin
Sickle cell disease	people of Afro-Caribbean and African origin
Hypertensive disease	people of West Indian and African origin

More information about some of these diseases and sources of further information are given below.

9.2 *Sickle cell disease*

The information in this section is taken from publications of the Sickle Cell Society and from articles by Elizabeth Anionwu, Head of the Sickle Cell Centre, Willesden General Hospital.

Prevalence

Sickle cell disease is a group of inherited disorders of haemoglobin in the red blood cells. As mentioned above, it is found in people originally from the equatorial belt where malaria is or was common. Possession of the sickle cell gene gives protection against some forms of malaria. In Britain sickle cell disease occurs mainly in people from Africa and of African descent, i.e. Afro-Caribbeans, and also, though less commonly, in people from the Middle East, the Mediterranean and South Asia. **It has been estimated that there are at least 3,000 people with sickle cell disease in Britain.**

Symptoms

The first symptoms of sickle cell disease usually appear after the age of three to six months. They include swelling of the hands and feet, pain in the joints, abdomen and chest, anaemia, and susceptibility to bacterial infections. Older children may have delayed puberty and be prone to leg ulcers and bed wetting. The painful sickle cell crises may be set off by dehydration, infection, strenuous exercise or sudden changes in temperature. Patients may require immediate hospitalisation to prevent or deal with these crises. **Sickle cell crises can be fatal unless urgent medical attention is given.**

Management

Sickle cell disease is usually diagnosed in childhood through blood screening, or because the child has a history of, for example, episodic pains, frequent infections and anaemia. However, there are milder manifestations of sickle cell disease and sickle cell thalassaemia (see 9.3 below) which may not be recognised until adolescence or even middle age. In these cases, aches and pains may be attributed to 'growing pains', arthritis or rheumatism. In some cases failure to diagnose the disease may lead to incorrect treatment or no treatment at all.

Because of the variability in manifestation, some people with sickle cell disease do not know that they have it. For them there is a real danger that a sickle cell crisis may be precipitated if, for example, they have an anaesthetic for dental treatment or surgery, or when they are pregnant.

Anyone of African or Afro-Caribbean origin who has not previously been checked for sickle cell disease must be given a blood test before anaesthesia or when they become pregnant, so that special medical precautions can be taken to ensure their safety.

There is as yet no cure for sickle cell disease, so its management must aim to reduce or prevent known complications, to treat problems and symptoms as they arise, and to provide long-term counselling and support. Although children are extremely vulnerable, more are now surviving into adulthood.

Sickle cell trait

The gene that carries sickle haemoglobin is recessive. People with one ordinary haemoglobin gene and only one sickle gene are said to have sickle cell trait. **This is not an illness and has *no* symptoms**; they are carriers of the disease, but they do not have it. However, if two people with sickle cell trait (i.e. two carriers) have children, there is a one in four chance that each child will have sickle cell disease. **It is estimated that about one in ten of Britain's African and Afro-Caribbean population has sickle cell trait, that is, is a carrier of sickle cell disease.** About one in 400 of the same population has the disease.

Screening and counselling

People with sickle cell disease, and their parents and families, require **clear and practical information on managing the condition and, as far as possible, preventing crises.** They also need skilled and sensitive long-term support to help them cope with the various difficulties and emotional pressures they experience, and to ensure that their practical and economic needs are met.

I remember the last time I went in, this was just before Christmas this year, and I was going to have a blood transfusion, and you know, when she examined me she looked into my eyes and said 'It's a pity the students aren't here, it would be a good sight for the students', and I felt, you know, like a bit of meat that they are just learning off. But there again, I can't really blame them, because it's not a white man's disease, and they are not really going to go that far to cure black people if their people ain't concerned. That is the way I see it.

Young woman with sickle cell disease

The communities at risk also need general information about sickle cell disease, how it is inherited and what it is. Screening facilities should be provided for all possible sufferers or (symptomless) carriers at certain crucial stages: for women during pregnancy who may have a mild and therefore undiagnosed type of sickle cell disease; for new-born babies at birth; and for all possible sufferers before anaesthesia for dental treatment or surgery. Screening should also be provided on demand for anyone who wishes to find out whether they have sickle cell disease or the trait gene. Counselling and education must be provided for anyone found to have sickle cell disease or trait, so that they understand its implications for themselves and for their future choices.

People phone me up in a real state and say 'Can you help me? I've just had a test done at the hospital and they've told me I'm sickle positive. What does it mean?' They phone up from all over the country, they're really scared. And I have to say to them, 'Go back to your hospital and ask "What do you mean when you say I'm sickle positive? Do you mean I have sickle cell disease or sickle cell trait?" Then phone me back and I'll explain it all.' Sickle positive doesn't tell you anything, it just frightens people. And often the health worker who's told the person they're sickle positive doesn't know what it means either, whether it's the trait or the disease. She's never had any training or information, nor any help with how to counsel. Incredible. We're talking about such a serious disease, and a diagnosis that's so common among the Afro-Caribbean community.

Sickle cell worker, Brent

The most commonly used blood tests for the diagnosis of sickle cell disease, the sickle test and the solubility test, are both rapid methods of indicating the presence (positive) or absence (negative) of haemoglobin. However, a 'sickle-positive' result does not differentiate between sickle cell trait and sickle cell disease. **Many people have wrongly been given the impression that they have sickle cell disease because they have a 'sickle-positive' result.** It is more likely that they just have sickle cell trait, though this can only be finally ascertained through haemoglobin electrophoresis, which is the most important and reliable blood test used in diagnosis.[2]

As with any genetically carried disease, it is as important after testing to tell people that they do **not** have or carry the disease as that they do.

 Since sickle cell disease is genetically carried, crucial issues about pre-pregnancy screening and genetic counselling also arise and are currently being debated. Some of the issues are discussed in 9.3 below.

A recent survey in a health district in North West London with a large black community showed that only two out of the 58 health visitors and school nurses interviewed correctly understood the possible significance of a sickle positive result. Twenty-one thought that it meant that the person definitely had sickle cell disease.

It's unbelievable that nothing is being done in any kind of systematic way to help people with sickle cell disease or trait. That's one of the problems I have in trying to get health workers to think about it. They feel that if the incidence was really as high, and the disease really as serious as I say, somebody would have done or be doing something about it. So they don't believe me.

Sickle cell worker

They know I have got the disease but they don't really know too much about it, and I don't think, this is just my personal view, I don't think they're interested because it's not a white man's disease, and I mean, from once it's not a white man's disease, I can't see them really digging into this thing to get any knowledge out of it, you know, because it is black people, and it's black people's problem.

Young woman with sickle cell disease

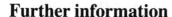 As a first step towards an effective service for those who have sickle cell disease the Health Service must become **much better informed** about the disease, its implications and management, and the needs of sufferers and their families. For an example of one such successful project see Chapter 10.

Further information

If you want to find out more about sickle cell disease, some sources of information are suggested at the end of this Chapter.

9.3 *Thalassaemia*

Thalassaemia is a genetic disease affecting the haemoglobin in the red blood cells, and occurring particularly among people from the Mediterranean area, including Cyprus, Italy, Spain and Portugal, and also from North Africa, the Indian subcontinent, and the Far East.

The **disease** is called **thalassaemia major**. The **carrier state**, in which a person has one ordinary and one thalassaemic gene, is called **thalassaemia minor.**

Prevalence

In Britain there are about 300 people with thalassaemia major: half of these are of Cypriot origin and the other half of Indian or Pakistani origin. About fourteen babies with thalassaemia major are born in Britain each year.[3]

It is reckoned that about one in seven people of Cypriot origin, one in twelve people of Greek origin, one in twenty people of north-west Indian origin, and one in one thousand people of English origin have thalassaemia minor and so are carriers of thalassaemia.

Thalassaemia major

Thalassaemia major generally becomes evident in affected children when they are **between six and eighteen months of age.** They become **severely anaemic and, if not treated, die of infection or cardiac failure** before they reach the age of six.

Treatment in Britain consists of **monthly blood transfusions**, accompanied by **daily subcutaneous infusions of an iron-chelating agent, desferrioxamine**, to prevent damage to the liver and the heart. Under this regime patients may live a relatively normal life for many years.

Thalassaemia minor

Thalassaemia minor, the **carrier state**, in which there are **no ill effects or symptoms except for occasional mild anaemia**, can be detected by a blood test.

If two people with thalassaemia minor have children, there is a one in four chance that each child will have the disease, thalassaemia major. A foetal blood test can diagnose a foetus with thalassaemia major, and the option of terminating the pregnancy can be offered to the parents.

Screening and counselling

In Britain thalassaemia has until recently mainly been noted in the Cypriot communities, and diagnosis and counselling facilities are being developed in the London area, where the majority of Cypriots in Britain live. Now that there is a large Asian British population, the number of thalassaemic Asian births is increasing, and screening and counselling facilities are also urgently needed for the Asian community.

There has been a good deal of discussion about the question of screening for thalassaemia and other genetic diseases, such as sickle cell disease, cystic fibrosis, haemophilia, and Tay-Sachs disease. **Some people have advocated mass screening of all those who, because of their ethnic origin, might be carriers.** Screening of schoolchildren has also been suggested.

There are however, many difficulties inherent in screening for a recessive inherited disease. Mass screening during childhood may seem an attractive alternative, but in fact can cause very serious problems: recessive inheritance is difficult to understand; children and their parents may not understand the idea of a healthy carrier and may worry about possible imminent onset of the disease; for some adolescents information about a 'fault' about which they can do nothing may be traumatic. They may feel labelled or branded for life. Extensive counselling and support may be needed to help with this; such counselling is not and is not likely to be generally available. In an already racially charged atmosphere, singling out one racial or ethnic group of school children as having 'faulty' genes may create major problems and tensions.

Researchers in North London concluded that 'mass screening for haemoglobinopathy is unjustified, at least in this country'. They advocated that there should be a programme of general health education about genetic diseases and their implications; that diagnostic facilities should be provided for potential sufferers or carriers of hereditary diseases on demand and at particularly crucial times, such as during early pregnancy; and that diagnosis must *always* be accompanied by counselling.[4]

Another study, again by researchers based in North London, and working with a Cypriot community, found that people were generally unaware that they personally might be affected by thalassaemia, but that most people were very ready to accept the advantage of screening facilities once they realised.[5] The researchers stressed that it is as important to tell people that they *do not* have or carry a hereditary disease, as that they do. If people are not reassured they may remain extremely worried and anxious.

The study found that thalassaemia screening is currently carried out in three main ways:

1. In ante-natal clinics during early pregnancy. Women in at-risk ethnic groups are tested by a blood test. If they are found to be carriers their husbands are tested too. If both parents are carriers the couple is offered ante-natal diagnosis and selective abortion (up to 22 weeks' gestation) if they wish.

The vast majority of couples wish to know of their risk, but all find this form of screening traumatic and would prefer to know before starting a pregnancy. In any case, our findings here and elsewhere do not suggest that all at-risk couples are being detected in ante-natal clinics, and the danger of couples being missed seems to be directly proportional to their distance from Central London.[5]

2. Incidentally, when people are admitted to hospital for other reasons. However, even though routine blood tests may show thalassaemia major or minor, the diagnosis and its implications are not always passed on to patients or their GPs. Whether they are or not seems to depend largely on the knowledge, concern and time of the clinician involved.

3. By self-referral for screening. In the Cypriot community this is happening because of increasing general awareness of the disease, due to publicity both in Cyprus and in Britain.

The request is often made about the time of marriage and screening at around this time seems to be ideal, for, with good counselling, the knowledge obtained is usually used calmly and responsibly. Presentation is to the general practitioner in the first instance, but many members of the at-risk community are better educated about thalassaemia than their general practitioners. No-one in this group [under study] was diagnosed or counselled by their general practitioner. The one woman who actively approached him for information failed to obtain any, and her efforts finally started her on the way to iatrogenic iron overload, the only fatal complication of thalassaemia trait. Similar experiences with other couples presenting for screening makes it clear that most general practitioners do not yet regard genetic counselling as part of their role.[5]

As with sickle cell disease, it is essential that all health workers should understand the nature of thalassaemia, its symptoms and management, and the needs of sufferers and their families.

Other hereditary anaemias

As well as **sickle cell disease** and **thalassaemia**, which are the most common, there are other hereditary anaemias about which health workers need to be informed: these include, for example, **Haemoglobin E**, which affects mainly people of Far Eastern and Bangladeshi origin, and **Haemoglobin C**, found mainly in the Afro-Caribbean population. Although these are harmless in themselves, they can cause serious illness if combined with a sickle or thalassaemia gene.

The only ethnic group among whom hereditary anaemias are not or are very rarely found is Northern European. Anyone of non-Northern European origin may have or may be a carrier of a hereditary anaemia.[6]

Possible sufferers and carriers should be screened on request or at crucial times, such as before or during early pregnancy and before operations or anaesthesia; they should be given a clear explanation of the results of the screening tests and should be advised or counselled as necessary.

Because of the severity of some of these anaemias, and because they are genetically carried, with all the implications of this for parents and couples who wish to be parents, it is obviously as important to tell people after any screening that they do *not* have the disease or the trait as to inform them that they do.

Further information

If you want to find out more about thalassaemia and other hereditary anaemias, further sources of information are suggested at the end of this chapter.

9.4 Hypertension and cerebrovascular disease

Research shows that **hypertension and cerebrovascular disease are more common among British people of African and Afro-Caribbean origin** than among other ethnic groups. Hypertension has long been recognised as a major black health problem in the USA.

Prevalence in Britain

Statistics of mortality rates in Britain between 1970 and 1972 in different ethnic groups show that people born in Africa have 4.5 times, and people born in the West Indies up to 6.6 times, the mortality rate from hypertension and cerebrovascular disease of people born in England and Wales.[7] Studies also show that in Africa and in the West Indies people living in urban areas suffer from higher blood pressure and higher rates of cerebrovascular disease than people living in rural areas.

People of African and Afro-Caribbean origin in Britain tend to have higher blood pressures than other ethnic groups, and higher rates of hypertension-related mortality. They are more prone to strokes than white people, but far less likely to have heart attacks. It also appears that at a given level of blood pressure people of African and Afro-Caribbean origin are more likely than white people to suffer a stroke.[8] In contrast Asian groups in Britain seem to have higher rates of heart attacks than either white or African and Afro-Caribbean groups.[7]

There are several factors which, singly or in combination, affect blood pressure. These include **age, dietary salt intake, alcohol consumption, stress** and, probably, **obesity**. Blood pressure rises with age in some people. This factor has a genetic component and may also be associated with dietary salt intake. Stress raises blood pressure in the short term, but it is not clear if it also has a long-term effect. Smoking is not a cause of high blood pressure, but when combined with high blood pressure is associated with an increased risk of coronary heart disease.

It seems clear that sensitivity to the different factors which might cause high blood pressure varies from individual to individual, and also between different ethnic groups, though it is not yet clear why this is so.

Drugs

An investigation of the effects of drugs commonly used to lower blood pressure suggests that there are also **differences in the way that hypertensive patients of different ethnic groups respond to the different drugs commonly used to lower blood pressure.** Because of physiological and other differences between ethnic groups a particular drug may be more or less efficacious or toxic and may produce different or more severe side effects.

Implications

The implications of all this for health workers are major: it is important to be alert to the **greater possibility of dangerously high blood pressure among people of African and Afro-Caribbean origin** and to ensure **proper screening.** Such preliminary screening can be economically and effectively done by general practitioners. Where necessary, suitable measures should be taken to bring the pressure down. It may also be **important to consider the patient's ethnic group when choosing an anti-hypertensive drug,** so as to ensure that the patient gets the most effective medication in the right dose and with the fewest side effects. **Health education programmes** should be directed at those communities and groups at greatest risk of coronary heart disease, strokes and high blood pressure.

Reactions and responses to many drugs vary between ethnic groups; **more research is needed on ethnic differences in disease patterns and in reactions to commonly used drugs. What information there is should be more widely disseminated and included in all training programmes.** Until this is done health workers will be inadequately equipped to offer competent health care in a multiracial society.

Further sources of information

Further sources of information are suggested at the end of this chapter.

9.5 *Rickets and osteomalacia*

The quotations and much of the information in this section are from *The Rickets Report.*[9]

Surveys over the last twenty years have shown a significant incidence of rickets and osteomalacia, particularly among **Asian groups** in Britain, and among **housebound elderly people of all ethnic groups.**

As well as the elderly, those at greatest risk include infants, children up to the age of five, adolescents, and pregnant and lactating women.

Rickets (the name given to the disease if it occurs while bones are still forming) and osteomalacia (the name given to the condition in adults) are caused by a lack of Vitamin D, but the precise combination of factors that leads to dangerously low levels of Vitamin D is not yet clearly understood.

Symptoms

Children and adolescents with rickets are **weak and irritable**. They may become **bow-legged or knock-kneed and waddle when they walk**, or even become unable to walk. Their **wrists and ankles may ache**. Their **arms, skulls and ribs** may also be affected. The correction of severe deformities caused by rickets requires surgery and several months in hospital.

Osteomalacia leads to **listlessness, aching bones**, and **weakness of the muscles**. Babies born to mothers with osteomalacia can be very ill.

In the **elderly, osteomalacia** also leads to **fragile brittle bones**, increasing the danger of fractures.

People with subclinical or mild rickets or osteomalacia may develop a severe form of the disease at crucial times, such as during growth spurts or pregnancy.

Prevalence

Estimates of the prevalence of rickets and osteomalacia among Asians and other communities in Britain vary. The Report of the DHSS Working Party on Fortification of Food with Vitamin D estimated that in the Midlands and the north of England about 1 Asian in 100 under 16 years of age suffers from rickets, and about 1 in 250 in London. Although people of Asian origin make up about 1–2 per cent of the total British population they account for at least 70 per cent of those cases serious enough to need hospital admission (excluding cases of osteomalacia in the elderly).[9]

More detailed local surveys indicate that the incidence is far higher. In 1976 a study in Glasgow found that 1 in 20 Asian children had rickets.[10] In 1973 it was estimated that 1 Asian in 10 had rickets or osteomalacia,[11] and in 1976 that 1 Asian child in 40 will have gone into hospital with rickets by the time he or she reaches adolescence.[12] It has also been estimated that as many as a quarter of all Asians, and half of all Asian adolescents, are affected by subclinical signs of rickets.

Sources of Vitamin D

Vitamin D can be obtained by the **action of sunlight on the skin** or from **dietary sources**. From recent research it appears that **sunlight is the most important source**, but that dietary Vitamin D can tip the balance in marginal cases.

Natural dietary sources of Vitamin D include oily fish, liver and eggs. In addition, due to the incidence of rickets among the British population in the 1930s, margarine has been artificially fortified with Vitamin D in Britain since the 1940s.

As far as sunlight is concerned, it is not clear how much is required, whether the weak sunlight of the winter and spring in Britain is effective in synthesising Vitamin D, or whether darker skins may filter out some of the essential ultra-violet rays in weak sunlight.

The quantity of dietary Vitamin D required to make a significant difference to the level of Vitamin D in the blood is also not known. Further there may be other genetic, metabolic, or other factors which combine to increase the risk of rickets or osteomalacia in certain families or groups.

The debate over fortification of suitable foods

It is thought that 60 per cent of British dietary intake of Vitamin D now comes from fortified margarine and eggs, though many white British people have a dietary intake of Vitamin D below that recommended by the DHSS.

Because margarine is part of a traditional British diet and not normally eaten as part of an Asian diet, Asian people, though equally in need of Vitamin D, do not benefit from the government's policy of mandatory fortification of all domestic margarines.

This, in combination with other social and environmental factors which may affect the amount of sunlight people get, such as the British climate, living in inner-city areas with no gardens or parks, staying indoors because of social isolation or even fear of racial harassment, may explain the higher incidence of rickets and osteomalacia among Asian people.

Strong arguments have been put forward for the fortification of a food which is normally eaten in the Asian diet (unlike margarine, which is not). The best arguments seem to be for the fortification of chapatti flour, which is eaten by about 95 per cent of the British Asian population, but in 1980 a DHSS Working Party of the Committee on Medical Aspects of Food Policy (COMA) rejected all ideas of fortification.[13]

Current DHSS policy is to recommend **vitamin supplements** for children under five and for pregnant and lactating women in all ethnic groups. The DHSS has also supported a **health education campaign** to inform Asian communities about rickets and osteomalacia and possible methods of prevention. **Critics of this campaign have been concerned that it gives the erroneous impression that Asian diets are inferior and that Asian people are to blame for the prevalence of rickets and osteomalacia in their communities** (see also 12.1 below).

A further point to be borne in mind (and this applies to all health education campaigns) is that people might be made to feel that their problems are of their own making. In attempting to educate people about a healthy diet it is unfortunately only too easy to create this impression. This is especially so when the programme is directed at a minority ethnic group, and one that may already be the butt of racism. British Asians could all too easily be seen – by themselves as well as by others – as somehow to blame for the condition that 'education' is purportedly going to cure. This is a clear danger in a campaign about food habits and health: people can be made to appear ignorant, conservative and wedded to outmoded traditions. To create such an impression would be especially unwarranted in the case of Vitamin D in the British Asian diet. If non-Asians in Britain have higher dietary Vitamin D intakes, it is not because they are more knowledgeable about nutrition but because the government chose to fortify margarine rather than just rely on educating people about the vitamin content of a tin of pilchards. The DHSS press release on the campaign tells us: 'Asian families must thoroughly understand why it is that in a country with a different climate and different ways of living care must be taken to ensure that groups such as children and mothers receive correct nourishment.' That may be true. But how many people reading that will be aware that non-Asian parents do not have a better understanding, and that they give their children a fortified food (margarine) without realising it? If this were stressed, it would help to avoid any impression that the problem is 'ignorance' on the part of ethnic minority groups. . . .

Food habits are deeply embedded in cultural mores and for many people they are also a reference point for self-identity in what they find to be an alien culture. To seek for change in this area of people's lives should not be done without good reason. But if people think of the majority British way of doing things as 'normal' and 'right' they will not realise such reasons are needed. Such ethnocentrism must not only be avoided but also countered and challenged explicitly if it is not to persist in influencing people's thinking.[9]

Further information

Some further sources of information about rickets and osteomalacia are suggested at the end of this chapter.

Notes

1. Milunsky, Aubrey, *Know Your Genes*, Pelican, 1977.
2. Anionwu, Elizabeth N., 'Sickle Cell Disease' *Health Visitor*, Vol. 55, July 1982.
3. Modell, B., Ward, R. H. T., Fairweather, D. V. I., 'Effect of Introducing Antenatal Diagnosis on Reproductive Behaviour of Families at Risk for Thalassaemia Major', *British Medical Journal*, 7 June 1980.
4. Rossiter, Mary A., Solomon, Maria, *et al.*, letter in *British Medical Journal*, 6 Sept. 1980.
5. Mourzouras, M., Ioannov, P., *et al.*, 'Thalassaemia as a Model of Recessive Genetic Disease in the Community', *The Lancet*, 13 Sept. 1980.
6. *Report of a WHO Working Group on the Community Control of Hereditary Anaemia*, World Health Organisation, 1981.
7. Marmot, M. G., Adelstein, A. M., Bulusu, L., 'Cardiovascular Mortality among Immigrants to England and Wales', *Postgraduate Medical Journal*, Dec. 1981.
8. Stamler *et al.*, 'Hypertension: The Problem and the Challenge', in *The Hypertension Handbook* Merck, Sharp and Dohme, 1974.
9. Sheiham, Helena, and Quick, Alison, *The Rickets Report* Haringey Community Health Council, 1982.
10. Goel, K. M., Sweet, E. M., *et al.*, 'Florid and Subclinical Rickets among Immigrant Children in Glasgow', *The Lancet*, 1976, pp. 1141–45.

11. Preece, M. A., Ford, J. A., *et al.*, 'Vitamin D Deficiency among Asian Immigrants to Britain', *The Lancet*, 1973, pp. 907–10.
12. Ford, J. A., McIntosh, W. B., *et al.*, 'Clinical and Subclinical Vitamin D Deficiency in Bradford Children', *Archives of Disease in Childhood*, Ch. 51, 1976.
13. Dept. of Health and Social Security, *Rickets & Osteomalacia*, Report of the Working Party on Fortification of Food with Vitamin D, Committee on Medical Aspects of Food Policy, HMSO, 1980.

More information

Other aspects of variations in patterns of illness are considered in the following sections:

1.2 **The organisation of the health services**
1.5 **Current health care policy**
2.5 **Health service policies: Allocation of resources for screening specific illnesses**
2.8 **Practical action: Policy**
5.2 **Communication difficulties for ethnic minority patients**
10.3 **Developing new services: Sickle cell disease**
12.1 **Basic training: Ethnic differences in patterns of illness and Reactions to drugs**
13 **Health education**
14 **Local needs: guidelines for doing your own research**
14.4 **Things you need to know: Patterns of illness**

Useful addresses

The organisations below provide information and support for patients and professionals.

The Sickle Cell Society
c/o Brent Community Health Council
16 High Street
Harlesden
London NW10 4LX
(01-451 3293)

The Sickle Cell Centre
Willesden General Hospital
Harlesden Road
Willesden
London NW10
(01-459 1292 Ext. 235)

UK Thalassaemia Society
107 Nightingale Lane
London N8
(01-348 0437)

Audiovisual materials

See 15.3 Training resources for health workers and other professionals on working in a multiracial society, especially the section on health under audiovisual materials.

Further reading:

See the reading list in Chapter 16:

16.9 **Patterns of illness,** including sections on
   Sickle cell disease
   Thalassaemia and other hereditary anaemias
   Hypertension and cerebrovascular disease
   Rickets and osteomalacia
   Mental health

Part 3: The health services

Part 3: The health services

How far are the health services meeting the needs of people from ethnic minority communities? What can ethnic minority health workers contribute, and what is their present position in the health service? Do training programmes equip health workers to work in multiracial communities, or do they emerge from training with professional values that are culture-specific and inappropriate in a multiracial society? Do health education programmes enable black people to have a greater degree of control over their own health, or do they simply undermine confidence by trying to change behaviour deemed 'unhealthy' by professionals? Some of these questions are considered in Part 3.

Chapter 10: some examples of **health service initiatives in response to identified needs;** health care needs that may not be met by existing services; practical ways to demonstrate need; factors for consideration when deciding on appropriate responses.

Chapter 11: the role of **ethnic minority staff in the National Health Service** and the need for positive action to ensure equal opportunity in employment.

Chapter 12: how **health worker training** may be failing to meet the practical needs of health workers in a multiracial society; questions and suggestions for developing more appropriate training; professional values that may be 'colour-blind' or 'culture-specific'.

Chapter 13: the gap between current **health education** theory and the message of health education campaigns 'aimed at' ethnic minority communities; practical considerations when designing health education programmes/information resources.

10 Responding to need

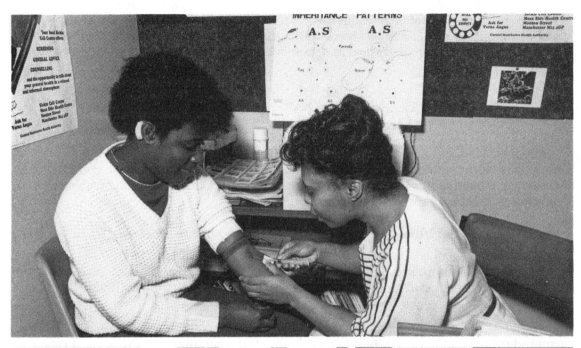

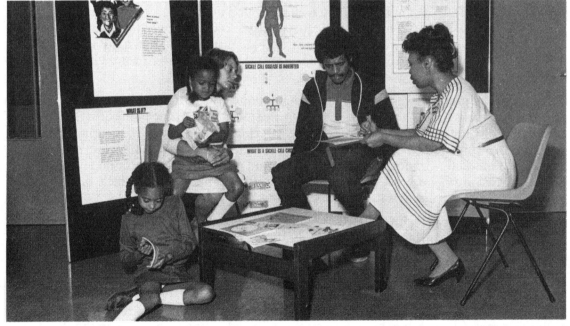

Introduction

This chapter looks at how the health services are responding to some of the needs discussed in earlier chapters, and describes some specific initiatives to improve the delivery of services. The needs we have so far outlined call for action at two levels:

- **to improve access to existing services**
- **to develop new services which are appropriate to need and culturally acceptable.**

The first section deals with the question of establishing evidence of need. The second section discusses some of the reasons for low uptake of existing services, and describes some examples of projects to tackle the difficulties. In the third section, four projects to provide new services are described in detail.

10.1 *Demonstrating need*

Small-scale studies and surveys are a valuable way of using original research to establish evidence of need and to influence the planning of services. Some suggested guidelines for doing this kind of research are outlined in Chapter 14. One such study which was eventually successful is described below.

Study of the use of GP facilities for Chinese restaurant workers in London

In 1976, the Community Health Council for Kensington, Chelsea and Westminster North East District carried out a survey into the use of existing GP facilities by Chinese people living and working in Soho.[1]

Until 1975 a Cantonese-speaking doctor had held a surgery in the area which catered for the needs of the Chinese population, but when this surgery closed it was not replaced. The Community Health Council found in their survey that, as a result, many Chinese people did not have adequate access to GP care in the area where they lived and worked. Many were travelling inordinate distances to find a GP who would accept them onto a list. About three-quarters of those interviewed would have difficulty communicating with a non-Chinese-speaking doctor.

Part of the problem was that there were not many GPs in the locality, and that their lists were small. Part of the problem was the need for an afternoon surgery: the majority of Chinese in the area work in the catering trade, with working hours from 8 a.m. to 3 p.m. and 6 p.m. to midnight. Part of the problem was language: most of the residents and work force are immigrants from peasant villages around Hong Kong. Most are Cantonese-speaking and about three-quarters speak little or no English. Some are not literate in their own language.

The Community Health Council argued that this picture is unlikely to change, because socially aspiring and second-generation Chinese tend to move out of the area, and vacancies in accommodation and the work force are taken by new migrant workers, usually from peasant backgrounds. Many first-generation restaurant workers are unlikely to learn English effectively, if at all.

The Community Health Council produced a report, based on the survey, arguing the case for a Chinese-speaking doctor to be allowed to open a practice in the West End. This was submitted to the Medical Practices Committee, the government body which determines the number of GPs who work in an area, based on the size of the population. Although the Committee agreed with the conclusions of the report, it did not accept these as adequate grounds for allowing an additional GP practice in the area.

Eventually, after lengthy negotiation, Kensington, Chelsea and Westminster Family Practitioner Committee and the Community Health Council worked out a solution which fell within the Medical Practices Committee's regulations. The original Cantonese-speaking doctor had closed his Soho surgery because he had been running it as part of his single-handed practice in Wandsworth. The Family Practitioner Committee persuaded him to apply for a partner and re-open a surgery in Soho. A second Chinese-speaking doctor was accepted by the Medical Practices Committee as a partner in this existing practice. In 1978 a Chinese GP surgery was opened in Gerrard Street, Soho, to the benefit of other local residents as well as the Chinese community.

The Community Health Council survey is important in two ways. First, it is an example of research into the views of an ethnic minority community about health service provision. Second, it demonstrates a way of using original research to change the status quo, and find a solution to a problem of access.

10.2 *Improving access to existing services*

Studies have demonstrated that patients who most need health services often make little use of them.[2] This is true for a significant proportion of the ethnic minority population. Possible reasons are:

- **lack of information** available to patients about the range of health services and how they work;
- **material circumstances** which prevent patients from using a particular service;
- **lack of understanding among health staff** about ethnic minority patients' expectations of the services;
- **communication difficulties** such as language differences and confusion over patients' names;
- **aspects of the service which are unacceptable to patients** because of social, cultural or religious conventions.

Some initiatives to meet these needs and improve access to services are described below.

Lack of information

Feedback from the recent DHSS rickets campaign, and audience reaction to the BBC-TV series 'Speak for Yourself' showed that **a large proportion of people who don't speak English as their first language have considerable difficulty in getting information about how the health services work**, what help and support are available for particular problems, and what benefits they may be entitled to.

'Your rights to health' project

In response to this need the BBC and the Health Education Council collaborated on a project to improve the availability of information to non-English-speaking communities. In 1982 the BBC produced a series of television advertisements, in twelve community languages, for a booklet published by the Health Education Council called *Your rights to health*, also available in twelve community languages.

As well as NHS care, the booklet includes information on health services provided by local authorities and by the Department of Health and Social Security in the form of welfare benefits. It aims to summarise what is available and what may be available in each district. It starts with information on who is entitled to use the services, who is responsible for running the services and providing health care, the GP's role in providing access to other services, and patients' rights on consent and confidentiality. This is followed by sections on specific services and situations (for example medicines, dentists and opticians, health and work, maternity services), which incorporate information on relevant welfare benefits.

Although welcomed as a step in the right direction, the booklets have come in for criticism from some quarters. Some people find them dense and difficult to read; many non-English-speakers have been unable to find out where to get hold of them; some critics feel there should be much more emphasis on patients' legal rights and what to do if you have a complaint or wish to change your GP.

For further information about the *Your rights to health* booklets, contact your local Health Education Department.

Patients' material circumstances

Patients may find it extremely difficult to make use of certain services because of material circumstances, such as shiftwork, transport difficulties, lack of money, lack of interpreters, and problems in arranging childcare. An Asian woman living in south Leeds in 1979 described her problems in getting to hospital ante-natal clinic appointments:

The hospital is two bus rides from where I live. My husband's on a three-day week at the moment, but he has to take the morning off work to come with me, because I don't speak much English and there aren't any interpreters at the hospital. I get a neighbour to look after my three children because there's nowhere for them to play at the clinic and I know it upsets the nurses to have them running around. We gave up going by bus because it can take an hour each way. It can take two or three hours at the clinic sometimes. If we go by taxi my husband gets back to work sooner and loses less pay. It still costs us about £25 a visit in taxis and lost wages. My husband brings home £45 for a three-day week.

Bengali mother

These sorts of difficulties are of course shared by all low-income families, black and white alike, although lack of language may exacerbate the difficulties for some ethnic minority patients.

One way of resolving the constraints like transport and childcare problems is to provide more facilities such as hospital buses and hospital crèches for outpatients' children. Another way is to **resite services like hospital out-patient clinics, that high-risk patients may find inaccessible, so that they become** *more* **accessible.**

The Sighthill project

One of the most striking examples of such an initiative is the pilot ante-natal care scheme set up at the Sighthill Health Centre in Edinburgh.[3] This was an exercise **to locate ante-natal care in the community** by setting up a health care team which was a partnership between GP, consultant obstetrician, hospital and district (community) midwives and health visitor. The GP led the team, which was able to provide a high standard of ante-natal care within a local health centre in an area of the city with a high perinatal mortality rate. The scheme achieved a dramatic reduction in the number of 'defaulters' (women missing appointments) and most significantly, in the perinatal mortality rate.

If nothing else the Sighthill experiment shows that services *can* **be made more accessible without reducing standards, and** *can* **reach patients most in need with difficult material circumstances. It is to be hoped that this precedent will encourage initiatives to take greater account of patients' circumstances in other areas of health care.**

Lack of understanding about patients' expectations

Health workers may not properly understand some patients' expectations of the health service. If a patient's experience and way of life are very different from those of the health professional his expectations of health care are also likely to be different. **The health worker may feel the patient needs treatment for which the patient sees no necessity** (for example, family planning services). **The patient may make unexpected (and apparently 'unreasonable') demands on services for good reasons of which the health worker is unaware.** For example, the patient who presents at a hospital outpatients' department with apparently minor symptoms, such as a temperature or headache, may be seriously worried because he associates them with the onset of life-threatening diseases such as typhoid or cholera which are serious risks in his country of origin.

Training in Health and Race project

In an effort to increase the level of knowledge and awareness among health professionals working with multiracial and multicultural communities, the Health Education Council and the National Extension College launched a three-year training project in 1982, to initiate and develop training courses and materials on aspects of health care in a multiracial society for different groups of health professionals.

There has been considerable demand from health staff at all levels for the training courses offered by the Project, but **it is clear that a small-scale project (a team of eight) of limited duration cannot meet the needs of health workers in all disciplines in all parts of the country. More positive commitment and action are required from those bodies responsible for training policy**, and by individual trainers responsible for curriculum innovation, if all health staff are to be properly equipped with the knowledge and awareness they need to provide effective care.

For more information about Training in Health and Race, contact:

Training in Health and Race
18 Victoria Park Square
London E2 9PF
Tel: 01-980 6263

Communication difficulties

Language

Over 200,000 adults in Britain speak English only slightly or not at all. Yet some health authorities with a high proportion of non-English-speaking patients have little or no interpreting provision.[4] This means that in some cases patients are not getting access to services, because they cannot explain their problems, and health staff cannot effectively perform vital tasks such as diagnosis, history taking, counselling, and giving instructions for treatment.

There are some circumstances in which only the skills of a trained interpreter can resolve complex or delicate communication problems. But there is a great deal that English-speaking health workers can do to make services more accessible by improving their own skills in communicating with patients whose English is not very fluent. (See also Chapter 5.)

Beating the Language Barrier course

In 1979 a local teacher of English as a second language (ESL) in Brent designed a course for Brent and Harrow Health Education Department to help health workers communicate better with patients. The aim of the course was to help health workers to assess the amount of English that clients speak and understand, to modify their own language so as to be more easily understood, and to compensate for lack of a common language by using supplementary means of communication. The course was first piloted for a group of health visitors and special care baby unit nurses from Brent; it was then modified and another course run for health visitors and school nurses from Harrow.

This course represents only one of a growing number of initiatives in different parts of the country. **There are experienced ESL teachers in most towns and cities who, if approached, would be able to provide the necessary skills and expertise to design and run communication courses for English-speaking health staff.** But the Brent course is one of the few that is more widely available as it has now been produced as a **Trainers' Manual**.

For further information contact:

Ann Casey
Health Education Officer
Brent and Harrow Health Education Service
Neasden Hospital
Brentfield Road
London NW10 8EY

Different naming systems

The naming systems of Asian, Chinese, Vietnamese, Cypriot and other minority communities in Britain are different from the traditional British naming system. In many areas health staff are given no guidelines on how to deal with these systems in identification and record-keeping. The result is that **ethnic minority patients tend to experience more delay, confusion and irritation from health staff because records cannot be traced, and names called out are not recognisable to the person they belong to.** When names are muddled there is a real risk of giving medicine or treatment to the wrong person.

DHSS/King's Fund Project

A three-year project jointly funded by the King's Fund and the DHSS has produced a series of training packs called 'Asians in Britain' for health staff working with patients from the Asian communities. The first pack in the series, *Asian names and records*, provides comprehensive training material on the origins and naming systems of the three main Asian communities in Britain. For further details about the pack contact:

> National Extension College
> 18 Brooklands Avenue
> Cambridge CB2 2HN
> Tel. 0223 316644

Unacceptable aspects of the service

Certain aspects of existing services may not be acceptable because of patients' religious, social or cultural beliefs. For example:

- Many Asian women do not wish to be examined by a male doctor, for religious reasons.
- Patients unused to a traditional British diet find it difficult to cope with food from the standard hospital menu.
- For some patients (e.g. strict Muslims, Hindus, Buddhists, Rastafarians, Jews), some or all foods in the normal hospital diet may be prohibited for religious reasons.
- In many cultures, a mother and her new-born baby traditionally stay at home for a month or six weeks after the birth. This is seen as a safety precaution and some women will not attend appointments at the post-natal or child health clinic until this period is over.
- Some people from South East Asian countries, such as Vietnam, believe that it is harmful to health to have blood taken from the body for blood tests. People may be deterred from seeking treatment if they believe they will be subjected to repeated blood tests.
- In many cultures women believe there can be long-lasting ill effects from immersing the body in water in the period immediately after childbirth. In some cases, ethnic minority women have discharged themselves from post-natal hospital care because staff have insisted that they bath, rather than washing or showering.

It is clearly not just a lack of knowledge that makes it difficult for some patients to get access to, or make use of, the services that are currently available. It may be necessary to make changes in existing services or develop new provision which takes into account the material circumstances and culture of the local population. It may also be necessary to develop new services to cater properly for specific needs which are not being met at all by existing provision.

10.3 *Developing new services*

Some health authorities are already attempting to develop more accessible and appropriate services, in a variety of ways. Three local initiatives to tackle unmet needs are described below.

Sickle cell disease

A recent survey has indicated that there are approximately 3,000 cases of sickle cell disease in Britain.[5] According to a Manchester report:

The lack of routine screening, incomplete recording and follow-up of cases, and inadequate knowledge of the condition among health professionals suggests that this number is probably an underestimation.[6]

(Detailed information about sickle cell disease can be found in Chapter 9.)

Brent Sickle Cell Centre

The information in this section is based on two articles written by Elizabeth Anionwu SRN, HV.[7,8]

In 1979 Brent Health District set up the Sickle Cell Centre specifically to provide information and support for families affected by sickle cell disease. **The Centre came into being as the result of action by various groups of people in Brent, including health workers, patients and their families, local people and the Community Health Council, who were all concerned about the lack of support for sickle cell sufferers in both the health services and the community.** In 1979 this activity culminated in the setting up of the first Sickle Cell Information, Screening and Counselling Centre in Britain and the transition of a local self-help group into a national charity called the Sickle Cell Society.

The need for such a Centre was highlighted by the work of a local consultant haematologist and health visitor, who found **a lack of information about the condition, little awareness among patients or staff, misconceptions about the genetics involved, no continuity of care and no uniformity of treatment for sickle cell sufferers.**

It soon became evident that it was health workers (e.g. doctors and nurses) who were actually creating confusion because they did not understand the results of various tests. As a result they inform people that they have 'sickle cell' or are 'sickle positive' without sorting out in advance whether the result is sickle cell trait or sickle cell disease. There is a crucial difference; sickle cell trait is not an illness unlike sickle cell disease.[8]

The Centre is run by a health visitor who attends the haemoglobinopathy clinic (for conditions such as sickle-cell anaemia and thalassaemia) organised twice monthly by the consultant haematologist. Several sessions of her week are devoted to home and hospital visits to affected individuals. Her responsibilities include genetic counselling, health education and liaising with other agencies, such as schools and housing departments.

People can come to the Centre for information and blood tests without a letter from their doctor – a radical concept in Britain. For the first three years it was the only Centre of its kind in Britain. During this time nearly 1,000 people visited it for blood tests and information, many coming from much further afield than Brent. Many more have telephoned or written in to the Centre; most refer themselves and a few are sent by health workers.

The health visitor who runs the Centre describes the needs that the Centre is trying to meet:

Frequent hospitalisation, uncertain prognosis, and the inability to be of any help during a painful crisis can cause immeasurable stress in the family. The parents sometimes experience guilt in having produced a child with sickle cell disease. Other emotions such as anger, hostility, fear and frustration may all be present in various members.[7]

Early diagnosis means that parents can be advised and supported before the child develops symptoms. Prompt medical attention can be provided once it is known the child has sickle cell disease and follow-up is arranged through the paediatric sickle cell clinic. I can inform them about the activities of the Sickle Cell Society in case they may wish to join or support their events.

Since March 1982 I offer counselling to all pregnant women found to have sickle cell trait following routine blood tests at Central Middlesex Hospital. Partners are also invited to this session and offered blood tests if they wish. Over 90 per cent of women and about 70 per cent of their partners attend. ***This excellent response dispels the myth that black people are poor clinic attenders. It shows that if the services match their need the uptake will be good.*** [our emphasis][8]

The Centre has close links with the Sickle Cell Society, which is now a national voluntary organisation. Its objectives include assisting affected families, promoting greater awareness about the condition among the public and the health professions, and raising funds for research. In 1982 the Society received its first major grant from the DHSS, and there are now branches in North East London and Birmingham, and an affiliated group in Manchester. It is hoped that more local groups will be set up, as they provide valuable support for families, both as a social group and through fund-raising activities. But the work of the Centre and Society is still underfunded, and the workers of both organisations feel there is little room for complacency. **Most of the recommendations put forward in a 1981 publication called** *Sickle Cell Disease – the Need for Improved Services* **have yet to be implemented.**[9]

For more information contact:

Brent Sickle Cell Centre
Willesden Hospital
Harlesden Road
London NW10 3RY
Tel. 01-459 1292
ext. 235

Sickle Cell Society
c/o Brent Community Health Council
16 High Street
Harlesden
London NW10 4LX
Tel. 01-451 3293

Gypsy health needs

The law says that Gypsies may only stop on official sites, but some local authorities still provide no sites at all, even though they are legally required to. There are about 9,000 Gypsy families in Britain and the lack of official sites means that over half of them are always illegally parked, often by the roadside. **Because these families are constantly being evicted and moving from one unofficial site to another, it is impossible for them to get access to regular health care.** There is no chance to complete a course of immunisation, to receive ante- and post-natal care, or to follow through a long-term treatment. **In some cases traveller families are made to feel unwelcome in local health centres and clinics and a significant number are refused treatment.**[10]

These and other needs emerged in two reports prepared by the Save the Children Fund (SCF).[10,11] SCF is only one agency among many who are concerned about the difficulties Gypsy and traveller families face in getting access to health care because of their mobility.

Save the Children mobile clinic

As a first step towards improving the availability of care, the Save the Children Fund has set up **a mobile clinic which takes medical care to the families**, usually at the roadside, but also at the annual Gypsy fairs in Cambridgeshire and Cumbria. The clinic gives **immunisation and tests children's hearing, vision and development. Mothers receive ante- and post-natal care. The staff treat minor ailments and refer serious cases to hospital.** When the medical officer manning the clinic is trained in **family planning**, this facility can also be offered to families who want it. An important part of the work is introducing both the authorities and Gypsy families to the idea of a mobile clinic. A tape–slide programme has been produced to explain to Gypsy families what happens at local clinics and why. The programme deals with the importance of ante-natal care, post-natal care and nutrition. It also deals with the desirability of breast feeding, and bottle-feeding techniques for mothers who are unable to breast feed. Other topics include immunisation and safety on sites, particularly where toddlers are concerned. Gypsy families are featured in all the visual material. Further tape–slide programmes have been produced to explain developmental testing of young children and the family planning services.

Although the SCF mobile clinic represents a positive step in the right direction, **many people feel that more health authorities themselves should be adopting a positive 'outreach' policy**, either by use of a mobile clinic, or preferably, by having a health visitor or similar health worker with special responsibility for Gypsy families in a given area, visiting sites regularly and building up trust and confidence. In areas where local health staff are sympathetic and have worked to build up contact with traveller families, access difficulties are gradually being overcome. **But most health authorities have a long way to go to develop services which can effectively meet the needs of traveller families without being intrusive or interfering in the travellers' way of life.**

SCF has carried out a survey of health authority provision to meet the needs of Gypsy families.[11] The report focuses on good practice in those authorities who are identifying and meeting need, in the hope that others will follow. It concludes with recommendations about ways of improving the delivery of health care to Gypsy families.

For further details about the SCF project contact:

Ann Bagehot
National Gypsy Liaison Officer
Save the Children Fund
17 Grove Lane
Camberwell
London SE5 8RD
Tel. 01-703 5400

Kit Sampson
Health Liaison Officer
SCF Mobile Clinic
Laxfield
Woodbridge
Suffolk
Tel. Ubbeston 231

Maternity services to reach ethnic minority women

Some groups of ethnic minority women, and especially non-English-speaking women with young children, may have particular difficulty in using the existing health services. For many, the maternity services are likely to be their main point of contact with the NHS; many are likely to be in the high risk category and, as we discussed in Chapter 3, many are particularly vulnerable to isolation and loneliness.

Hackney multi-ethnic women's health project

This project was set up in response to the needs of non-English-speaking Muslim women having babies at Hackney Mother's Hospital, most of whom are from rural Southern Europe and Asia. The aims of the project are:

- **to improve the physical health of non-English-speaking women and babies (many of whom are in the high risk category);**
- **to develop a support system which will help mental health;**
- **to reduce racial tension in the hospital;**
- **to help hospital staff understand the special needs of this group.**

In 1980 three workers were appointed to work with ante-natal and post-natal women at the mothers' hospital Their duties include:

- interpreting;
- organising and supervising interpreters for additional languages and clinics;
- advocacy – the workers are expected to speak on behalf of women and make sure they are aware of the options open to them and understand the implications of agreeing to treatment;
- health education – particularly nutrition and hygiene education and education in how to use the health service;
- education of health workers to increase their awareness and understanding of the culture, economic conditions and health problems of non-English-speaking women;
- advising the health service about the specific changes needed to enable the service to respond to identified needs.

Despite some initial apprehension about the project on the part of hospital staff, the workers are now welcomed to the wards to sort out, for example, family planning problems, food difficulties and baby feeding problems. **They have gradually tried to shift the belief that it is the women who cause problems for the hospital to one of accepting that the hospital presents major problems to the women.** The workers have been trained by midwifery tutors to interview and fill in booking forms for non-English-speaking women.

As a result of the project, medical staff have tried to resolve the problem of Muslim women being examined by male doctors. It is now policy that, whenever possible, a woman's request to be seen by a female doctor is respected, and only female medical students accompany the doctor. Project workers have also alerted health staff to the dangers of over-estimating the comprehension of second language speakers: in several cases women who had been given rubella vaccines thought they had been given Depo-Provera. They had understood 'You *must* not get pregnant for three months' as 'You *cannot* get pregnant. . . .'

Medical staff now arrange clinic appointments so that women speaking the same language all come to the same clinic. This frees the workers from the need to attend all clinics, and gives them time to develop group education. They are also collecting available mother tongue health education literature and materials and identifying the gaps with a view to producing their own materials.[12]

Since the Hackney Project began, a similar project, the Maternity Services Liaison Scheme, has been started by Tower Hamlets Health Authority.

For further information about these projects contact:

Fedelma Winkler	Liz Smart
City and Hackney Community	Maternity Services Liaison Scheme
Health Council	Montefiore Centre
210 Kingsland Road	Deal Street
London E2 8EB	London E1
	Tel. 01-377 8725

10.4 Practical action

This chapter is by no means a comprehensive survey of ethnic minority health care needs and responses. **There are many other areas of need we have not touched on**, and there are certainly unmet needs that are not properly catered for in present local policy and practice.

Policy

The 1976 Race Relations Act allows bodies such as the NHS to take positive action in various ways to establish **equal access and opportunity for disadvantaged racial groups**. (See the section on Equal Opportunity Policy in Chapter 11). This is likely to involve:

- **Actively consulting with black organisations, community groups, community representatives and ordinary people.** (The local CRC does NOT necessarily represent a true cross-section of community interests.)

- **Making access to existing services as simple, straightforward and understandable as possible, and improving services where necessary.**

- **Being sensitive to black experience and cultural factors.**

- **Promoting a wider understanding of ethnic minority health needs among all staff.**

- **Using staff whose own experience will enable them to forge real links, establish good communication and build trust.**

In July 1979, as part of a comprehensive programme to redress inequalities in the provision of services (as well as in employment opportunities), Lambeth Borough Council adopted a series of administrative procedures that could usefully be applied by health care planning committees[13]:

- **Health authority members, officers and committees could be asked to automatically consider the racial dimension when making decisions.**

- **Officers and committees might be asked to include a consideration of the following factors when producing reports:**
  1. Whether or not provision of services/facilities would **benefit** deprived racial groups and in what way.
  2. Whether or not the provision of services/facilities **took account of the different and specific needs** of black groups (e.g. culture/language/customs, etc.), and how these differences would be catered for.
  3. Indications of **take-up or participation** by deprived racial groups in services/ facilities provided by the Health Authority (in the presentation of service statistics/data, etc.).
  4. Whether or not provision would be **non-discrimatory** (either intentionally or otherwise), provide equality of opportunity, improve race relations.

- All report-writing staff could be asked to ensure that appropriate **comments be included in future reports**, so that the **needs of ethnic minority groups are considered prior to decision-making.**

Individual practice

There are various ways in which individual health workers can play an important part in creating awareness of unmet needs and influencing decisions at policy level:

- Writing **reports**.
- Writing **articles** in professional journals and local papers.
- **Initiating or supporting relevant pieces of research:** for example, a small-scale survey of patients' views of health service for a student dissertation; a phone-in programme in community languages to monitor people's expressed health needs. (See also guidelines for doing your own research in Chapter 14.)
- Gathering your own **statistical evidence** of particular need **from your caseload.**
- Building up **useful contacts** with local ethnic minority community organisations and individual people, **encouraging and supporting community campaigns** on health issues.
- Finding out about **examples of good practice** in other areas.

Notes

1. Kensington Chelsea Westminster & N.E. District Community Health Council, *Study of Use of GP Facilities for Chinese Restaurant Workers in London*, 1976.
2. See for example Townsend, Peter and Davidson, Nick, (eds), *Inequalities in Health: The Black Report*, Penguin, 1982, Chapter 4: Inequality in the Availability and Use of the Health Service.
3. McKee, Ian, 'A new look at ante-natal care', *World Medicine*, September 21, 1977, pp. 72–79.
4. *Asians and the Health Service*, Wandsworth Council for Community Relations, 1978.
5. Diaz, H., 'UK News Round Up: The Scourge of Sickle Cell Anaemia' *Weekly Jamaica Gleaner*, September 1980
6. *Sickle Cell Disease in Manchester*, Manchester Community Health Group for Ethnic Minorities, 1981.
7. Anionwu, Elizabeth N., 'Sickle Cell – Menace in the Blood' *Nursing Mirror,* 20 July 1978.
8. Anionwu, Elizabeth N., 'The Sickle Cell Centre and Sickle Cell Society – Community Health Initiatives in Brent' (unpublished manuscript), 1983.
9. *Sickle Cell Disease: The Need for Improved Services*, Sickle Cell Society, 1981.
10. *The Health of Traveller Mothers and Children in East Anglia*, Save The Children Fund, 1983.
11. *Gypsy Children and Their Health Needs*, Save The Children Fund, 1979.
12. Winkler, F. and Yung, J., 'Advising Asian Mothers' *Health and Social Services Journal*, 9 October 1981.
13. Ouseley, Herman *et al.*, *The System*, Runnymede Trust and South London Equal Rights Consultancy, 1982, p. 25.

More information

Most of this book is concerned with specific health needs that are not necessarily met by existing services. If you are primarily concerned with responding to needs in your local area the most useful starting point is probably:

14 **Local needs: guidelines for doing your own research**

Other sections that may be useful are:

1.3 **Poverty and racial inequality**
1.4 **Poverty and access to health care**

2.5–2.8 These sections deal with various aspects of **discrimination, health, and health care policy and practice**

3 **Migration and health**, especially
3.4 **Coping with the British health care system**

5 **Communication**, especially
5.6 **Practical action: improving communication across a language barrier**

6 **Working with families and individuals** looks at different family systems and how health care should take account of family organisation

7 **Health beliefs and practices**, especially
7.2 **Expectations and experience of the health services**
7.4 **Working with different health beliefs and practices**

8 **Foods and diets**, especially
8.7 **Practical action: giving nutritional advice**
8.8 **Food in hospitals and institutions**

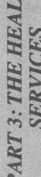

9 **Patterns of illness** sets out detailed information about ethnic variations in patterns of illness

13 **Health education**

Further reading
See Chapter 16: Reading list
16.10 Responding to need.

11 Ethnic minority staff in the National Health Service

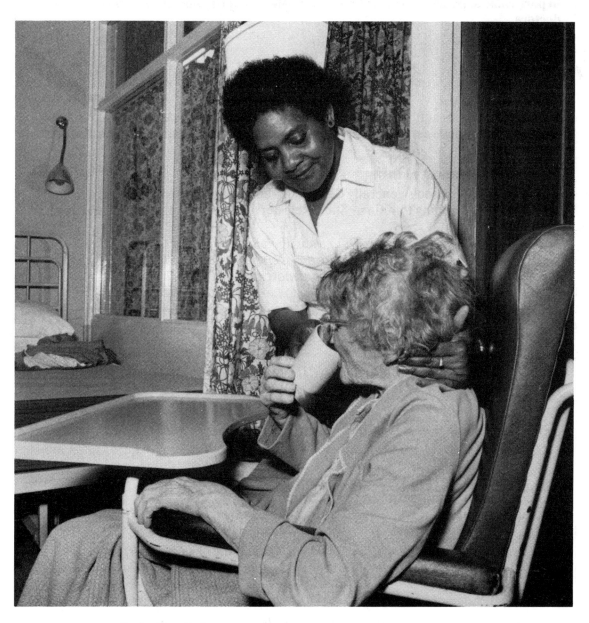

Introduction

One group of health workers whose potential contribution to multiracial health care has been consistently undervalued are the ethnic minority staff working in the NHS.

This chapter looks at some of the factors which influence the way in which black health workers are recruited by the health service. We also look at the differences in the distribution of white and ethnic minority staff within different sections of the NHS, and in particular at policies and practices which affect minority nurses, health visitors and doctors.

11.1 *Nurses*

During the 1960s and 70s, a significant proportion of nurses were recruited from overseas, from the West Indies, Africa, Singapore, Malaysia and other Third World countries.

Recruitment and training

British nursing schools generally demand **higher academic qualifications** from overseas nurses wishing to train as State Registered Nurses than from native British students.

I came over from Jamaica in the 70s to train as an SRN, with three A levels. I realised when I started the course that it was only the overseas nurses who had A levels. Some of the other girls in my intake had O levels but most only had CSE's.

Afro-Caribbean nurse

TRIBUNALS
Sister Dora School of Nursing

On 13 December 1982, the Birmingham Industrial Tribunal registered the settlement of a complaint by Mr Yim Choong Chong against the Sister Dora School of Nursing, which is controlled or managed by Walsall Health Authority.

Mr Chong was 31 in February 1982 (the date of the incident complained of), and was born in Malaysia of Chinese parents. He came to live in the UK in 1970 and trained as a mental nurse at Claybury Psychiatric Hospital in Essex. He qualified as a Registered Mental Nurse in December 1973, and subsequently worked at the West Suffolk Hospital Psychiatric Unit at Bury St Edmunds; and the De-la-Pole Hospital in Hull, where he was a Staff Nurse, providing full nursing care to geriatric female patients who were either schizophrenic or severely demented. The Home Office removed the time limit and conditions attached to his leave to enter the UK in November 1975 and, by February 1982, his application for British Nationality had been with the Home Office for about one year.

Shortly after his appointment to the De-la-Pole Hospital, Mr Chong decided to seek to qualify as a State Registered Nurse to improve his career prospects. He wrote to some 80 Schools of Nursing. Eight of these sent him application forms, which he completed and returned. Of these, two subsequently wrote that they were unable to offer him a place; two rejected his application on the grounds that his educational qualifications did not meet the required standard; one stated that he would have to sit a further examination before he could be considered; two offered him places on their State Registered Nurse training courses, one of which he accepted; and one (the Sister Dora School of Nursing) wrote to him on 10 February 1982:

'Dear Mr Chong,
Thank you for your completed application form and copies of your certificates.

I regret to inform you that I notice from your form that you are of Malaysian Nationality and in the present state of the British labour market, it is not my policy to consider anyone who does not hold full United Kingdom citizenship. I am afraid, therefore, I am unable to help you.

Yours sincerely
S Green (Miss)
Director of Nurse Education'

After receiving Miss Green's letter of rejection, Mr Chong contacted Hull Citizens' Advice Bureau who referred him to the Commission for Racial Equality.

The Commission provided him with legal representation and agreement was reached on terms of settlement, in which the respondents:

– *admitted that they discriminated against Mr Chong on the grounds of his Malaysian Nationality, contrary to the 1976 Race Relations Act;*

– *apologised to Mr Chong for doing so;*

– *undertook not to commit acts of discrimination contrary to the 1976 Race Relations Act in future;*

– *undertook to pay Mr Chong £500 as compensation for the injury to feelings they acknowledged he had suffered.*

CRE *Employment Report* September 1983

In the early 1970s **most overseas nurses were channelled into State Enrolled Nurse training**. In 1972, 9 per cent of all NHS nurses came from overseas, but they made up 20 per cent of the total number of SENs working in the NHS.[1]

Overseas nurses as a proportion of all nurses in 1972[1]

	percentage
All nursing staff	9
Senior nurse managers	1
Charge nurses/sisters	4
Student nurses	14
Midwives	15
Pupil nurses	20

Often nurses who were offered SEN training were not made aware, until it was too late, **of the differences between SRN and SEN qualifications; the SEN is not recognised as a nursing qualification in most countries outside Britain, and so is of little practical use to overseas nurses who wished to return home after training.** In a survey of 365 overseas learners published by the Royal College of Nursing (RCN) in 1979,[2] nearly half said that their UK qualifications would not be recognised in their home countries.

With increasing unemployment the situation is becoming worse. There is now practically no recruitment of nurses from abroad. In addition, evidence suggests that the recruitment policy of some schools of nursing may work to the disadvantage of black school-leavers in this country, in a number of ways.[3]

For example, many nursing schools now impose entry requirements far higher than those deemed necessary by the General Nursing Council (GNC). The GNC Entrance Examination is comparable to four 'O' levels but some schools of nursing demand six 'O' levels at one sitting, without apparently relating this to job performance. Racial disadvantage built into the education system means that a significant proportion of young black people are not obtaining 'O' level results comparable with other school leavers. Black students who meet the minimum requirement stipulated by the GNC may be excluded from nursing schools which demand higher qualifications. If these additional qualifications are not *necessary* for the job, this constitutes indirect discrimination. (See 2.2.)

A common fear of recruiting organisations is that changing discriminatory policies will 'lower standards'. In this example, such an argument is based on ignorance of what racial disadvantage in education means. It does not necessarily mean that black school leavers are less intellectually capable than white ones; it means that for a significant number of black students academic achievement is not an accurate reflection of intellectual ability. What is called for is an alternative form of assessment that is geared to the needs of the job and is fair to *all* applicants; this does not constitute a lowering of standards.

Once in training, **ethnic minority nurses are often encouraged to specialise in low status disciplines** such as **geriatrics** and **mental subnormality**. According to GNC figures nearly one third of overseas learners are in psychiatric and mental handicap nursing[4].

When I was being trained the black girls were sent to do the geriatrics option and the white ones to do obstetrics or community options.

Promotion for black nurses is only ever possible in the low status disciplines such as geriatrics. It is very rare that you find a black nurse running or even staffing on surgical wards. This seems to be reserved for whites.

Afro-Caribbean nurses

Promotion

In a recent study undertaken by the Polytechnic of North London, *Migrant Workers in the National Health Service*, it was found that **Irish nurses were more likely to have reached grades of ward sister, nursing officer or senior nursing officer than their English counterparts, whereas the Afro-Caribbean nurses were less likely.**

Ethnic origins of senior nursing staff at one London hospital[5]

Ethnic origin	Ward sister Nursing officer Senior nursing officer %
British	20
Irish	35
West Indian [Afro-Caribbean]	10
South East Asian	20
Other	15
	——
	100

This pattern cannot be explained by the length of time Afro-Caribbean nurses have spent in the job, because in general they came to this country earlier and form a more stable workforce than, for example, nurses from Malaysia and the Philippines. The Afro-Caribbean nurses in the sample were on average older than either the British or the South East Asian nurses, so the lack of promotion is not explained by the length of time they have been qualified.

This report was based on a small sample, but it demonstrates the need to examine the possibility that **direct and indirect discrimination may be occurring.** It is possible that part of the explanation lies in the **stereotyping** of different ethnic groups. One hospital administrator interviewed in the report remarked that South East Asian nurses were considered hardworking and compliant, but Afro-Caribbeans were seen as uncooperative and even 'bolshy'.[6] How far promotion is affected by this type of stereotyping could only be established by further research.

Work permits

Once they are qualified, **overseas nurses have to apply for a work permit, which can be a lengthy process, making some health authorities reluctant to employ overseas nurses at all** and making it very difficult for them to change jobs.

One very real area of worry and anxiety experienced by every overseas nurse learner has been illustrated clearly over the last two years. That is, the Home Office status of an overseas nurse whilst in training, as compared with his/her situation once qualified and subsequently employed. Whilst in training the overseas nurse has permission to stay in this country as a student, despite being an employee of the NHS. Once qualified, the Home Office require that Department of Employment permission must be given to the hospital before the same individual may continue employment within the NHS. Each time a trained overseas nurse changes his/her job, the potential employing authority must apply for another Work Permit. This involves nurse managers in lengthy and often confused negotiations with local Employment Offices (Job Centres) for several weeks – sometimes months – before Permission to Work (Work Permit) is granted. Meanwhile the overseas nurse is neither student nor worker, is placed in great insecurity, is unable to commence employment or even leave the country for a holiday without the necessary extension of permission to stay (dependent on D. of E. approval of Work Permit) stamped in his/her passport. Again, the Work Permit nightmare has arisen following high levels of UK unemployment.[7]

Nursing and cultural conventions

In many multiracial areas there is a clear need for more nurses who speak the language and share the background of the local ethnic minority community.

However, the national nursing bodies and most District Health Authorities have done little to develop an equal opportunities policy in nursing, or to look at ways of overcoming the factors which deter some potential students from taking up a nursing career. For example:

- Many Asian girls feel that **religious convention requires them to wear trousers**, for reasons of modesty. Although the regulations regarding nurses' uniform have changed to take account of this, this has not been much publicised and potential Asian applicants may not be aware that trousers are permitted.

- Some Asian girls may also be **apprehensive about nursing male patients** during training, since close contact with strange men is felt to be socially unacceptable in many Asian families.

- Orthodox Jewish young people may be deterred by the **requirement to work on the Sabbath** (i.e. Friday evening to Saturday evening).

- Some young people from ethnic minority communities may be put off by the **catering arrangements** in living-in accommodation during training, where it is frequently impossible to buy or cook the food they like to eat.

There is no choice of food and they have pork quite often which I don't eat. I've lost so much weight which I just can't put on again.

Mauritian nurse

Our cooking has its problems. Our colleagues don't like the smell and we don't like to cook certain foods; sometimes they can be quite rude. It's very difficult living in a community.

Malaysian nurse[8]

- **Some careers guidance advisors** who are aware of these difficulties actively **discourage ethnic minority students** (and Asian girls in particular) interested in nursing, rather than exploring the implications properly with each individual. This means that some potential students are never given the chance to consider nursing as a serious option.

The RCN report mentioned above identified other aspects of nursing that can conflict with the beliefs and conventions of some ethnic minority nurses from overseas (see Box, below).

TRIBUNALS

KINGSTON & RICHMOND A.H.A.
Nurses' uniform indirectly discriminatory

In January 1980, 18-year-old Tajwinder Kaur, an English-born Sikh, was offered a place on Kingston and Richmond Area Health Authority's pupil-nurse training course. In discussing the matter of uniform with Mr Miller, Senior Tutor with the Authority, she explained that the custom of her community required her to wear trousers and forbade the wearing of skirts, but that she would be willing to wear trousers of specified design and colour under a nurse's dress. Mr Miller told Miss Kaur that this would constitute an infringement of uniform policy and would not be acceptable. Miss Kaur could not accept their alternative suggestion of wearing thick tights and, after further correspondence, the offer of the place was withdrawn.

Miss Kaur accordingly brought an action with CRE assistance under section (1) and she alleged indirect discrimination under section 1(1)(b) that the Area Health Authority were applying a requirement such that the proportion of persons of her racial group (Sikh/Punjabi/Indian) who could comply with it was considerably smaller than the proportion of persons not of that racial group who could comply with it, and which the Area Health Authority could not justify on non-racial grounds. She was represented at the Tribunal by Mr Kuttan Menon, the CRE's Senior Legal Officer.

It was alleged not that there had been any intention to discriminate, but that indirect discrimination had nevertheless occurred. In reaching its decision, a London Industrial Tribunal examined the Area Health Authority's independent uniform policy, which it found by implication forbade the wearing of trousers, but not for reasons of hygiene. The Tribunal also considered evidence that Rochdale Area Health Authority allowed the wearing of trouser suits as part of nurses' uniform to encourage girls of Asian origin to apply for nursing posts. It held that insistence on the wearing of a uniform exclusive of trousers was a 'requirement or condition' within the meaning of the Race Relations Act. It also held that the Sikh community constituted a racial group within the terms of the Act, and that the proportion of Sikhs who could comply with the uniform requirement was lower than that of other racial groups; the requirement was therefore to Miss Kaur's detriment. The Tribunal also found that the requirement was discriminatory against Miss Kaur as a Punjabi and Indian.

As to the requirement being justifiable, the Tribunal decided unanimously 'that it is more than convenient, and is reasonably necessary, for the respondents to have a requirement that nurses (including trainees) should wear a uniform on the wards', but 'that the requirement in its present form is (unintentionally) discriminatory and that the respondents can find some other and non-discriminatory method of achieving their object'. A recommendation was made that within six months the respondents should cease to impose any condition which requires every female nurse to refrain from wearing trousers on the wards.

CRE *Employment Report* April 1981

NHS Feedback
Nurses uniform

There has been an interesting footnote to the case of Tajwinder Kaur v Kingston and Richmond Area Health Authority (see 'Employment Report' April 1981 p. 9).

The General Nursing Council has issued an Approved Instrument under their powers conferred by the Nurses Act 1956/69, stating that in future 'enrolled nurses shall while working wear any uniform required by the person or Authority by whom she is employed'. A similar amendment to the regulations was also made for registered nurses.

This effectively repeals the regulation used as its defence by Kingston and Richmond Area Health Authority. Uniforms are now a matter for local clarification.

It is to be hoped that this will take into account the appropriateness of attire for Muslim and Sikh nurses.

CRE *Employment Report* July 1982

Overseas Nurses – Training for a Caring Profession[9]

Different cultural attitudes and practices form a complex, almost indefinable area of need. So much is dependent upon the type of family and socio/religious background as to the degree of difficulty any one individual will experience during adaptation and adjustment to a new environment. As with colloquialism and British customs, religious and cultural attitudes may contribute to a sense of disharmony and isolation, but, even worse than this, may lead to compulsory involvement in practices totally forbidden by culture or religion:

Death – at home when one menstruates you are not allowed to go near a dead body. They don't take those sort of things into consideration. You're very reluctant to do some things but you have to – there's no choice. (Malaysia)

*Diet – eating beef – I'm not supposed to but I **have** to. There's no choice. (Malaysia)*

We are not used to swearing, drinking or smoking. Back home we are taught not to do these things. But here it's part of socialising. (Malaysia)

It was a long time before I got used to coming back late – at home you don't go out after 6 p.m. and it's very strict. (Mauritius)

Religious – having to serve pork, etc. to patients when it is forbidden by my religion. (Mauritius)

Religion – things like Buddhist beliefs. We have 15 days of celebration over Chinese New Year and during that time we're not supposed to have contact with death and disease. My parents are very strict Buddhists. (Malaysia)

Nervous about going to a male ward but I was too shy to say anything at the time. (Malaysia)

Jokes relating to the environment and society I don't always understand. (Zimbabwe)

Going to pubs, etc. – when I first came it was very hard. (Mauritius)

I have difficulty accepting the morals of the people here. Freedom of thought and speech is also different here to Malaysia. We're not used to it. (Malaysia)

Parties – if we don't go we feel very old-fashioned but if we go we don't really enjoy the party because it's so utterly different to what we're used to from home. (Indonesia)

Abortions. Touching dead people. My family are superstitious about this. (Malaysia)

*The point being made here is not that exceptions should be allowed for all the variations that may arise, but that **opportunity should be given, firstly to enable overseas learners to discuss their attitudes, beliefs and experiences, within informal tutorial groups, preferably with an input from British learners in the same set. Secondly, that ongoing dialogue should be encouraged, where the learner may feel able to explore freely the anxiety and distress which arise from ward situations and day-to-day living.** In this way a sensitivity and awareness towards the cultural needs of overseas learners can be developed and put to practical use in enabling the individual to adjust in a less threatening environment.* [our emphasis]

In addition to the need for **proper counselling and support**, some of the difficulties outlined in the report could be overcome, at least in part, by a little more **flexibility in the regulations and planning of nursing bodies, nursing schools, catering departments, etc.** and a more **positive approach by careers advisors, nursing managers and nursing**

163

tutors. It is neither necessary nor desirable that ethnic minority communities should remain under-represented in the nursing profession. Ethnic minority nurses clearly have an important role to play in the effective delivery of nursing care, and should be represented at *all* grades in the nursing profession, not simply the lowest.

Attitudes to ethnic minority nurses

The recruiting and interviewing policy of some nursing schools increases the likelihood that ethnic minority nurses will be under-represented on training courses.

One black nursing officer told me that she is excluded from the interviewing panel when the applicant is black. What kind of logic is that? Should all white nursing officers be excluded from interviewing white applicants?

Postgraduate nursing researcher

Whether or not there is a deliberate intention to discriminate against black nurses on the part of nursing management, many strongly feel that they receive less favourable treatment than white nurses throughout their training.

In my year there were seven black girls. Six of us came over to enter nurse training and one was already living here. By the end of three months we were left with only three. One girl was allowed to come all the way from the Congo . . . after two weeks she was told her academic qualifications were not acceptable and she had to leave the course and return home. After the first preliminary test another three girls (two from Mauritius and one from Ghana) were told to go and do SEN training as they were not up to standard.

Even academic performance is not recognised. At the end of my SRN training I was the best student of the three intakes during my year. This should be a gold medal. That year, however, no gold medal was given since 'the standards were not high enough'. I was offered £5 because, as the nurse tutor explained – 'the cash will come in handy for you girls going back home'. The girl who was second was offered a silver medal, inscribed.

Afro-Caribbean nurses

11.2 Health visitors

There are few health visitors from ethnic minority communities, and the Asian population is particularly under-represented in the profession. **Until very recently there has been little positive effort to recruit people from ethnic minority backgrounds to health visiting. One or two District Health Authorities now advertise for health visitors with specific qualifications, such as an ability to speak Urdu, but this kind of positive action is very new and unusual.**

One of the reasons for the current situation is that successful entry to health visitor training depends on the applicant having had a British education, and being familiar with British academic techniques. Successful applicants have to cope with culture-specific intelligence tests, and be able to write essays according to British academic conventions.

Although statutory bodies in other fields (for example, education authorities and social services departments) are beginning to recognise in their recruiting policies that **appropriate experience is a far more relevant qualification for working with multiracial communities than conventional academic techniques**, this is slow to happen in community nursing. As a result, many ethnic minority nurses with considerable experience are excluded from health visitor training because their written English or essay writing techniques are not acceptable.

I did my health visitor training in the early 1970s. I remember doing the intelligence test for entry to the course and realising that some of the questions depended far more on familiarity with European climate and culture than actual intelligence. There was one question, 'In autumn squirrels gather . . .' and then four words to choose from, one of which was 'nuts'. I'd never seen a squirrel, I had no idea what the gathering habits of the squirrel were.

Afro-Caribbean health visitor

Health Visiting

تیمارداری کے لیے جانا

ਬੀਮਾਰ ਨੂੰ ਪੁੱਛਣ ਲਈ ਜਾਣਾ।

તંદુરસ્તીની તપાસ માટે મુલાકાત

স্বাস্থ্য পরিদর্শন

The Nursing Career with a Difference -

As a qualified Health Visitor, you'll know all about that important difference — the never-ending variety of people you meet every working day. Shouldering their problems isn't easy, of course, but it's one of the most vital areas of health care today.

Here in Sandwell we're made more than ever aware of this fact through our large immigrant population. We have many people needing skilled help, and few enough hands to provide it. That's why we're looking for more people like you — SRNs with midwifery or obstetric experience and the Health Visitor Certificate or Diploma. We would particularly welcome applications from speakers of Bengali, Gujerati, Punjabi, Urdu or other Asian languages.

We place the greatest emphasis on prevention rather than cure; if you share our views why not come along and see us at work?

We can then give you all the facts about working full or part time in Sandwell, about our generous £178 initial uniform allowance and £118 annual renewal, about car allowances and possible help with car purchase.

For further details please contact Mr. G. Roberts, Divisional Nursing Officer (Community) Sandwell Area Health Authority, Shaftesbury House, High Street, West Bromwich, West Midlands. Tel 021-525 7611.

SANDWELL AREA HEALTH AUTHORITY

81/11/47

---

13. The bare trees made a lacy pattern against the (summer, empty, wide, blue, wintry) sky.

19. The mellow November sun came streaming into the room. The sky was bright and there was a genial (dampness, warmth, breeze, cold, sun) in the air. It was almost like a morning in May.

26. The old man walked into the wine cellar and looked for his cherished bottle of (medicine, lemonade, paraffin, claret, liquid).

33. History has known several cases when a mode of thought has seized the imagination of a vast majority of the intelligentsia, as existentialism has today in France; hence the great (imagination, eagerness, caution, fear, popularity) with which a true philosopher approaches such highly popularised philosophies.

Selected questions from intelligence test for entry to Health Visitor Course at Manchester Polytechnic in 1975.

Attitudes to health visitors

There is evidence to suggest that, rather than recognising the positive value of proper ethnic minority representation in the profession, health visitor course tutors sometimes demonstrate clear prejudice against black applicants.

For example, two black nurses who had been unsuccessful in their applications for places to train as health visitors were asked to describe, for a research study, what had happened at their interviews:

I was asked at one point during the interview, 'Some white families might object to a coloured health visitor – how do you feel about that?'

One of the interviewers said to me, 'You West Indians are hard on your children and you could improve your own values before going into health visiting, or you might inflict them on your clients.'

The researcher who spoke to these nurses made this comment:

These two remarks reflect some of the common attitudes within the health service establishment towards ethnic minority health workers. The assumptions are, firstly, that caseloads are made up only of white families and, secondly, because the cultural values of some black people are different from white norms they are therefore inferior values as well.

You can argue that in asking the question about white families not liking black health visitors, the interviewer was trying to be honest and present the applicant with a realistic view of the difficulties. But you can't take that remark in isolation. How often are white applicants asked how they think being white will affect their work with black families . . . how often are they asked how effective they think they will be when they don't know anything about the lifestyle of the black families they'll meet, and possibly won't speak the client's language? Black applicants probably have a deeper understanding of the needs of black families, but how often are they asked what positive contribution they can make as black health visitors?

The second comment appears to be based on straightforward prejudice against Afro-Caribbeans, and the applicant was naturally offended. Do white health visitors never impose their own values on clients, or are white health visitors supposed to be value-free?[10]

11.3. *Doctors*

In 1977, about a third of all doctors in the UK came from overseas, according to a survey carried out by the Policy Studies Institute (PSI).[11] The majority (i.e. about 80 per cent) of overseas doctors are black, and doctors from the Indian sub-continent make up by far the largest proportion of this group (about 18.5 per cent of all doctors).

Distribution

Because many overseas doctors return to their country of origin after a period of training in Britain, the survey found a **much higher proportion of doctors from overseas working in hospitals (38 per cent) than in general practice (20 per cent).**

Specialisation and career prospects

Within hospitals, the general pattern is that **overseas doctors are over-represented in the lower medical grades** (registrar, senior house officer) and **under-represented in the higher grades** (senior registrar, consultant).

Overseas doctors as a percentage of all doctors in 1975[12]

	percentage
All doctors	35
Consultants	14
Senior registrars	28
Registrars	57
Senior house officers	60

Overseas doctors are also **over-represented in the least popular specialties**, such as geriatrics and mental illness. Most of those who have managed to reach the grade of senior registrar or consultant are to be found in these specialties. It is far more difficult for overseas doctors to reach the position of consultant in popular specialties such as general surgery.

Overseas consultants according to specialty in 1975[12]

	percentage
All specialties	14
Geriatrics	34
Mental illness	19
General surgery	9

Overseas registrars according to specialty in 1975[12]

	percentage
All specialties	57
Geriatrics	85
Mental illness	64
General surgery	52

Overseas doctors are **under-represented in rural areas, and in teaching hospitals**. In 1977 only 19 per cent of ethnic minority doctors who qualified overseas were working in a teaching district compared with 45 per cent of British qualified doctors.

Training opportunities

This has implications for the training and career prospects of overseas doctors, as teaching hospitals generally offer wider training opportunities and, especially in London, may have lighter workloads. Greater prestige is attached to teaching hospitals and to particular specialties within them. Overseas doctors whose experience is limited to non-teaching hospitals are at a disadvantage when competing for jobs against doctors who have worked in teaching hospitals, according to the PSI survey. Results indicated that, consistently, **black overseas doctors had to make more job applications before being successful than white overseas or British doctors.**

Attitudes to ethnic minority doctors

The individual experiences of several doctors are quoted in the PSI report, including those of an Asian doctor who is unusual in that he is now a consultant in a teaching hospital:

Dr. Vengat first qualified as a doctor in India, but then came to Britain and immediately took the British MB examinations. He is, therefore, a British-qualified doctor who nevertheless had his basic training in India. Dr. Vengat speaks English perfectly, and as a young doctor was already well-qualified. As a junior doctor he had some difficulties, nevertheless, in getting suitable training jobs, although these difficulties were overcome, and he finally completed an impressive training programme. It was at this point, when he began to apply for consultant posts, that he encountered serious difficulties. He made 18 or 20 applications, and was shortlisted seven or eight times without success. He was beginning to become desperate and to apply for posts which his consultant thought were quite unsuitable. At this point, he was shortlisted for a consultant post by a selection committee which contained two doctors with whom he had previously worked – he had collaborated with one of them on a scientific paper. Through these contacts he found out how the committee had discussed his application. It emerged that the superintendent of the hospital flatly refused to appoint him, saying that the matron would not work with an Asian consultant. No appointment was made. Someone who heard about this case offered Dr. Vengat a locum job as consultant at his present hospital; he was later appointed a substantive consultant.

Dr. Vengat said that if he had had difficulties in finding a job as consultant in spite of the fact that 'my training had been first class, I had done all the very top jobs and had done research', then other overseas doctors with lesser qualifications and experience must have had still greater difficulties. Although the period of his greatest difficulties was ten years ago, he thinks that 'in some ways it is more difficult now'.[13]

The PSI survey found that **about half the overseas doctors interviewed felt they were likely to receive unequal treatment from selection committees because committee members wrongly put a lower value on the qualifications of overseas doctors, or**

167

believed they were less competent to practice in the UK. Although the majority of those doctors who regarded unequal treatment as inevitable did not interpret it as evidence of racial discrimination, the survey points out:

Under the law, a systematic tendency to undervalue overseas qualifications or the competence of overseas doctors might well amount to racial or ethnic discrimination, but overseas doctors are not knowledgeable about the law, and this is not the category of thought which they spontaneously apply in this context. They may also hesitate to commit themselves (when talking to a white British interviewer) to judgement which roundly condemns others and is humiliating to themselves.[14]

11.4 Caught in the middle – the status of ethnic minority staff

Ethnic minority staff often feel caught in the middle of a situation which is not of their making. **Many feel that they are undervalued, and sometimes exploited, because of the way services are organised in the NHS.** This in turn leads to contradictions in their relationship with other staff, and with patients, that tend to create further frustration and resentment.

On one hand, there is no doubt that the participation of sympathetic ethnic minority staff from the local community is of enormous benefit in the effective delivery of health care to that community.

- They are likely to understand the social and cultural conventions of the community and have a good sense of the most appropriate approach in questions of health care.

- Individuals and families are likely to be far more receptive to health care and advice given by someone from their own community whom they trust and respect, and with whom they can communicate properly.

- Other colleagues working with patients from ethnic minority communities can gain valuable understanding and practical expertise by drawing on the insight and experience of health workers from those communities.

But set against this is a lack of recognition, both at an organisational level and among other colleagues, of the potential value of ethnic minority staff. In addition, black health workers often have to cope with the prejudices of other staff and patients towards black communities; some of this prejudice is inevitably directed at them personally.

White professionals who train, supervise or work with ethnic minority colleagues need to be aware of some of the difficult contradictions they face working within the NHS.

Professional blacks are treated as rare specimens by most of their white colleagues. I am no exception. Generally speaking, racist humour is used to make simple conversation and reactions to these generally leaves us, the black individuals, feeling guilty that we have challenged them. It is a continuous process that those blacks like myself, who have moved up (in a manner of speaking) in society, have very often to contend with the labels that not only do we carry 'chips on our shoulders', but we are over-sensitive to racial issues. No one cares if after a hard day's graft the extent of my social pleasures are limited simply because blacks are not allowed; no one cares if I am a professional when I go to the shops and a white employee has no desire to serve me; no one cares if as a black professional, I wish to buy a house in a particular area of the city, when the estate agents would suggest alternatives; and no one cares when as a black professional I question the educational output that is being given to my children and to many of the young people I work with. To white society all that is irrelevant for if I have made it then everyone else can. It confirms their belief that racism is a figment of our imagination and that the benevolence of white society, indeed of British society, is so bountiful that no one should feel they are disadvantaged. To most professional colleagues, the question of colour and discrimination is a theoretical base and is expressed in the fact that society is constructed in a number of classes. It is very difficult for them to imagine that my colour and those of many black, capable individuals, is used as a weapon against us. The fact that we communicate in a common language and that we share loves for the theatre and for other middle-class orientated values, automatically gives them every right to eliminate colour in any discussion.

Black British man[15]

Relationships with colleagues

The expectations and attitudes of other staff towards ethnic minority colleagues tend to be contradictory.

- Ethnic minority staff (and particularly overseas doctors) are often **regarded by colleagues as less competent and less qualified even though there is no objective evidence to support or refute this belief.**

- Some ethnic minority staff are frequently called upon to act as **interpreters** for patients who do not speak English. In doing so **they provide a skill and a service that other colleagues cannot**, but in many cases **they are expected to do this on a voluntary basis and in addition to their normal workload.**

- Paradoxically, it is regarded as **unethical for ethnic minority staff to spend too much time with patients from their own ethnic group**, despite the fact that they may be the only members of staff who can communicate with such patients. Other staff tend to discount the fact that on a hospital ward, for example, **minority patients (particularly non-English-speakers) are often ignored and isolated, and need this kind of support** from staff who *can* communicate with them.

- At the same time, **it is not desirable that ethnic minority staff should always be identified with, or work solely with, patients from their own community if they do not wish to**. There are several projects in existence where ethnic minority workers have been appointed with special responsibility for a particular minority community in order to redress inequalities in the delivery of care. One such worker pointed out the difficulties in this role.

It is not so much the principle as the inevitable reaction of other colleagues if you have particular responsibility for a minority community. The danger is that you either come to be regarded with suspicion as a second-class health worker providing a service for a second-class community . . . or else you find that every problem relating to patients from that community is automatically referred to you, whether it's necessary or not. Some of my colleagues don't really believe there is a need to redress inequalities . . . they think ethnic minority patients are getting special treatment, and that's reflected in their attitude towards me.

Asian community health worker

Relationships with patients

Ethnic minority health workers sometimes face difficulties that other health staff do not in their relationship with patients:

- **Black staff inevitably encounter racial prejudice from some white patients.** Because ethnic minority staff are found in the lower grades, this means that in some areas a higher proportion of staff who come in direct contact with patients are likely to be black. Racially prejudiced patients inevitably notice this, and it is the black health workers who bear the brunt of their prejudice. Although this situation is the direct result of health service recruitment and training policies, **there is sometimes little support from managerial or senior nursing and medical staff for black staff in dealing with prejudiced patients.**

- Ethnic minority staff from the local community may be **under pressure** from patients in their own community who expect them to provide more help than they are able to. **If patients know a health worker as a friend or neighbour, they may feel he or she should represent them in contact with other health workers.** They may find it difficult to accept that the health worker's position within the health service hierarchy makes this impossible and would damage relationships with other staff.

- For various reasons ethnic minority staff may **resent being continually identified with patients** from the same ethnic group. For example, **the professional health worker may come from a completely different background and have nothing in common with patients from the local community:**

They're both 'European', but your average English consultant doesn't identify very closely with a farmer's wife from rural southern Italy . . . and yet the English consultant doesn't understand why his 'Asian' registrar can't communicate with his 'Asian' patient. He could be a Hindu doctor from south India and she could be a Muslim woman from the rural Punjab . . . they've got nothing in common, not even language.

Senior registrar

- In addition **ethnic minority health workers are of course aware of the generally low social status of ethnic minority communities in Britain.** Some may understandably wish to distance themselves from a patient group that is obviously held in low regard by some of their colleagues.

Coping with pressures

Individual staff cope with these pressures in different ways, but their reactions are often misunderstood by other health workers.

You can handle it in several ways. Some people feel that if you want colleagues to treat you as an equal you have to maintain a greater professional distance from patients than white staff do. You can't afford to become identified with patients from your own community because it undermines your own status. It's not in your interest to volunteer information to colleagues when it only confirms their view that you are different from them, so you just keep quiet if people ask about religion or diet or whatever. The reaction when you do try to explain is so often 'Ooh, how odd you are' and then you just feel a fool.

Asian nurse learner

If you try to question the assumptions of other colleagues or try to present an alternative viewpoint, people don't want to know, and if you ask too many questions you're regarded as a troublemaker, so a lot of nurses just keep their heads down and keep it bottled up inside.

Afro-Caribbean staff nurse

11.5 *Health Service policies and practices: practical action*

Policy and practice in many organisations are based on the assumption that equal opportunities already exist, and that there is no discrimination. However, research studies[16] have shown that policies and practices based on this assumption often work to the disadvantage of different racial and cultural groups, and are therefore discriminatory in effect.

In this chapter we have discussed some aspects of NHS policy and practice that affect the recruitment, training and job levels of ethnic minority health staff. There is clearly a need for Regional and District Health Authorities, examining bodies such as the United Kingdom Central Council for Nursing, Midwifery and Health Visiting and professional associations such as the British Medical Association to examine certain policy issues in more detail.

Policies and practices: points to check

- Are **greater demands placed on ethnic minority staff than on other staff doing the same job** (because of their interpreting skills, for example)? Is this recognised in bonus pay or time off in lieu, etc.?
- Are ethnic minority staff **over-represented on certain shifts?** If so, why?
- Are ethnic minority staff **under-represented in certain grades**, and if so what are the reasons?
- Are ethnic minority staff **over-represented in certain specialties?** If so, are there justifiable reasons?

- Are ethnic minority staff **encouraged to apply for jobs in areas for which they are particularly qualified** because of their background, experience, first language, knowledge of a particular community, etc.?
- Are ethnic minority staff **under-represented in selection for training programmes**, promotion, etc.?
- Do ethnic minority staff receive **consideration of their particular needs?** For example do catering facilities make provision for different **dietary patterns?** Do **holiday arrangements** allow for extended leave at reasonable intervals (e.g. every three years) so that staff can return home?
- Do **staff involved in interviewing and job evaluation receive proper training to avoid cultural bias** in interviewing and selection procedures?

Policies and practices which result in ethnic minority employees receiving less favourable treatment, intentionally or unintentionally, direct or indirectly, constitute unlawful discrimination within the terms of the 1976 Race Relations Act. In general the health services have been slower than other statutory bodies (e.g. Education Departments, Social Services, Housing Departments) in recognising the need to tackle the inequalities created by past discrimination and disadvantage.

A growing number of local authorities have adopted an **equal opportunity policy** as a useful framework for examining current policies and practices and are committed to making charges where necessary.

Although a number of Health Authorities describe themselves as Equal Opportunity Employers, only one, Liverpool Area Health Authority, had taken steps before re-organisation to monitor existing policies with a view to taking positive action.

Equal Opportunities Policy: what does it mean?

An Equal Opportunities Policy does not mean reverse discrimination in favour of black people. It represents a commitment by an organisation to ensure that its policies and practices do not result in any individual receiving less favourable treatment on grounds of sex, marital status, religious belief, disability, race, colour, or ethnic or national origins. **An effective Equal Opportunities Policy benefits *all* employees by establishing a fairer system for recruitment, training, work allocation, promotion opportunities, etc. and will ensure that *no* employee is disadvantaged by conditions or requirements that are not justified.** This is the principle; the practical implementation of this kind of policy change needs care and planning, and some of the details are discussed below.

Employment and delivery of services

An Equal Opportunities Policy is meant to apply not only to employees but to all individuals for whom the organisation provides a service. Within a District Health Authority this means looking at and analysing:

- **how jobs and promotion are offered**
- **to whom services are provided**
- **what facilities are made available**
- **how resources are allocated**
- **how training is organised.**

To be really effective an Equal Opportunities Policy needs to contain certain key elements:

- **a policy statement (see Box, below)**
- **training for all staff**
- **positive action to redress inequalities**
- **monitoring**
- **consultation with ethnic minority employees and trade union representatives at all stages.**

Policy statement

The employing organisation should set out a clear policy statement which can be brought to the attention of employees and users of the service. The statement should include:

- **recognition of past discrimination**
- **a commitment to redress inequalities**
- **a commitment to positive action.**

A sample policy statement

THE CITY AND EAST LONDON AREA HEALTH AUTHORITY (TEACHING) EQUAL OPPORTUNITY POLICY

1. *The City and East London Area Health Authority (Teaching) is an Equal Opportunity employer. No job applicant or employee will receive less favourable treatment on grounds of sex, marital status, religious belief, disability, race, colour, nationality, or ethnic or national origins. Therefore no employee will be disadvantaged by conditions or requirements which cannot be shown to be justified.*

2. *There may be certain posts which under the provisions of the Race Relations Act 1976 and Sex Discrimination Act 1973 will carry a Genuine Occupational Qualification; these will however be few and the need for such a classification will be determined at regular intervals and whenever such a post falls vacant.*

3. *It is acknowledged that it is essential to remain on guard against some of the more subtle and unconscious varieties of discrimination which may not easily be identified and that these may result from general assumptions about the capabilities, characteristics, and interests of minorities which may influence the treatment of individuals or groups.*

4. *Induction courses for new employees shall include a reference to the Authority's policy on equal opportunity.*

5. *Any employee who considers that he or she is suffering from unfair treatment on the grounds of sex, marital status, religious belief, disability, race, colour, nationality, or ethnic or national origins, may raise a complaint through the agreed procedure for dealing with individual grievances.*

6. *This policy will be reviewed by the Area Personnel Officer in the light of changing legislation or guidance from the DHSS, the Equal Opportunities Commission or the Commission for Racial Equality, through the established joint consultative machinery.*

7. *It is recognised that to ensure that this policy is fully effective it will be necessary to introduce personnel procedures that will guard against inadvertent discrimination. In endorsing this policy the AHA(T) authorises its officers to prepare and implement such procedures, subject to appropriate joint consultation.*

Training for all staff

Unless the policy is carefully explained to staff, people may misunderstand the aims, or feel suspicious or threatened by the proposed changes. Training should be provided to explain to all staff the implications of the policy, and how and why procedures will change.

A good training programme would contain the following elements:

- it should be **workplace-based**, preferably looking at casework and examples from within the department whose staff are being trained;
- it should provide information about **the law on direct and indirect discrimination**;

- it should emphasise that staff have a **personal responsibility** to eliminate discriminatory practices;
- it should make clear what **the consequences** will be for individuals who continue to discriminate.

Positive action to redress inequalities

The 1976 Race Relations Act allows training bodies, employers and trade unions to take positive action in various ways to establish equal access and opportunity for disadvantaged racial groups. Below are some examples of what positive action might mean:

- *It allows special measures to meet the special needs of ethnic minorities, for example language training. (Section 35)*
- *It allows special courses for ethnic minorities under-represented in particular jobs. For example a training body can give special courses in areas of social work to ethnic minorities to allow them to qualify for community work. (Section 37)*
- *Employers can give special training where ethnic minorities are under-represented. For example: One company had a number of Asian supervisors with the experience for promotion to posts where Asians were under-represented, but where Asians did not have a knowledge of the specialised language needed to get on the training course. The company organised special language training courses to help the Asians qualify for promotion training. No discrimination was allowed in promotion selection. The Asians were being equipped to go for promotion on a basis of equal opportunities with white colleagues. (Section 38(1)(2))*
- *Trade unions are allowed to give special training where members of ethnic minorities are under-represented and can encourage them to take advantage of opportunities to hold posts. For example a number of unions produce training courses in languages other than English to encourage participation by the ethnic minorities who speak those languages. (Section 38(3), (4) & (5))*
- *The Act allows any of these special measures to be advertised.*[17]

Monitoring

Unless policies and practices are carefully monitored, there is no way of knowing whether discrimination exists, or whether positive action policies to remove discrimination are working.

But monitoring procedures must be agreed in consultation with the relevant trade unions and ethnic minority representatives; if it is not set up as a cooperative exercise, it is likely to create suspicion and resentment about why the information is being collected. This may seriously damage relations with staff and relations between the health authority and local minority communities. These are aspects of the exercise that need to be considered:

- There should be clear agreement between the health authority, trade unions and ethnic minority communities involved about **confidentiality** and who has access to records.
- There should be clear agreement about **the aims of monitoring**, aspects of employment and services to be monitored, and the scope of **positive action** to be taken as a result.
- Employees and service users should be **clearly informed** (for example, by letter or leaflet) about the reasons for monitoring.
- Monitoring should be done on a basis of **self-classification** according to categories which are acceptable to ethnic minority employees and service users.

Consultation

An Equal Opportunities Policy should only be implemented after **discussion and with the agreement of trade unions, and ethnic minority employees and service users.** Consultation should take place at all stages to ensure that policy changes are appropriate to local circumstances and acceptable to the ethnic minority communities involved.

The Commission for Racial Equality has produced a series of information leaflets for employers on Equal Opportunity Policies, Positive Action and Monitoring. These are listed at the end of the chapter.

Individual practice

We discussed earlier in this chapter the kinds of pressures ethnic minority health workers can face in their relationships with colleagues and patients, and the reasons why they may not wish to be singled out because of their ethnic origin, or associated with patients from the same background.

On a personal level, white colleagues who work with ethnic minority health staff have a clear professional responsibility to help change this climate to one in which ethnic minority staff feel their background, experience and insight are recognised and valued by other colleagues, and their contribution seen as an essential and positive element in the effective delivery of health care.

White health professionals in a training or supervisory role have a key part to play in changing the current climate. The checklist below provides suggestions which can be taken up immediately in the day-to-day working situation.

- Look at the organisation of team meetings, case conferences, etc. to find ways in which the **participation** of black staff can be encouraged. For example, consider putting 'multiracial and multicultural aspects of care' on the agenda at all relevant meetings.

- Whenever possible, invite local ethnic minority health staff and community workers, etc. to **speak** at seminars and conferences in order to present a multiracial perspective.

- Take up the interests of black staff and find out whether there are **special needs** for canteen, social or cultural facilities; religious holidays; extended leave arrangements, etc.

- Ensure that ethnic minority health staff are **informed about and encouraged to apply** for training programmes, promotion opportunities, etc.

- Look at areas in which ethnic minority staff may need **support and counselling** in coping with aspects of health care that conflict with their own beliefs and cultural conventions.

- Some black health workers feel reluctant to speak out at meetings or seminars, often because of lack of confidence or experience, or fear of hostility. Consider whether a **working group or support group for ethnic minority workers only** might be appropriate in some circumstances.

- Encourage all staff to accept that **racial and ethnic differences** can be significant in health care and **should be recognised positively rather than ignored**.

- **Seek advice and information** from ethnic minority colleagues wherever appropriate, and encourage other colleagues to do the same.

- **Make it clear to all staff that attitudes or actions based on racial prejudice are unprofessional and unacceptable in the workplace**.

Notes

1. Thomas, M. and Williams, J. M., *Overseas Nurses in Britain: A PEP Survey for the United Kingdom Council for Overseas Student Affairs*, Political and Economic Planning, Broadsheet 359, 1972, p. 6.
2. Walsh, Susan, *Overseas Nurses – Training for a Caring Profession?*, C.H.A.N.N.E.L., 1979. (The Royal College of Nursing's overseas advisory service C.H.A.N.N.E.L. was incorporated into CHAT, a new personal advisory service for all nurses, in 1980.)
3. *Ethnic Minority Hospital Staff*, Commission for Racial Equality, 1983, p. 8–9.
4. Hicks, C., 'Racism in Nursing', *Nursing Times*, 5.5.82 and 12.5.82.
5. Doyal, L., *et al.*, *Migrant Workers in the National Health Service*, Polytechnic of North London, 1982, p. 74.
6. Doyal, L., *et al.*, *Migrant Workers in the National Health Service*, Polytechnic of North London, 1982, p. 75.
7. Walsh, Susan, *Overseas Nurses – Training for a Caring Profession?*, C.H.A.N.N.E.L., 1979, paragraph 12.
8. Walsh, Susan, *Overseas Nurses – Training for a Caring Profession?*, C.H.A.N.N.E.L., 1979, paragraph 28.
9. Walsh, Susan, *Overseas Nurses – Training for a Caring Profession?*, C.H.A.N.N.E.L., 1979, paragraphs 43, 44.
10. Baxter, Carol and Grant, Joan, *Nursing in Manchester: The Black Experience*, Community Health Group for Ethnic Minorities (Manchester), forthcoming.
11. Smith, David J., *Overseas Doctors in the National Health Service*, Policy Studies Institute, 1980.
12. *Doctors from Overseas: A Case for Consultation*, Commission for Racial Equality/Overseas Doctors Association, 1976, p. 11.
13. Smith, David J., *Overseas Doctors in the National Health Service*, Policy Studies Institute, 1980, p. 175–6.

14. Smith, David J., *Overseas Doctors in the National Health Service*, Policy Studies Institute, 1980, p. 172.
15. Husband, C., *'Race' in Britain: Continuity and Change*, Hutchinson, 1982, p. 181.
16. See for example, two studies which look at local authority policies:
    Ouseley, Herman, *et al.*, *The System,* Runnymede Trust and South London Equal Rights Consultancy, 1982.
    Young, Ken and Connelly, Naomi, *Policy and Practice in the Multi-Racial City*, Policy Studies Institute, No. 598, November 1981.
17. *Equal Opportunities – Black and Minority Ethnic Workers; A Pack for Negotiators*, National Union of Public Employees (London Division), 1981, Section 6.

More information

This chapter has discussed equal opportunities policies as a framework for improving the employment position of ethnic minority health staff. The corollary to equal opportunity in employment is of course equal opportunity in access to services. Service provision is discussed throughout the handbook, but the following sections may be particularly useful:

1.5 **Current health care policy**
1.6 **Developing a multiracial approach**
2.5 **Health service policies**
2.6 **Professional practice**
2.7 **Health workers' attitudes and expectations**
2.8 **Practical action**
7.4 **Working with different health beliefs and practices** and especially **Practical action**
8.8 **Foods in hospitals and institutions**

Chapter 10: **Responding to need**
Chapter 12: **Health worker training and professional values**

Further reading

See reading list in Chapter 16:
16.11 **Ethnic minority staff in the National Health Service**

12 Health worker training and professional values

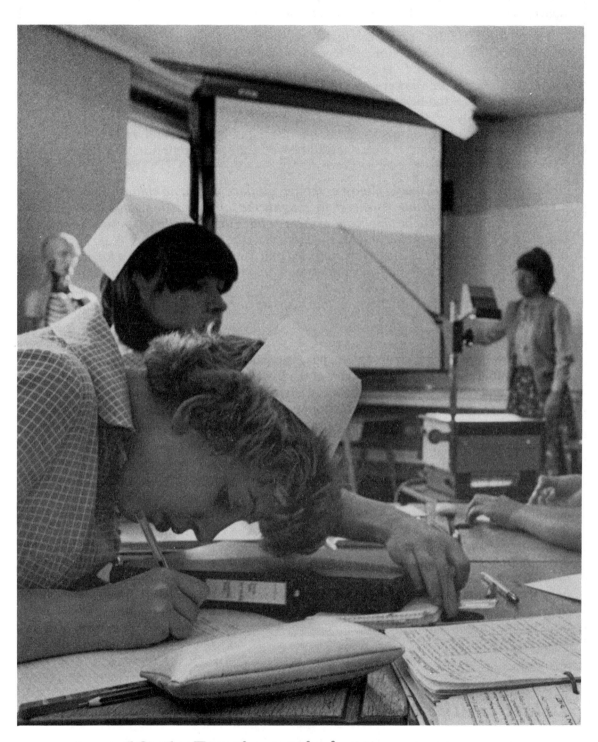

12.1 Basic training
12.2 In-service training for working in a multiracial society
12.3 Professional values

Introduction

This chapter considers how current training programmes may be failing to prepare health professionals adequately to work in multiracial communities. Sections 1 and 2 focus on the basic and in-service training needs of health staff and the final section analyses the culture-specific nature of some current professional values. Throughout the chapter there are practical questions and suggestions which tutors and trainers can use to help them review current training philosophy and develop new, more appropriate courses based on multiracial principles.

The National Health Service is largely responsible for the professional training of its own staff – initially in schools, colleges and on the job – and then continuously through in-service training. **At present most training seems to be based on the expectation that health workers are going to work with patients from a fairly uniform Anglo-Saxon Christian-oriented culture.** Nurses, doctors and other health workers learn about family relationships, diet and nutrition, practical care, admission procedures, interpersonal relationships, bereavement, last rites, and a whole host of other things, in ways which assume certain shared cultural assumptions and patterns of behaviour.

In the classroom we are taught almost as though the patients had no culture; I suppose it's assumed that we and our patients share roughly the same ideas and values and way of life so we don't need to be taught about them or have them mentioned – we'll understand a lot without being taught. But that's not true, and as soon as we go back onto the wards we – or I at least – feel confused and lost because there are a lot of patients whom I don't automatically understand, and whose background and way of life I don't share, and so I feel I can't look after them properly. We seem to get little or nothing in the classroom, for example, that helps us care properly for people from minority groups.

English student nurse

Up to now little more than lip-service has been paid to the idea of training staff to accept the multiracial and plural nature of the British population and to work equally effectively and sensitively with patients and clients from all ethnic groups. If ethnic minorities are mentioned at all during training courses, they are often categorised as a special and separate problem group, like the disabled or the handicapped, outside the scope of 'normal' practice.

When I was training we had an outside speaker who came in to talk about 'Asian patients'. He talked mainly about the difficulties that Asian people cause in hospital: eating different food, showering instead of bathing, wanting their families to visit, causing all kinds of problems. There was also a bit of discussion about how long we would have to put up with all this kind of thing, when we could expect them to be completely westernised. The whole feeling was that Asians were a problem, an unfair drain on us and on the Health Service. Nobody ever said anything about our equal right to health care, the fact that we live here and work here and pay our taxes, and should have rights too, in this society. I just sat in the corner and kept my mouth shut. I was so angry and confused I didn't know what I could say. Anyway, they were all so busy disapproving they wouldn't have listened. That was all we had on Asian patients.

Asian SRN

12.1 Basic training

A recent informal survey of ten schools of nursing in urban areas confirmed that, where the presence of minority groups was acknowledged at all, it was by a token two or three hours. In a two-year training course for community physicians only one hour was devoted to a discussion of ethnic minority health needs.

This token approach is inadequate in many ways:

- **It sends a clear and official message to trainee health workers that minority groups are regarded as marginal, outside and apart from the normal mainstream areas with which health workers can be expected to concern themselves.** Ethnic minority groups are not seen as part of the British population, but as somehow extraneous to it. Provision for ethnic minorities is therefore not one part of the whole package of varied provision necessary for the different groups within society, but something extra, special, and by implication less deserved. Health workers who base their actions on these attitudes cannot provide nor, as managers, plan a fair service for minority groups.

- **It teaches one set of norms and values as though they were universal, and does not prepare trainees to understand or respect others as equally valid.** As a result people in Britain with minority cultures, different religious and ethical beliefs, different conventions about hygiene and modesty, different diets and different family networks, may not be understood or readily accepted by health workers. Lack of understanding may result in a reluctance to accommodate their needs and wishes.

- **It does not give health workers the specific skills or information they need to work effectively with members of minority groups.**

At a practical level

Health workers need to know, for example, about

- different **dietary patterns** and how these may affect provision and dietary advice;
- different **religious beliefs and practices** and their implications for health care;
- how to recognise important **physical symptoms** of, for example, fracture, sprain, jaundice and cyanosis in all racial groups, not just on white skins;
- and how to give **practical care to terminally ill patients** of different religious groups.

During an orthopaedic lecture the nurse tutor said that the signs and symptoms of a fracture were pain, swelling and redness. I commented to her that dark skins would not appear red. The whole class looked at me disapprovingly and the tutor just brushed off my comment as being irrelevant. The only time that ethnic differences were recognised was in a derogatory sense. We were taught that Asians brought TB to this country. Minority groups were also regarded as lacking in hygiene. My attempts at questioning these statements were always met with hostility. I was labelled as racist and eventually just kept quiet about all this.

Afro-Caribbean nurse

Diagnostic skills and skin colour

Recognising overt physical signs and symptoms is an important part of doctors' and nurses' diagnostic skill. Significant changes on brown or black skins may be much more difficult to recognise than those signs which health workers have been trained to recognise on pink skins. Failing to recognise the different physical signs of some conditions may have serious or even fatal consequences. Unless health workers are aware and informed about the possible variation in important physical symptoms, black patients face a real risk of getting less competent and less effective health care.

When my second baby was three days old I noticed that he was slightly jaundiced. I mentioned this to the paediatrician who replied 'I can't tell with you coloured people.' You see I have been a midwife myself and know the dangers of untreated jaundice. So when the jaundice got worse I mentioned it on two more occasions to him and got the same reply. I completely lost trust in all the staff. I just felt that they did not know how to look after me or my baby. After this I would not leave my baby alone, not even to go to the toilet – not even to go to sleep. I would not even let them hold him or give him a drink. I became so frightened and distrustful of them even after years of having worked with these same people. I just felt they were incompetent and that because of them my baby was at risk.

Afro-Caribbean health worker

Most experienced nurses working with patients of different races have learnt to recognise physical changes in different skins: in a case of cyanosis for example, black skin does not go obviously blue but becomes darker and the change may be more difficult to detect. Changes in lip colour are also difficult to detect. If staff are not confident of their ability to detect cyanosis in a black patient through observing obvious physical changes it is most important to check the mucous membrane inside the mouth. Because of the diversity of possible skin colours and of possible signs of, for example, pallor, jaundice or tumours, **training should stress the importance of careful**

observation geared to individual patients. It should emphasise the need to take extra care with darker patients in whom skin colour changes are often far less obvious. It may be necessary, for example, to look for colour changes in lighter areas of skin, such as the conjunctiva, palms and the inside of the mouth in a dark-skinned patient.

Ethnic differences in patterns of illness

There are important variations in patterns of illness among different ethnic groups. These are considered in detail in Chapter 9.

I remember the only times racial variation was mentioned, it was for something negative. We were told for example that 'VD is more common in black people'. Another comment I remember about hyperptylinisation – over-production of mucus in the mouth. We were told 'it mainly affects black people because of poor oral hygiene'. Well I get it and there's nothing wrong with my oral hygiene. Whenever cross-cultural references were made it was always something negative, never positive, and always cast in terms of 'We do this and it's the norm, but they. . . .'

Afro-Caribbean health worker

Reactions to drugs

Dosages of drugs tested and found to be effective on white patients are almost always used as the norm for prescribing practice, and are treated as universally applicable. In fact, people of different racial groups may react very differently to certain drugs and dosages.[1] Some drugs may, for example, be more effective or have fewer side effects with some racial groups than with others. Health workers, and in this case particularly doctors and pharmacists, must be informed about such variations in order to give equally effective health care to all groups in society.

At a conceptual level

Health workers need to consider, for example,

- different **family and support systems** and their implications for health workers;
- different possible **expectations and use of health services;** expectations of maternity care;
- issues such as the **nature of culture, cultural adaptation and maintenance**;
- the implications of health work in a multiracial society;
- the **position and experience of minority groups** in this society and their likely implications for health and for health care needs.

In order to avoid the implication that minority groups are marginal or abnormal, these issues mus⸴ be built in as an integral part of the curriculum, not tagged on at the end as a special subject. For example, discussion of nutrition and diet should routinely cover the dietary habits of all groups, minority as well as majority. It should recognise the validity of the different dietary traditions now represented in Britain. Unless their training explicitly recognises the plural and multiracial nature of British society, health workers are unlikely to recognise and accept it in their own practice.

The usual approach to basic training ignores the existence of racial prejudice and racial disadvantage which crucially affect the health status and needs of minority groups.

In ignoring them it may also imply that they are irrelevant and can even appear to condone them. White trainees, in particular, need to examine the roots and effects of racism in Britain and the existence of personal and institutional racism inside the NHS as well as in wider society. They need to become aware of how racism and deprivation affect the health status and the lives of people in minority groups.

Minority group patients and clients cannot be separated from the physical and social environment in which they live; they are not blank sheets when they come through the clinic or hospital door. If they have had bad experiences of health workers or of other white people and institutions, this is bound to affect their attitudes towards and expectations of health workers and health service provision.

Growing up in a society where white is the norm, and white is good, and where white people hold the power to enforce this system of values through all institutions, reinforced by the media, and even through language, nurses must begin to understand how this has affected them as individuals.[2]

180

In a society which is institutionally racist, policy decisions and their implementation can have no neutrality. They will either perpetuate racism or counter it. Most people in the caring professions are concerned, by the very nature of having chosen the field of work, to adopt practices which do not serve to reinforce racism. However the emotive nature of the subject has meant that white people have been reticent to openly and honestly discuss the issues. [3]

When I am working with a group of health workers of different races I ask them to talk about how they feel about themselves and about their colour. The black nurses always talk about how they have had to deal with racism in their personal and professional lives, how it feels to be a black person in this society, the pressures and the negative attitudes they face, the amount of hurt they experience. They also talk about how good they feel about the strength and mutual caring of black people, that when they meet other black people, they feel a kinship, a sharing of experience, if you like a kind of bond because of what they have all been through. And when I ask the white nurses 'And how does it feel to be white?' there's often just silence. They often have never thought specifically about being white, it's so normal they've never thought about it except in relation to their black patients, and it isn't of any particular significance to them.

Trainer

Questions to think about

Does basic professional training in your District prepare trainees to work with a multiracial population?

You may like to consider the following points:

- Does the training generally assume a universal white norm (often unstated), or **are white values and ways clearly presented as one of many possible and equally valid options** that exist in British society?

- Is the multiracial nature of British society **built into the content of the whole course** or are ethnic minority issues limited to a few sessions, often at the end?

- Are trainees given the **practical knowledge** they need to work effectively in a multiracial society?

- Are **social and economic factors** given as much consideration as cultural factors in assessing the needs and health status of different groups?

- In what contexts are ethnic minority groups mentioned in training? What **general attitude** is conveyed towards ethnic minorities and their needs? Positive? negative? open? grudging? respectful? derogatory?

- **The implications of 'equal treatment for all' are not the same in a plural and multiracial society as they are for a monocultural population.** Are these implications discussed in training? Are the needs and wishes of minority groups considered as valid as those of the white majority?.

- What **sources of information** do trainers and tutors use to find out about the characteristics and needs of ehtnic minority communities? How **reliable** are they? How do trainers and tutors try to ensure that their sources are as **accurate** as possible?

- Are **negative and prejudiced comments** about black people or ethnic minority groups **challenged** or allowed to pass in training sessions and elsewhere?

- Are issues of **racial prejudice, racial discrimination and negative attitudes and behaviour** towards minority groups and their cultures **discussed openly** in training?

- Are the **views and experiences of ethnic minority trainees listened to with respect**, and taken into account? What **support** are they given?

- What steps can be taken to make **all basic health worker training more appropriate** to the needs of a multiracial society?

We found in our research that there was a real resistance to discussing these issues, to talking about colour, about black people. There was a tradition of often very well intentioned and polite colour-blindness among white people which tended to filter out any discussion of race and which generally led to inaction. There was a feeling that talking about race and issues surrounding race, even to black people, or perhaps

181

especially to black people, was embarrassing and offensive. Pointing out to black people that they were black and that you'd noticed it was impolite. Now why would it be impolite to point it out if white people didn't in fact feel that it is slightly shameful to be black? And that's the root of it. It seems that even well intentioned colour-blindness hides somewhere a deeply held prejudice about black people, a racial prejudice.

White race relations researcher

12.2 *In-service training for working in a multiracial society*

Few health workers have been prepared by their basic training specifically to work in a multiracial society. There is therefore an urgent need to provide them with opportunities in the form of in-service training to discuss the crucial issues outlined above and to fill in important gaps in information and understanding.

Like basic training, in-service training cannot and should not aim to fill in a whole series of information gaps, nor to teach people a series of facts about all the different minority groups in the area in which they work. **Its aim is to bring people to a level of understanding, sensitivity, and awareness from which they can go on to develop and learn for themselves.**

Working in a multiracial society: some aims and objectives of in-service training

- to enable trainees to **understand and accept the multicultural and multiracial nature of our society** and to work effectively within it.

- to give trainees **practical information** that will enable them to do a better job.

- to **relate information to trainees' real needs and problems** as health workers in different disciplines.

- to provide a **structured opportunity** for trainees to think through and discuss the implications of working with patients from different ethnic groups, and of providing equal and appropriate care to all sections of the population.

- to enable trainees to **question and rethink their existing expectations and assumptions, views, and conclusions** about ethnic minority patients.

- to enable trainees to **understand their own culture-based values and assumptions** and how these affect their understanding of people from other cultures and groups.

- to enable trainees to **see and accept differences and similarities** in culture, lifestyle, background and experience, and to work with ethnic minority patients **in a more informed and positive way.**

- to **prevent stereotyping and generalising** about ethnic minority groups, and to enable trainees to see and work with ethnic minority patients as **individuals**.

- to **counteract**, and to enable trainees to counteract, **racist myths, stereotypes, propaganda; to identify and correct misinformation** picked up from the press, through the grapevine, etc.

- to **make trainees aware of how personal, institutional and societal racism operate**, and how they affect ethnic minority patients and their families[4].

It is often very difficult to step back and look at one's own cultural and ethnic background. This may be particularly difficult if an individual has always been part of the majority culture in the area and thus hasn't had to consider personal beliefs as only one of a number of acceptable alternatives or to develop a racial and ethnic identity. . . .

If health workers will take the time to examine their own attitudes, beliefs and practices concerning health, illness and medical care, as well as exploring those of the cultural groups with whom they are working, they will understand much more clearly the basic areas in which conflicts and disagreements lie. They will then be in a better position to begin an examination of which personal beliefs and attitudes are simply 'cultural baggage', and not useful or desirable within the local situation.[5]

Possible topics for inclusion in training courses

Topic areas can be used as starting points for assessing trainees' level of knowledge and awareness, filling in some basic essential facts, getting trainees to examine their own attitudes and assumptions, and discussing possible differences and their implications for health worker practice.

Below is a list of suggested topic areas:

The local picture	e.g. local ethnic minority communities; patterns of settlement related to employment, housing etc.; local information.
Migration and health	e.g. immigration: history and causes; legislation; cases; effects of laws and administration on families in Britain; contribution of immigration debate towards picture of black people as a 'problem'; the experience of migration and effects on health; environmental and social pressures for migrant families.
Racial inequalities in health	e.g. socio-medical disadvantage; unequal access to health care; indirect discrimination in the structure of health care institutions; racism within the health service.
Names	e.g. keeping records efficiently; addressing people correctly; recognising other things from names.
Religions	e.g. the main beliefs and practices of Hinduism, Sikhism, Islam, Judaism, Rastafarianism, etc. as relevant; their practical implications for health workers.
The family	e.g. family values; minority group families in Britain; concepts of responsibility, individuality and joint effort; male and female roles; expectations of children, the elderly, the sick.
Food and diets	e.g. religious restrictions on diet and their implications; traditional diets of various ethnic groups; providing or advising on food in hospital; giving effective dietary advice.
Health care	e.g. possible experiences of health care; ante-natal and maternity care; expectations, fears and worries; suggestions about effective practice.
Language and communication	e.g. languages spoken locally; awareness of the effects of speaking little English; ideas on improving communication despite language difficulties; using an interpreter well.[6]

Setting up in-service training

There are many possible models of such in-service training courses and a good deal of debate about which model is most effective. Here are some of the current areas of debate:

- How far should such courses focus on the practical concerns of health workers?
- If the central issue is racial prejudice and discrimination, must this be tackled before attention is given to more practical health-related issues?
- Who should run in-service training courses?
- Who should receive training and how?
- How long should courses be?
- How effective is training for junior health workers, when it is generally senior health workers and administrators who decide the ethos and policy of an institution?
- How can senior health workers and administrators be reached by training?
- Can training without the accompaniment of appropriate policy changes and clear support from above achieve anything?

Here is one trainer's approach to the in-service training of nurses:

In order to train nurses to cope with diverse patterns of behaviour and cultural assumptions they have to be given a basis of information about possible differences and variations.

183

At a very practical level they need facts to fill in the gaps in their knowledge: they know which of the foods that occur commonly in the British diet contain iron; they need to know what foods that a vegetarian Hindu woman is likely to eat contain a significant amount of iron, then they can discuss usefully with her what she eats and discuss whether she could increase her intake of certain iron-containing foods. They know a married British woman may be very reluctant to remove her wedding ring. To cater for this they usually arrange to tape it before an operation: if they can't they know that it may be important to explain why and to assure the woman that her ring will be kept safe and will be put back on her finger again as soon as possible. They need to know whether any of the religious minority groups are likely to feel equally strongly about other jewellery or items of clothing, and what to do. Then they know to check with patients and can avoid removing any item that the patient feels strongly about, and if it must be removed they can discuss sympathetically with the patient what it would be best to do before operations, etc. They know that many British women wish to have their husbands with them when they are in labour. They need to know that in some groups women may prefer a mother or a female relative. Then they can discuss with any woman whom she would like to have with her and make the companion welcome accordingly.

All along it is not a question of stating definite differences, but of sketching possibilities and discussing the implications of possible differences for health care to be sensitive and practical.

This kind of information is not however an end in itself. There are too many ethnic minority communities in Britain for nurses to be fully informed about the culture and way of life of each. And any generalisations are of course inadequate. Also ethnic minority communities are changing and adapting all the time; a young person born and brought up in Britain is likely to have different values and beliefs from his or her parents who came to Britain as adults. Religious beliefs and practices will be more important to some people than to others. Traditional ways may be more important to some than to others.

The giving of information has therefore a greater and far more important aim than the mere transferring of facts, however sensitively done. Information about other cultures is a tool by which people may come to a general acceptance of difference.

Most people grow up believing that the ways they know and understand are right and best. 'A good mother is the same all over the world, a family is a family is a family . . .' and we all know what a family should be like. But that isn't true. What makes a good mother, or a good husband, or a good marriage, or a good family, varies from culture to culture. This is a difficult lesson to learn, particularly in such emotional areas. But nurses need to accept that Britain today is a multiracial society, which means a society in which many cultures and systems of belief co-exist, and will continue to co-exist as separate parallel systems. To provide proper care for everyone in Britain, different beliefs and ways of life and values must all be catered for in their own right. If nursing and medicine provide health care in a way that is only appropriate to people of the majority culture, they cut other groups off from a vital resource to which they have every right.

This is a difficult lesson to learn and a very much more difficult lesson for nurses to act on. Nurses are, as part of their job, continually having to assess people's needs, abilities, state of mind, need for support and help, etc. In a multicultural society they need to be able to suspend many of their own automatic culture-based criteria and apply the criteria of the particular person in front of them. In order to do that a nurse needs first of all a real understanding of what culture is and what it means to herself and to her patient or client. She needs to be able to put herself very sensitively in someone else's shoes. She needs to accept other people's ways of being and of doing things as equally valuable, equally right and equally worthy of respect – and for anyone, from whatever culture, that is a difficult lesson fully to take on board.

In practical terms, I find that the best way to do it seems to be to learn a good deal about one particular ethnic minority group. About practical things, about values and beliefs – and to get inside the internal logic of a completely different culture. To do this one has also to examine and identify a lot of features of one's own culture. And this is part of the learning process. By becoming aware that one has a culture oneself, and by identifying some of its rules and norms (most of which as part of a majority one has never had to identify but has always taken for granted as right and normal and universal) and comparing them with other rules and norms which other people hold equally valuable and normal, one begins to be able to step away from one's own culture a little and to identify it as one system, but only one of many. True, it is the system to which one is vitally and irrevocably attached, but that does not make it in any way superior to others, only different and probably personally preferable.

In effect this training process is about unlearning what is sometimes called 'cultural racism' – in other words unlearning a set of unconscious assumptions we grow up with that our way, the Western way, the white way, is the best way of doing things. If I personally choose to live in a certain way, that is fine – but if I then treat people from other cultures who live differently as though they are backward, or inferior because of that difference – that is a kind of racism.

Current research in Britain and the United States seems to show that a training approach that contains many and varied elements is most effective:

- **Each trainee brings different perceptions and experiences to a training session, and each trainee responds to different material and methods.**

- **To be most effective training courses should contain a mixture of information, discussion, role play and other informational and experiential techniques.**

- **The content must be related to what the trainees have said they want to find out about and wish to use.**

- **It must come from a source credible to the trainees.**

- **Trainees' attitudes and long-term behaviour are most likely to change when there is clear commitment to an improved service from senior management.**[7]

If the current attitudes in our hospitals are all that we wish them to be, then the more student nurses are exposed to them, the quicker they will adapt themselves. If they are not then we are in great difficulty; we can expose the students to what are held to be desirable attitudes outside the hospital . . . but when they meet the 'real' nursing staff, the people actually doing the nursing, they will experience great conflict, and on balance are likely to change to conform to the values of those with whom they are now working.[8]

Questions to think about

If the basic training of health workers practising in inner city areas has not equipped them to work with a multiracial population, then special in-service training is needed. Here are some practical questions to consider relating to the current debate about the most appropriate and effective forms of in-service training in this field:

- What will be the overall **aims and objectives** of an in-service training course?

- How will the aims and objectives be **modified** to suit the needs of the people being trained?

- Is it more effective to have a group of trainees **all from one profession** or to have a **multidisciplinary** group?

- If important emotional and personal issues are going to be discussed, what is the **maximum number** of trainees desirable?

- Should all the trainees be of **equal status** in their professional hierarchy? Will differences in hierarchy inhibit more junior staff?

- How much **time** will you need or can you arrange to have?

- Will your trainees be of **different racial groups?**
  If they will, will you have a closer or different relationship to people of your own racial group than to people of other groups?
  Will you find this difficult?
  What will you do about it?

- How are **minority group trainees** likely to feel during sessions?
  How can you use and support their experience and understanding?
  How can you ensure that they feel able to voice their reactions to what is said and

to intervene if they feel that derogatory or racist things are being said?
How can you **support** them if white trainees are hostile and negative either to them personally or about ethnic minority groups or clients in general?

- How can you **create an atmosphere in which all trainees can voice their feelings**, frustrations, worries, and negative views without fear of disapproval? Prejudices and negative views can only be tackled constructively if they are brought out into the open and can be openly discussed. Otherwise they are likely to remain hidden. Trainees who feel that their views and conclusions are disapproved of or that they cannot ask certain questions that genuinely worry them are likely to become angry and frustrated and to become more hostile towards members of other groups.

- Who will **plan** the course?
How can members of the minority groups concerned be involved in planning and running the course?
How can you ensure that their views are given proper weight and attention?
How will you identify the training needs of trainees?

- How will you decide the **balance between the different strands** of the course?
How much **practical information** will you include?
How much will you include on **issues of cultural pluralism, cultural differences, cultural awareness** etc.?
How much will you include on **socioeconomic factors** affecting the health and experience of minority groups? How much will you include on issues surrounding **racial discrimination and prejudice?**
How will you decide the balance between **different methods** on the course, e.g. formal inputs by yourself and by outside speakers, open discussion, case studies, role play, films, video, etc.?
What kind of **experiential material** can you build into the course to enable trainees to experience and identify with some of the feelings of black people in a predominantly white society?

- What would you consider a **successful** course?
How would you **evaluate** it?
What can you do to ensure that the **benefits of the course are maintained** once people are **back at work?**

- What kind of **follow-up** will there be?

12.3 *Professional values*

Professional values, like any other values, reflect the attitudes and ideology of the society from which they spring. In her book *Transcultural Nursing*, Madeleine Leininger, an American nurse-anthropologist, looks at the health professions as a distinct 'subculture' within American society, and examines some of the values that underpin professional practice in the USA[9]. She suggests that **through professional training, nurses and other health workers acquire a set of attitudes, beliefs and practices which are culture-specific. These 'professional norms' tend to reflect the values of white middle-class and professional society as a whole.** But, suggests Leininger, it is not necessarily good professional practice to expect such norms to be valid for all social groups. Professional values are often applied automatically and unconsciously, but unless they are re-examined, health workers are in danger of imposing their own culture-specific values on patients from minority communities, resulting in inappropriate action and the possibility of wrong decisions.

Below is a discussion, based on Leininger's article, of some of the values that underpin professional practice in Britain:

- **optimal health**
- **equal care**
- **individual care**
- **achieving and doing**
- **cleanliness**

- **time orientation**
- **technology/automation**
- **engineering medicine.**

Optimal health

The role of health professionals is, of course, to help their clients and patients achieve the best possible health for their individual circumstances. **But there is a tendency for health workers to assume, because they are specialists in health care, that the priorities they set out for patients to achieve optimum health are the only right ones and logical ones, and that patients whose priorities conflict with professional advice are not behaving in a rational or logical way.** This is not necessarily true. For example, the Bengali woman quoted in Chapter 2 decided not to attend ante-natal clinic appointments because of the economic costs and the difficulty of arranging childcare. This was not an 'illogical' response. The perceived benefits of attending the ante-natal clinic in the interests of possible future well-being, were outweighed by the constraints of her present circumstances.

People's expectations of 'optimal health' are also influenced by past experience and previous availability of health care. What is considered 'normal' in one society may be considered 'abnormal' in another. For example, a recent study of one Asian community in Britain suggested that some Asian families were used to treating mild attacks of malarial fever at home, and only expected to call in a doctor for the most serious attacks.[10] Health workers should be prepared for the fact that things they see as major disruptions to 'normal' health may not be seen in the same way by all patients.

Equal care

A mother is a mother . . . I treat all my patients exactly the same, regardless of their colour.

Health Visitor

Democratic societies are based, at least in principle, on the ideal of social equality. **It is a basic premise of health care in Britain that in theory patients with similar needs should receive equal care.**

But treating everybody equally is not necessarily the same as treating everybody equally well. Different groups and individuals have different needs and it is generally accepted that a crucial part of good health care involves providing a service tailored to individual needs. Treating a non-ambulant patient as if he could walk is manifestly ridiculous. It is equally ridiculous to treat a patient who doesn't speak English well as though he could, or to ignore the fact that a patient is black and pretend he is white.

Providing the same service to all in the face of differing needs is not an equitable service.[11]

Applying the same criteria to all patients does not necessarily result in an equal distribution of resources or care, **the inverse care law means that disadvantaged groups are likely to require not the same, but more resources than other social groups**, to redress existing inequalities.[12]

Individual care

Western societies place great emphasis on the individual. The individual is seen as the primary social unit in that individual rights and responsibilities take precedence over obligations to the family. **Health care in Western societies is centred on the individual; health education campaigns and other preventive health initiatives are based on the assumption that the individual is responsible for his own health, as opposed to health being a collective responsibility.**

In other cultures, more emphasis may be given to the social reasons underlying a person's illness. **People from ethnic minority communities in Britain may have grown up in a society where the way of life is based on joint effort, where the sick person is seen as part of a wider social group**, and where the whole family, or village, may become involved in the diagnosis and treatment of illness. Health workers may need to re-examine their ideas about **confidentiality** and the **excluding nature of the conventional one-to-one relationship between professional and patient.**[13]

Achieving and doing

Western societies place great value on material achievement through individual effort. The Protestant work ethic and the drive to increase productivity are part of the same emphasis on material wealth. **In the West the poor are often regarded as lazy, incompetent or unproductive, when the real cause is a lack of resources and exploitation. Many health workers are beginning to realise that a way of life that attaches most value to consuming material goods and achieving material status is not necessarily the most healthy.** For example, diet and urban living in industrialised societies tend to produce a higher level of heart disease and stress-related illnesses than village life in Third World countries.

Cleanliness

Hygiene and cleanliness are of course essential in maintaining health. But **many health workers find it difficult to accept that people from other cultures may follow principles of hygiene and cleanliness which are different, but equally valid.** For example, in some cultures the English are considered dirty because they immerse the body in bath water and then sit in their own dirt for half an hour; the practice of washing dishes in a bowl of water that is already polluted from washing earlier dishes, without rinsing off either the water or the detergent, is considered very unhygienic in cultures where dishes are always washed under running water.

Nevertheless, both the media and health professionals often consider 'poor' working-class people and 'foreigners' as 'dirty'. **Dirt may be seen as the prime cause of disease, while other causes such as overcrowding and low levels of nutrition, the results of poverty, are overlooked.** For example, it has only relatively recently been acknowledged that there is no necessary connection between lice and dirt. The most scrupulous personal hygiene cannot eradicate lice, if, for example, a child is in contact with other children carrying lice at school. In fact, lice stand a better chance of survival on a clean head than a dirty one.

Health workers may need to re-examine their beliefs about cleanliness and dirt, and consider whether the prevailing white middle-class ideas about cleanliness are in fact as hygienic as they might be.

Time orientation

Western society is obsessed with punctuality.

Malaysian nurse

The Western obsession with timekeeping and punctuality is reflected in the spread during the 1970s of the **appointment system** in general practice, and in the frustration felt by medical, nursing and clerical staff when patients fail to keep their appointments, arrive late or turn up on the wrong day. In theory the appointment system is intended to make access to treatment quicker and easier for patients. In practice patients' experience of the appointment system may give them the opposite impression. **It is not surprising to find that patients who have grown up in a village society where bureaucratic administration, timekeeping and appointment systems are not a part of normal life, see little purpose or sense in the way the appointment system operates in reality.**

Technology and automation

The importance of technology and automation in industrial production is reflected in an increasing emphasis on technology and automation in health care in Western countries. Large sums of money are invested in high-cost 'technological' medicine (for example, heart transplant units), often at the expense of preventive health care in the community, even though many argue that high-cost curative medicine is less cost-effective in the long term than measures to maintain health and prevent illness in the first place. **In Third World countries such as Bangladesh, China, Mozambique and Vietnam, the emphasis is on developing a comprehensive system of low-cost, community-based, preventive health care for the whole population, rather than on** curative technology which can only help a limited number of people. **Many health professionals now believe that there should be a similar shift of emphasis in British health care.**

'Engineering' medicine

The current Western model of health care concentrates very much on physical symptoms and problems; medicine is based on an **'engineering' approach** to the body, where each part or function is dealt with in isolation; the patient and his condition are treated as if he were in some way not part of, and not affected by, the real world and environment in which he lives. There is increasing dissatisfaction with this approach and health workers are moving towards a more **holistic approach** to health care. Nursing is moving in this direction with the adoption of the Nursing Process, which stresses the need to care for the whole patient, not just his physical condition, and to assess the needs of each individual patient in terms of his long-term physical and emotional needs, his environment, his economic circumstances, his family and social life, and so forth.

Building diversity into professional practice

In assessing the health care needs of patients in a multiracial society it is clearly essential to take into account factors that crucially affect individuals such as race and the experience of discrimination, income, housing, and other linked environmental factors, as well as sex, age, religion, etc. Ethnic minority patients may have different needs from white majority patients, both as individuals and as a group. **The effective professional is one who is equipped with knowledge and appreciation of diversity in values and beliefs; who can use this awareness to look critically at her own cultural values, and to assess more objectively the strengths and weaknesses of the existing system of health care.**

Notes

1. Overfield, Teresa, 'Biological Variations: Concepts from Physical Anthropology', in Henderson, G., and Primeaux, M., *Transcultural Health Care*, Addison-Wesley, 1981, pp. 279–86.
2. Homans, Hilary and Satow, Antoinette, 'Integration or isolation?' *Journal of Community Nursing*, Oct. 1981.
3. Homans, Hilary and Satow, Antoinette, 'Fair service for all' *Journal of Community Nursing*, Feb. 1982.
4. *ILT and NHS Awareness Training*, National Centre for Industrial Language Training Working Paper No. 34, 1982.
5. Brownlee, Ann Templeton, *Community Culture and Care: Cross-Cultural Guide for Health Workers*, C. V. Mosby, 1978, pp. 244–5.
6. Adapted from *ILT and NHS Awareness Training*, National Centre for Industrial Language Training, Working Paper No. 34, 1982, p. 6.
7. Shaw, John, 'Training methods in race relations within organisations: an analysis and assessment', *New Community*, Vol. 9, No. 3, 1981.
8. Bendall, E., 'A nursing dilemma', *Nursing Times Occasional Paper*, 1971.
9. Leininger, Madeleine, *Transcultural Nursing: Concepts, Theories and Practices*, Wiley Medical, 1978.
10. Ashton, J. O., *Health Patterns in the Asian Population of the Dewsbury District of Kirklees AHA and Their Implications for Health Education*, Health Education Dept., Leeds University/Leeds Polytechnic, 1978, (dissertation for Diploma in Health Education).
11. Statement from Wandsworth CCR quoted in *Racial Equality and the Health Service*, Camden Committee for Community Relations, 1983.
12. Hart, Julian Tudor, 'The Inverse Care Law', *The Lancet*, 27 February, 1971, p. 412.
13. For an example of the wider relationship between practitioner, patient, and the patient's social group in another culture, see McLean, Una, *Magical Medicine: A Nigerian Case Study*, Penguin, 1977.

More information

Tutors and trainers seeking more detailed information about specific aspects of health care may find the following chapters particularly useful:

5 **Communication**
6 **Working with families and individuals**
7 **Health beliefs and practices**
8 **Foods and diets**
9 **Patterns of illness**
13 **Health education**
15 **Sources and resources**
16 **Reading list**

Further reading

See Chapter 16: Reading list
16.12 **Health worker training and professional values**

13 Health education

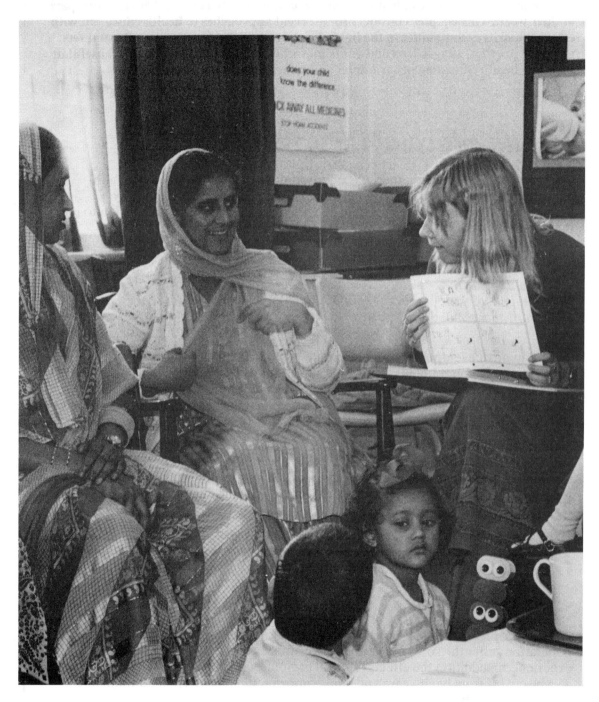

Introduction

Current health education theory emphasises that the overall aim of health education is to enable people to make rational and well informed decisions about habits and practices that may affect their health. It also enables them to begin to take greater and more conscious control over the health care and information they receive, and over some of the external factors which may influence their health. It is increasingly recognised that all health workers are or should be health educators, but many hospital and community staff have only limited opportunities to reflect on and develop this part of their work. This chapter considers some recent approaches to health education with ethnic minority communities in the light of current health education theory, and sets out some practical suggestions and guidelines which health workers may find useful in planning health education programmes and information resources.

13.1 Health education: current thinking

Current health education theory is questioning the traditional idea of health education campaigns and is becoming more orientated towards **community development approaches** which enable communities to define and take action to meet their own needs.

A caricature of an ineffective health education programme would be a campaign devised by health professionals to 'mend the ways' of the public by instructing them to do something that they cannot reasonably or easily do, or even have a positive wish not to do, and do not know why they should. The problem is, there are campaigns like that, or at least, there have been.

Health education officer

Community development programmes require of health educators a good deal of time, effort and commitment. They require sensitivity, willingness to listen and to take direction from non-professionals, willingness to learn and to give up one's authority and the security of one's status, and willingness to give up preconceptions and dearly held beliefs and procedures.[1]

Community-based approaches are also inevitably never as neat and well marshalled as those which can be organised from the top; this may mean that the health educator is put under pressure from those in authority because a community-based programme seems slow to take off, messy, disorganised, split or unproductive.

13.2 Health education and ethnic minority communities

A higher proportion of people in ethnic minority communities than in the majority population suffer the socio-economic disadvantages that adversely affect health, and experience in addition the effects of racial prejudice and discrimination. They may also be cut off from health care and health information by barriers of unfamiliarity, language and culture.

Appropriate health education programmes, while they are not always able to remove some of the more fundamental causes of ill-health, can enable people to make more informed choices about their health and health care, so giving them greater control over their own health and well-being.

But it is essential to ensure that any health education programmes aimed at minority communities are genuinely enabling to members of those communities. There is a real risk that programmes may be based on disapproval, or may aim to eradicate or change a pattern of behaviour because it is different, or outside the majority norm. (See Chapter 4.)

There was a lot of worry when we first began to realise that a lot of the Asians coming here were vegetarian. The feeling was that the sooner we could get them to start eating a British-style diet the better. There was even a feeling that if they started to change their diet it was in some way a sign of good will, you know, that a good immigrant gives up those old ways and learns better ways here. I remember talking to a health visitor who had 'good' Hindu families and 'bad' Hindu families. The 'good' ones gave their children meat and a lot of English foods, the 'bad' ones didn't. At that time health education for Asians often meant trying to get them to wean their babies onto English tins, especially things like chicken dinners.

Health education officer

Community-based nutrition education should not focus on changing people's bad habits. Rather, it should try to recognize and strengthen those food habits and traditions that are healthy.[2]

Minority communities are particularly vulnerable to this kind of approach, because much health education may be planned and given to them by people who do not know very much about their daily lives and choices, or understand the basis of them. It is only too easy to pick out behaviour in an unfamiliar community which does not fit in with a health worker's own expectations, and which is therefore regarded as undesirable or unhealthy.

It is obviously vital to increase awareness of racism within health education units and to be alert and critical of health messages aimed at various ethnic groups. This is particularly important in the case of campaigns for behaviour change where the change may well be in the direction of white middle-class values. It is perhaps necessary to examine carefully the issue of behaviour change when planning any health education activity. Is a change of behaviour necessary or appropriate? It may be more appropriate to provide opportunities for people to take control of their own health decisions.[3]

In addition, in a general climate of racism and hostility, **minority communities may see even the best intentioned programmes aimed at them as derogatory and racist, trying to force them to adopt white majority norms and ways.** This was for example, a major problem with the recent DHSS rickets campaign.

 The main criticism of this campaign was that the government should have opted to fortify foodstuffs used by the Asian community, as it did with the white population during the war (Chapter 9). Critics felt that in the form the campaign eventually took, the resounding message was 'Asian diets are inadequate'. The director of the campaign has repeatedly pointed out that the campaign did not aim to change Asian diets or cultural practices in any way, but rather to inform both health workers and communities about the problems of Vitamin D deficiency and possible solutions.

The aim was, however, consistently misinterpreted by many local health workers as an exhortation to make the Asian communities change their (implicitly inadequate) traditional diets.

The fact that the campaign was so widely misunderstood by those responsible for implementing it locally, and so open to criticism, emphasises the importance of very careful planning and consultation with local communities concerned. It also underlines the need to consider the wider implications of any health education programme aimed only or specifically at ethnic minority groups.

Successful health education programmes

Two successful health education projects concerned with ethnic minority health needs are ante-natal projects: Hackney Women's Health Project and Tower Hamlets Maternity Services Liaison Scheme[4].

Key elements of their success are:

- **Out-reach work**. Going out to make contact with women in the community, rather than waiting for them to come to a health service institution.
- **The involvement of health educators from, and of, the community**.
- **An informal, flexible and equal but supportive relationship between workers and clients**, rather than a formal, less flexible official or professional one.

- **Using word-of-mouth networks** to inform potential clients of the existence of the service and what it can offer.
- Offering women the help, support and information they **request** rather than **imposing** ideas of what they need.
- **Building community support** networks stemming from health-related matters, e.g. ante-natal groups, mother-and-toddler groups.
- Accompanying, supporting and acting as **advocates** for women in their contacts with the health service and health workers.

(See Chapter 10 for a full description of one of these projects.)

Questions to think about

Here is a list of questions to think about when considering health education programmes. It may also be useful in considering one-to-one health education:

- What is the **message** of your health education programme?
- Have you worked out a clearly defined set of programme **objectives** and a clear rationale?
- **How** have you decided upon the programme? **Why** do you think it is needed?
- Have **people from the communities** you are aiming to work with participated in developing the programme? Is it related to the communities' **perceived or proved needs?**
- Does the programme aim to enable people to make **better informed decisions** about their health and health care?
- Does it aim to enable them to **take more control over their own health** and the health care they receive?
- Will it help them to be more **confident in their encounters with the health service** and with health workers?
- Are the changes or solutions you suggest both **necessary** and **possible?** Have you checked this out with members of the community?
- Does your message imply **criticism** of the lifestyle of a particular ethnic group? Or the superiority of the ways of the white majority?
- **How much do you know** about the communities you are aiming to reach, and about their views and priorities? How can you **increase** your knowledge and understanding?
- Is the message of the programmes **acceptable** to the group you are aiming to reach? **Was it developed with and by people from that group?**
- Who is going to take the message to the communities? Can the health educator involved **communicate effectively** with the people you want most to reach?
- Have you considered possible **barriers to communication**, such as language, culture, age, sex, race, personality, attitude, status? How can you minimise or overcome these?
- Have you **tested** the effectiveness of your message and your medium?
- If you are planning to use written back-up material, have you **checked** it for **clarity, legibility, attractiveness?** Are the pictures clear? Will the people you are aiming to reach **identify** with the people and lifestyles illustrated in the material?
- How will you **distribute** any written material or leaflets?
- How will you **evaluate** the relevance and effectiveness of your programme? How can you get feedback on how it was perceived and how useful it was?
- Can you set up a **long-term** dialogue with people from local minority communities so as to learn more about their main health-related concerns?

We thought people needed information about vitamins and things. But when we went to ask people we met, groups at the gurdwara and the mosque, for example, we found that what they really wanted to know was how the health service works, what to do if they're not happy with their doctor, and even how to ask about certain health problems, you know, what the English name was.

Health education officer

A recent phone-in programme in London, in which people could phone in, in confidence, with health queries in Asian languages, found that the health worries mentioned were most frequently asthma, hay fever, and breathlessness (13 per cent of all questions); family planning, fertility, infertility and psycho-sexual problems (11 per cent); diabetes (11 per cent); general nutrition and slimming (not rickets) (8 per cent); and problems relating to mental health (8 per cent). In contrast most current medical literature on the health problems of Asian communities in Britain highlights rickets, tuberculosis and low-birth weight babies[5].

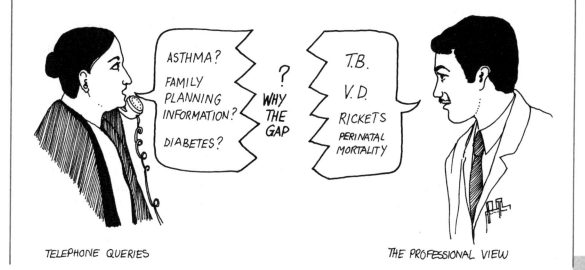

TELEPHONE QUERIES

THE PROFESSIONAL VIEW

13.3 *Written materials*

You may wish to use written or pictorial materials to back up your message. If no suitable materials are available you may need to design your own.

Questions to think about

Here are some questions to think about when choosing or designing suitable health education materials.[6]

- **Content:**
  Does the content reflect the interests and needs of the reader?
  Is it clear and unambiguous?
  Will the reader realise that the material is specifically aimed at his/her community?
  Is the information and advice based on the community's own way of life and habits or on those of the white majority?
  Is the community's culture presented in an accurate and positive way?

- **Readability:**
  Is the reading level suitable?
  Does the text use everyday language and expressions?
  Does it use short simple sentences? Straightforward grammar?

- **Layout:**
  Is the text cramped and confusing, or clear and well spaced?
  Is the information organised so that the sequence of reading is clear?
  Is the text laid out to avoid breaking words between lines?
  Where there are captions, is it clear what they refer to?
  Does the material look attractive? Is it well produced?

- **Illustrations:**
  Are the illustrations clear and simple? Are they of things with which people will be familiar or will recognise easily?
  Do they have a purpose?
  Are they culturally appropriate? Might they cause offence?
  Will your readers identify with the people and things illustrated?
  Are the illustrations realistic? Pictorial conventions (cartoons, speech balloons, perspective, symbols such as ticks, crosses, arrows, etc.) are often assumed to be a way of communicating visually with people who cannot read. In fact they are usually linked to the ability to read, and **people who cannot read may not be familiar with them.**

- **Typeface:**
  Is your typeface as clear and attractive as possible?
  Words or headings written in capitals are more difficult to read than small letters.
  A typeface which is cramped or too widely spaced will make reading more difficult.
  A fancy or unusual typeface will be more confusing than a simple one.
  Black type on white or pale paper is the most legible colour combination.

- If you are using material **produced by other people,** have you checked that it meets all the criteria listed above?

Translated material

- It may be important to produce translated material in order to reach communities whose first language is not English. **In most communities many adults who do not read or write in English will read and write in their own first language. If they do not, they are likely to have friends and relatives who read and write for them.** Clear, well translated health education material can be very effective.

A survey of literacy in 48 Bengalis and 42 Pakistanis attending clinics or community groups in Oldham was carried out, with approximately equal numbers of men and women. Among Bengalis 90 per cent of men and 52 per cent of women could read their mother tongue while the figures for reading English were 41 per cent and none respectively. Among Pakistanis 85 per cent of men and 77 per cent of women could read their own language but only 25 per cent of men and 4 per cent of women could read English. . . .

[The survey] indicates that work done in translating material into Bengali or Urdu is certainly worthwhile. This is particularly so for the women, most of whom cannot read English. Of those who can read both languages the overwhelming majority prefer their own language.

There is a large group of Urdu speakers who can read English 'a bit'. There may therefore be a role for materials written in simple English, in terms of both vocabulary and sentence structure.[7]

- **Do not underestimate the time you will need to get material translated:**
  Jenny Lo, of BBC Television's Continuing Education Department, estimated that getting translations of the booklets *Your Rights to Health* (see Chapter 10) took about three months. As far as possible the BBC used translators who were also community workers and who were aware of the needs and everyday modes of expression of the target group. They also used 'official' translators.

  Initial briefing meetings were held for several translators of each language. When the materials had been translated all the translators for each language met to compare and cross-check their versions against each other's. Disagreements and differences were discussed together and ironed out before a final version was produced.

  If you are starting from an English original, make sure that its meaning is crystal clear and that the language is as simple and straightforward as possible. A complicated or badly worded English text will almost certainly be made worse by translation.

- **An alternative approach is to discuss the main issues with members of a particular community and for them as a group to produce material in their own language.** Health workers who are members of the appropriate minority group may be very useful in ensuring that the health-related content is correct.

- **Many areas now have community printers who can typeset and print materials in different languages and alphabets.** Your local Community Relations Council should be able to give you the names and addresses of local community printers.

- **You will need someone to check the translated material once it is typeset.** A lot of hard work will have been wasted if the writing is upside down or if the wrong captions are under the wrong pictures. Remember that some languages, for example, Arabic and Urdu, are written from right to left, and Arabic and Urdu booklets and leaflets should start from what English people would regard as the back.

- **It is important for health workers to know exactly what any leaflets they give out say:** it may be possible to have the text or a summary of the main points in English on the back of the leaflet; it may be possible to insert a simple English parallel text in the main part of the leaflet (if this does not make the leaflet too crowded); it may be possible to provide each health worker with a complete translation on a separate sheet to keep.

- In all communities there are at least some people who read English. In many communities a large proportion of people read English either as their first language or as a second language. **The most desirable and useful course of action may be to produce identical leaflets both in the community's first language and in English, using the same illustrations, and conveying the same message as simply and clearly as possible in both languages.** The English-language version would meet the needs of English-speaking health workers. It would also provide a culturally appropriate leaflet for those members of the community who read English.

  If there is no translation on the leaflet itself, **don't forget at least to put the title in English somewhere and to say what language it is in.**

Questions to think about

- Do the people translating the content fully understand the aim of the material, the people you are trying to reach and the need for simple everyday language?

- Do you have a good working relationship with the translators? Will they discuss any problems and difficulties with you?

- Is the translation in the appropriate language? For example, some members of the Vietnamese community are completely bilingual and can read both Vietnamese and Chinese, but many read only one or the other. People from Pakistan who speak Punjabi as their mother tongue will generally read and write Urdu, the language of education in Pakistan. Sikhs from India whose mother tongue is Punjabi will generally read and write Punjabi written in the Gurmukhi alphabet.

- If you are using existing translated material, have you checked that it meets all the criteria outlined above?

Notes

1. For a practical introduction to the community development approach, see Henderson, P. and Thomas, D. N., *Skills in Neighbourhood Work*, George Allen and Unwin, 1980.
2. Werner, David and Bower, Bill, *Helping Health Workers Learn*, Hesperian Foundation, 1983, Chapter 25 p. 34.
3. Rossiter, Jane E., *Health Education and Minority Groups*, unpublished paper, Brent Health Education Unit, 1981.
4. For further information about these projects contact:
   Fedelma Winkler
   City and Hackney
   Community Health Council
   210 Kingsland Road
   London E2 8EB

   Liz Smart
   Maternity Services Liaison Scheme
   Montefiore Centre
   Deal Street
   London E1
   Tel. 01-377 8725
5. Webb, Penny, 'Health problems of London's Asians and Afro-Caribbeans', *Health Visitor,* April 1981.
6. Adapted from Mares, Penny, *The Vietnamese in Britain*, Health Education Council/National Extension College, 1982, pp. 143–4.
7. Learmonth, Alyson, 'Asians' Literacy in their mother tongue and English', *Nursing Times*, 28 February, 1980.

More information

For information about rickets and osteomalacia, see 9.5.
For more information about the issues surrounding the rickets campaign, see
'Inadequate culture' in 4.1: Cultural differences.

Communication skills in health education, see
5   **Communication**, especially
5.6 **Practical action: improving communication across a language barrier**

See 8 **Foods and diets**, especially
8.7 **Practical action: giving nutritional advice**

See 10 **Responding to need** for examples of health education initiatives, including a
description of Hackney Women's Health Project described in this chapter.

Health education in family planning, see 'Questions to think about' in 6.4 **Family
planning**

Research health education needs, see
Local needs: guidelines for doing your own research

Organisations concerned with health education and existing materials, see 15 **Sources
and resources**

Further reading

See the reading list in Chapter 16.
16.13 **Health education**

See also relevant publications on specific topics in reading lists for other chapters, e.g.
16.5 **Communication**
16.7 **Health beliefs and practices**
16.8 **Foods and diets**

Part 4: Resources

14 Local needs: guidelines for doing your own research

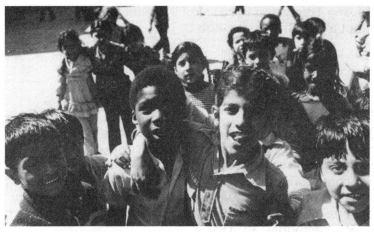
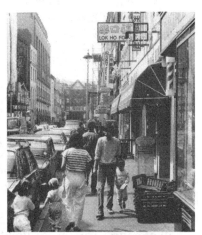
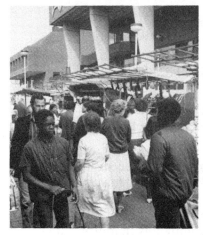
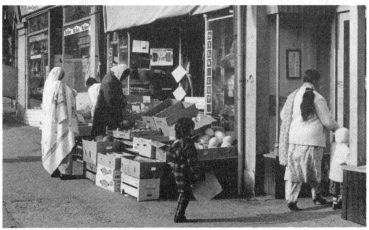

Introduction

This chapter outlines the importance of local research to ensure that health care interventions are effectively geared to the needs of local ethnic minority communities.

Some possible areas for research are suggested, followed by a discussion of methods and techniques for gathering information.

Some of the following sections are based on a summary of the main points in a chapter called 'Methods for Gathering Information' in an American book, *Community Culture and Care* by Ann Templeton Brownlee.[1] This summary has been heavily adapted to make it relevant to the British situation.

14.1 *Why local research is necessary*

The health and health care needs of different ethnic minority groups within the local population are likely to vary, depending on the circumstances surrounding migration and settlement. The subsequent changes in lifestyle, family grouping, patterns of employment, housing conditions, diet, etc. as well as the effects on the population of racial discrimination in housing, education, employment and other areas of life, all have a significant effect on health and health care needs. These needs will of course vary according to local conditions, such as:

- The kind of work people do and the health and safety risks involved.
- Local housing conditions, the size, age and quality of available accommodation, and environmental hazards.
- The presence or absence of community support networks and social focus such as religious centres, social clubs, etc.
- The availability of appropriate health care, which might mean whether the local ante-natal clinic is run by a male GP or a female midwife, and whether there are practitioners of traditional medicine working locally.

Local research is essential if planners and practitioners are to get an accurate and specific picture of local health needs. For example, the background and material circumstances of the Afro-Caribbean community in South London may differ considerably from those of the Afro-Caribbean community in Manchester. Health care interventions that are appropriate in Brixton may be completely inappropriate in Moss Side. Local research is also essential to clarify other factors that health workers need to be sensitive to:

- **Statistical information.** If such data is available it may be very inaccurate, as people are understandably reluctant to answer questions about ethnic origin or skin colour if they don't know why they are being asked. Only someone who knows the area and the local community can assess how accurate or useful the 'official' demographic data is likely to be.

- **Divisions within the local community.** Health workers need to be aware of the differences between, for example, Afro-Caribbean families from different islands in the Caribbean, or between Chinese and Vietnamese families in Vietnam, if they are to respond to individual needs in the same way that they are able to respond sensitively to differences between, for example, a young mother in Surrey and a Yorkshire sheep farmer.

- **Differences in length of settlement.** Needs will obviously vary according to how well established different sections of the local community are. Long-settled communities (for example, the Chinese in Cardiff and Liverpool-born blacks) are more likely to be suffering from the long-term effects of racial discrimination and inequality than from problems of language or unfamiliarity with the health services.

- **History of settlement of the local community.** The extent to which people within the local community identify with each other and are able to support each other in dealing with the common pressures they face, may depend on the circumstances in which settlement originally took place. Some communities, such as the Sikhs, have a long tradition of migration, and people have generally settled in the same town in Britain as other people from their own village or region back home. On the other hand, refugee communities such as the Chileans and Vietnamese were forced to migrate and had little choice in where they settled; some families and individuals may feel they have little in common with each other apart from their forced migration. Such communities may be more fragmented, and the psychological stresses they face may be greater, as a result of this experience.

- **Local networks.** Local research can identify specific community networks through which useful interventions can be made. It may be possible, for example, to identify a trade union branch, a religious centre or an influential group of older women that could be involved in the design and promotion of a particular health education programme.

14.2 *Who should do the research?*

Research can mean anything from informal discussion between a health visitor or community worker and the mothers they work with, to a large scale in-depth questionnaire survey involving a team of professional interviewers whose findings are turned into statistical data by a computer.

Both approaches are useful in different ways. The health visitor's or community worker's personal survey may well be of more immediate, direct and practical value to other health workers and members of the local community than a lengthier professional, highly structured research project which does not involve local people or the health professionals who work with them.

The best people to carry out the research are likely to be those who already have a good understanding of, and rapport with, people in the community, such as a local health worker and/or community member. If this is not possible it may be necessary to find other sources of help, perhaps a health education unit or staff or students from a university or polytechnic department.

It is essential that local health workers and community members retain control over what is to be researched; otherwise the research may lose its practical value.

It is also important that members of the community participate in the design and execution of research to make sure that it accurately reflects the felt needs of people within the community and not just the perceptions of 'outside' professionals.

14.3 *What general approach to take*

- **Look for shared experiences and similarities; don't just concentrate on cultural differences.**

  As we discussed in Chapter 4, focusing only on cultural differences can lead to a catalogue of 'bizarre' practices which probably do not help to develop any real understanding of the lives of people in the community and their health needs.

- **Don't start from the assumption that 'culture' is a problem.**

  The Black Report clearly shows that it is not culture but class disadvantage that is the primary cause of health inequalities. A significant problem, suggests the report, is that health service provision is generally geared to white middle-class cultural patterns and so tends to be less appropriate and relevant to the needs of other social groups.[2] This is the problem that local research should outline and explore.

- **Try to build up a composite picture of different social groups within the community.**

  Be careful of making generalisations and creating stereotypes; research should explore the differences and diversity within the community that are likely to be significant in health care.

- **Give proper consideration to the effects on health of social and economic disadvantage.**

  Research which does not take these factors into account may produce recommendations which are not practicable because the resources and options available to people in the community are limited.

- **Give proper consideration to the effects of racial discrimination and inequality.**

  Racism, as we discussed in Chapter 2, impinges on almost every area of life for black people. Any research to assess the health needs of an ethnic minority community must consider direct and indirect discrimination as a major contributing factor.

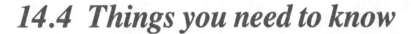

14.4 *Things you need to know*

The following sections contain suggestions about the kind of questions that health workers need to be able to answer if their work with local minority communities is to be effective. Fifteen possible areas of investigation are outlined.

- Migration
- Social and cultural background of the community
- Living conditions
- Local amenities and services
- Communication
- Language
- Family life
- Mothers and babies
- Health beliefs and practices
- Use of the health services
- Patterns of illness
- Care of the dying
- Foods and diets
- Maintaining dietary traditions in Britain
- Food in hospital.

This is by no means a comprehensive list of areas for investigation. We have not, for example, attempted to cover topics such as mental illness and the needs of the elderly. At the same time, individual health workers will obviously find some sections more relevant to their own discipline and areas of interest than others. A health visitor, for example, might decide it is more useful to confine herself to exploring some of the questions in the 'Mothers and babies' section.

The questions in each section are intended only as a starting point, to suggest possible areas for investigation. Some areas are likely to be pertinent to certain communities but irrelevant to others. There may be other more relevant questions that need answering, depending on the local situation. Later sections in this chapter may be helpful in deciding exactly what and how to investigate.

Material conditions

- What kind of housing do most people live in? Privately rented? Council? Owner occupied?
  What specific housing problems are there?
  How do housing conditions affect health?
  What housing improvements would improve health?

- Which industries do members of the community work in? What kind of jobs do they do?
  What are working conditions like?
  How long is the working week?
  How many people work on permanent night shifts?

What are the specific health and safety hazards in the workplace?
How do working conditions affect the state of health of working members of the community?

- What is the level of unemployment in the community? Is any age group particularly affected?

- To what extent does the community suffer from racial disadvantage or discrimination in housing, employment and education?
  How does this affect the state of health of the population?

Migration

- Is the community in question a migrant or settler population?
  Have people settled in Britain for a relatively long period, and perhaps permanently, or do members of the community come and go, dependent on work permits?
  How does this affect people's state of health?

- What were the original reasons for the migration?
  Have those reasons influenced why and where people have settled in the local area?
  Did members of the community choose to migrate or were they forced to?
  What additional pressures face refugee communities such as the Chileans and Vietnamese?

- What effects has migration had on the health of the community?
  For example, in what ways have changes in climate, housing, employment and standard of living affected health?
  Does life in Britain create health problems that members of the community have not previously had to face?
  If so, does this affect use of the health services by the community and/or health education needs?

- Is there a distinct community or are families and individuals geographically scattered and isolated?
  What community networks are there?
  What social facilities?
  What religious centres?
  Are there well developed community networks that could form the basis of, for example, a health education programme?

- What additional health care support, if any, do isolated members of the community need or want?

- Do members of the community originate from rural or urban areas in their own country?
  What additional pressures face people coming from rural areas?
  What additional information and explanation about health and health care in Britain may be necessary for individuals from a rural background?

- Have people experienced significant changes in status through migration that could affect health needs?
  For example, have women in the community had to cope with additional responsibilities or pressures because they have lost the support of other female relatives?
  Because they have left behind husbands or children?

Social and cultural background of the community

- What are the differences in the backgrounds of individuals and families within the community?
  For example, are there differences in ethnic origin? Religious affiliation? Social class? Educational background? Political sympathies?
- How important are these differences to members of the community?
  How are they likely to affect relations between families and individuals?
  Relations between you and different patients?

For example, political groupings within the community could affect the community networks you decide to work through in a health education programme.
Differences in ethnic origin could affect the language(s) you choose for translated information.
Differences in religious beliefs may include different dietary rules which will affect the type of nutrition advice you decide to give to different families within the community.

- To what extent does the religion of the community affect health care? What practical aspects of care may need to be adapted to conform with religious beliefs and practices?
  Are all health workers aware of these implications?

- What is the age structure of the population?
  How has it changed over the last ten years?
  Are new health needs emerging as a result of changes in the age structure?
  For example, are there appropriate daycare facilities, sheltered housing, etc. catering for the needs of the elderly from the minority community?

- How many people in the community are British-born?

- What is the 'normal' family structure within the community?
  What changes have taken place in the traditional family pattern as a result of coming to Britain?

- What differences are there between the health worker's expectations and the traditional pattern of child care?

- What is the traditional role of women?
  What changes have taken place as a result of coming to Britain?

- Who are the individuals with influence in the community, to whom people turn for help or advice?
  What informal word-of-mouth networks exist to gather and disseminate information about health and health care?
  Beware of self-appointed community 'leaders', but look out for individuals whom other people seem to look to for advice and support, the 'opinion-formers'. For example, there may be an older woman in the community whom young mothers consult about children's illnesses.

- What factors influence status within the community?
  What differences are there between the health worker's ideas about status and those within the community?
  How will this affect your relationships with patients?
  For example, the head of the household may expect to be involved in decisions about the patient's treatment. Failure to consult him or her may cause offence, damaging the health worker's relationship with the whole family.

- What is the incidence of racial abuse or harassment in the area?
  How are such incidents dealt with by the local police?
  What community support is there for families and individuals suffering racial harassment?
  How does it affect the mobility of vulnerable members of the community, such as the elderly, the isolated and mothers with young children?
  What effects does it have on the health of the individuals at risk?

- How far do the living conditions and financial means of members of the community affect their ability to follow treatment and advice about health care?
  Are the recommendations they receive practical?

Local amenities and services

- What are the local shopping facilities?
  Who in the family is responsible for buying food, clothing, etc.?

- What local nursery, playgroup and childminding facilities are there?
  Do members of the community know about them?

206

Do they use them?
If not, are there specific reasons that prevent people from using childcare facilities?

- What links are there between the schools and the minority community?
  Is there a multiracial approach to health education in schools?
  Are there any ethnic minority pastoral care staff?

- What social services support is available to the community?
  Does the local social services department employ ethnic minority social workers?
  If not, has the department applied for Section II funding in order to do so?

Communication

- What are the formal and informal channels of communication within the community?
  For example, is there a community newspaper?
  Who is important in the local grapevine?
  Do health education and preventive health programmes make full use of both formal and informal community networks?

- Who are the staff who act as 'gate-keepers', controlling communication between community and other health care staff?
  For example, receptionists and interpreters may have considerable influence in deciding what information does or does not reach medical and nursing staff.
  Are 'gate-keepers' properly trained to work with patients who face communication difficulties?

- Who are the opinion-formers within the community?
  Is it possible to identify members of the community with particular influence among certain groups?
  For example, a male community relations officer may be influential among businessmen in the community, but young women with children are more likely to turn to somebody's aunt for advice.

- What are the barriers (apart from language) that can prevent effective communication between health staff and members of the community? For example, how far do differences in social and economic status, sex, age, class, religion and cultural conventions create barriers between health worker and patient?

Language

- What is the first language spoken within the community?
  What variations are there in the languages or dialects spoken by different groups within the community?
  What percentage of the community speaks English?
  Which groups speak English only slightly or not at all?
  What are the determining factors: age? sex? others?

- How many people are literate in their first language?
  Literate in English?
  Which groups are not literate in either language?
  What are the determining factors?

- What are the languages spoken by health staff who come in contact with members of the community?

- What information is lost because health staff and community members cannot communicate properly with each other?
  What misunderstandings occur?
  What is the attitude of staff towards people who can't communicate well in English?
  How much does an inability to communicate with staff contribute to patients' stress and anxiety?

- What methods are currently used by health workers to communicate with patients who don't speak much English?

None?
Sign language?
Volunteer interpreters?
Paid interpreters?
What other solutions to communication difficulties could be used?

- What information is produced in the first language of the community?
  In written form?
  In the form of audio-cassette or tape–slide presentations?

- Do staff and patients have access to interpreters?
  What training is available to interpreters and health workers who make use of them?
  In what way should health workers change their style of communicating when working through an interpreter?
  How can the health worker ensure feedback from the patient when working through an interpreter?

- What words or concepts are difficult to translate into the first language of the community?
  Does medical terminology present particular problems?

Family life

- What are the similarities and differences between the health worker's ideas about family relations, family size, responsibility and authority within the family, and those of community members?
  In what ways should the health worker adapt professional practice to take account of these differences?

- What variations are there in the type of family group within the community?
  How many people have become separated through migration from other members of their family group?
  How does this affect the support offered by the family group?
  How much has family life been disrupted by immigration restrictions?
  What are the effects of separation on the mental and physical health of family members?

- Which families are related and what obligations are involved in the relationships?

- Is there any hierarchy among families in the community?
  Which families (if any) are most influential?
  Are there any conflicts or alliances between family groups that might affect community health work?

- What roles do father, mother, son, daughter, aunt, grandfather, etc. play in the family group?
  Who is in a position of authority?

- Who generally makes decisions in a typical family in the community?
  Who decides what to do when a family member is ill?
  If the patient is not the decision-maker in the family, to whom should the health worker direct questions, advice and instructions?

- Is illness regarded as an individual or a family matter?
  What actions does a family take when a member becomes ill?

- When one member of a family visits a GP or clinic, what role do other family members expect to play in the process?

- When a member of the family is admitted to hospital, what will be the effect on those left at home?
  What role will relatives expect or wish to play during the stay in hospital?

- What are a family's expectations of medical treatment?
  Should treatment be discussed with other family members apart from the patient?

Mothers and babies

- What differences are there likely to be between a woman's previous experience of childbirth and the procedures and routine in the British hospital where she will have her baby?
  What aspects of delivery and hospital care are likely to need explanation?

- Is every pregnant woman asked who she would like to have with her during labour and delivery?
  Will it be necessary to notify and get the agreement of the maternity unit concerned in some cases?

- Are there any special customs the family wish to observe concerning the birth of the baby?

- What role do other family members expect to play in the birth and care of the baby in the first few weeks?
  Who else in the household will be closely involved with care of the baby or any other children?

- What foods do women from the community traditionally eat during pregnancy? During lactation?
  What foods are considered beneficial?
  What foods are avoided?
  What variations are there in the traditional pattern?

- What weaning foods are traditionally used?
  What variations are there in the traditional pattern?
  What acceptable substitutes or alternatives are there for traditional foods that are not obtainable here, if any?

- How many children do women say they want?
  What are the views of other members of the community about ideal family size?
  What variations are there in views about family planning?
  Which methods are preferred and why?
  What doubts or anxieties exist about different methods and their effect on natural fertility?

Health beliefs and practices

- Have you talked to various families about their beliefs concerning cause, prevention, diagnosis and treatment of illnesses?
  Have you checked people's understanding of medical explanations and practices?

- What traditional beliefs and practices are beneficial to health?
  Should traditional beliefs and practices be changed?
  Are changes in health beliefs taking place already?

- Do members of the community divide illnesses into the same categories as the health worker (for example, 'physical' and 'mental' illness)? If not, what are the differences?
  Is this likely to influence the type of treatment that will be acceptable?

- Can you find out whether the treatment you consider most appropriate is acceptable?
  If it is not acceptable, what should you do?

- How does a sick person regard his illness?
  What does he consider caused the condition?
  What role does he expect the health worker to play?

- What illnesses does a family expect to treat without professional help?
  Who treats them, and how?

- Are there any traditional practitioners in the area?
  What kind of illnesses do they treat and how?
  How many members of the community refer to them?

209

- Do people go to traditional practitioners instead of their GP?
  As well as their GP?
  Only for certain types of illness?
  If so, which ones?

Use of the health services

- What differences are there between the local health services and the health facilities that newly arrived members of the community were used to in their own country?

- What are people's expectations of the health services?
  What is their previous experience of the effectiveness of Western medicine and health care?

- Do all members of the community know what health services are available and how to use them?
  For example, what mother-tongue information is available about
  - the function of different health professionals such as the health visitor, GP, midwife?
  - location of services?
  - welfare benefits?
  - special provision for groups such as the elderly, the handicapped?

- What kind of symptoms do people regard as particularly worrying?
  Do their views differ from those of the health worker?
  What are the reasons for these differences, if any?

- Do members of the community seem to prefer some types of medicine and treatment to others?
  If so, which?
  For what reasons?

- Should you change your own practice to better meet the needs and expectations of people within the community?
  What kind of adaptations could you feasibly make?

Patterns of illness

- Are there different patterns of illness within the community related to patterns of disease in the country of origin?

- Is the community more at risk from certain diseases because of ethnic origin?
  If so, what information and training is available to health workers about differences in prevalence of, for example, cystic fibrosis, sickle cell disease and thalassaemia among different ethnic groups?
  What information is available to members of the community?
  What screening facilities are available?
  What counselling support is available for those affected by such illnesses?

Care of the dying

Things you should check when caring for a dying patient from a minority community:

- Are there any special preparations, customs or ceremonies that the patient or his family wish to carry out?

- Where and how does the patient want to die?

- What role do other family members wish to play?

- In hospital, is it possible to discuss with the family and patient (if appropriate) what adjustments in hospital procedure would make things easier for them?

- Do other health workers need to be told about or prepared for customs and procedures that differ from their own expectations? For example, customs about laying out the body, ways of expressing grief, customs about mourning.

210

- Is there a member of the community with whom you can discuss what role the health worker is expected to play in case of a death?
  How and when to offer condolences?
  What other actions may be expected of you?

Foods and diets

- Which foods are most commonly eaten by members of the community?
  How are different foods prepared?
  What variations are there in ways of preparing the same foods?
  What is the nutritional value of foods prepared in different ways?

- What variations are there in the normal diet of families and individuals within the community?
  What variations are there in the normal diet of individuals within the same family?
  For example, are certain foods considered inappropriate for children?
  Eaten more by men than women?

- How many meals are eaten in a day?
  What foods do they consist of?
  What are the most common dishes?
  How are they prepared?
  What cooking methods are used?
  What, if anything, do cooking methods contribute to the diet?

- What do people think the ideal diet should consist of?
  What are the reasons for preferring some foods to others?
  What underlying beliefs and dietary rules influence food choice?

Maintaining dietary traditions in Britain

- Are changes really necessary in the traditional diet?
  Should the health worker press for change?
  For what reasons?
  In what circumstances?

- Do the diets of families in your area seem to lack any essential nutrients?
  If so, what are the likely causes?
  Lack of supply?
  Lack of information?
  Cost?
  Physical reaction to certain foods?
  Social or cultural restrictions on certain foods?

- If essential, what types of changes would best fit in with traditional food preferences and cause least disruption to the existing diet?

- What changes do you think will occur in the traditional diet as people adapt to life in Britain?
  Will this have implications for the incidence of health problems such as high blood pressure, heart disease and obesity?
  How can the development of harmful food habits be discouraged?

- Do people recently arrived in the area know where the best shops are for the kind of food they buy?

- To what extent have changes already occurred in the traditional diet of the families you work with?
  Which new foods do they use?
  Which foods are difficult to get hold of?
  How are these changes likely to affect the balance of the traditional diet?

- What variations are there in beliefs about, and use of, food therapy among members of the community?

- How much do people's traditional beliefs affect the dietary advice you give?
  How could advice be adapted to fit in with traditional food beliefs and practices?

Food in hospital

- Should relatives be encouraged to bring suitable food into hospital?
  What is the attitude of the hospital and hospital staff?
  Could eating arrangements for patients not used to the standard British diet be improved?
  For example, do facilities exist for storing meals brought in by relatives?

- Do ward staff discuss with individual patients which foods are acceptable or unacceptable when choosing food from the hospital menu?

14.5 How to start the research

Look and listen before asking and acting

Spend time getting to know people and letting people get to know you before you start asking questions. **It will take time for people to get to know and trust you;** if you rush in too soon asking questions and trying to change things you may upset and offend people; you may end up closing the doors you are trying to open.

The first time I went to visit a Pakistani family on my caseload they offered me a cup of tea so I sat down with them for 20 minutes. There were three women and their children in the house but we couldn't communicate; the only person with any English was a toddler of two. The older children were at school and the men were at work, but I somehow felt it was important to just sit down and be there, to let them know I wanted to be there and was ready to learn. On my next visit they were so welcoming. Some of my colleagues are in and out of the house without ever sitting down and being prepared to open up to their clients.

Health visitor

Find out how people from the community feel about being involved in a research study

Think carefully about the design of the research. If it is designed in such a way that people feel they are 'being studied' like zoological specimens, they may justifiably feel reluctant to contribute and resentful at being asked questions. There are two ways of involving people in research. One is to regard them as 'subjects' for study, the other is to **invite them to participate in the design and execution of the research**.

- Make sure that people understand what you are doing and why, and that they agree with the purpose of the research.

- Make sure you are not re-inventing the wheel by covering ground that has been researched before, or by interviewing people who have 'been researched' several times already.

- Try to involve people from the community in doing the research.

- Always give something back in return for information.

People naturally like to know the reasons for the research they are taking part in; they need to know that the information they are giving will not be misused and that the results will be of positive benefit to the community. It is important to let people know the outcome of the research, either by making available copies of the final report (or at least a summary), or by letting them know what action is taken as a result of the findings.

Find out whether there are any special rules or protocol that should be followed

It may be important to consult certain people, for example, community 'leaders', or the head of a family, in order to gain support for the research, and to avoid giving offence.

Find out before you start about the different political or religious factions within the community; if you approach the wrong group you may end up losing the support of the people you most wish to reach.

212

If there are strong conventions about contact between the sexes within the community, it may be thought inappropriate and even offensive for a male researcher to interview girls and women, and vice versa.

Put people before answers

The quality of answers you get to your questions is likely to depend on how much people know about you, trust you, like you or agree with what you're doing. There may be times when it is important to put aside the objectives of your research. For example, if as a result of your work you find youself being asked to help with a serious problem or crisis which is outside the range of your research, you cannot afford to walk away if you want to retain the respect and confidence of the people you are working with. There may be times when you need to modify the original objectives in the light of people's reactions to your questions. **If their replies do not fit in with the design of the research, you are probably asking the wrong questions and looking for the wrong answers.**

14.6 *Ways of gathering information*

There are various ways of gathering information; the most appropriate method will depend on what you want to find out. It may be useful to combine several of the methods outlined below.

Surveys

Collecting quantitative information, generally asking identical questions of a large number of people, usually to produce statistical data. (For example to find out how many local women missed ante-natal appointments, and how often.)

In-depth interviews

Interviewing a small number of people at length, asking open questions to obtain a free response, usually to gather qualitative rather than quantitative information. (To find out for example, *why* local women missed their ante-natal appointments.)

Observation

Looking and listening and, if appropriate, joining in with what's going on. For example, an invitation to a meal or a wedding would be a valuable opportunity to learn through observation and participation.

Secondary research

Looking at secondary sources of information about the community, such as academic research, local reports and surveys, television documentaries and press items.

Experimental research

Setting up a situation in which you can make changes and observe the results, usually comparing them with a situation where no changes have been made. For example, to assess the effectiveness of dietary advice in preventing rickets, a health visitor working in Southall in 1981 counselled a group of pregnant Asian women on the need to eat foods high in vitamin D.[3] The levels of vitamin D in the blood plasma of these women were compared with those of a control group who had received no dietary counselling. (The results suggested that dietary advice was not, in fact, effective in raising vitamin D levels.)

Case studies

Studying in depth various aspects of one person or situation, possibly combining some of the above methods.

Other possible approaches
- **Find someone from the community willing to work closely with you.**

If you do not come from the same background as people from the local community, or do not speak their language, it may be possible to find someone who does, who can explain, advise and help you to build up contact with other people in the community.

I learnt so much from working with one particular Afro-Caribbean colleague. If we were talking about a particular issue and I was on the wrong track she'd just say 'I know you don't mean it like that but what you're saying might offend a lot of black people because. . .'. She was very good at tactfully pointing out my mistakes; she taught me a great deal about working with black families.

White community worker

Be careful to find someone who is still in touch with, and trusted by, other people in the community.

We do have a liaison officer, an Asian woman, but I don't like to take her with me when I'm visiting some of my Pakistani clients. They don't like her, because she's from a well-to-do city family, you see, and doesn't really have any time for women from a village background. She likes to keep her distance, and she makes them feel it.

Health visitor

- **Get to know a wide cross-section of people from the community.**

  Talk to **patients** about their needs and their views of the health services.

  Get to know **people who are widely respected and considered 'wise'** within the community. Bear in mind that 'official' community leaders may only represent one interest group. Other people may, for example, turn to their local shopkeeper for advice; younger women may go to someone's aunt for advice about their children's health.

  Get to know **community workers** and **people involved in community organisations.**

  Talk to as many 'ordinary' people as possible, working men and women, women at home with children, pensioners, and young people.

- **Get involved in community activities.**

  Go out and see what it's like living in the area.

  If you get involved with what's going on, you can learn a lot by questioning as things happen.

  Learn from informal conversations over cups of tea.

  Find out how things work by asking people how they'd solve a particular problem or what they'd do in a particular situation.

14.7 *How to ask questions*

Explore people's attitudes towards questioning before you begin
People may be understandably suspicious or reluctant to give information to an outsider, for a variety of reasons. Until people get to know you, you may find it easier to learn from observation and informal questions than from asking direct questions.

Pre-test the questions you want to ask before starting out
Ask the opinion of people you know well from the community about the questions you want to ask. Check whether they will be appropriate and acceptable to other people in the community.

Ask yourself the same questions about your own culture to make sure you're not asking questions that are impossible to answer.

Health workers often ask me for information about traditional Asian diets. During a training session I once asked a group of white health visitors to describe the traditional British diet. The only thing they agreed on was that it couldn't be done – there are so many variables – age, sex, class, region, personal preference – the only things they could describe with absolute certainty were the foods that they and their families ate – and the variations were enormous.

Asian community worker

Learn interviewing techniques that are acceptable to the community

At the simplest level, conventions about things like eye contact and body language vary considerably between cultures, so that your behaviour might be misinterpreted if you do not follow the normal conventions of the community. You also need to be sensitive to other aspects of interviewing, for example:

- **Learn when to ask questions and when not to ask them;**
- **Learn what questions to ask and what not to ask.**

*White people are always asking black people where they were born, and how long they've been in this country. I suppose that kind of curiosity is meant to be polite interest. People don't realise how rude it is. You hear white people asking questions like this: 'Where are you from?' 'Manchester.' 'No, I mean where are you originally from?' 'I was born in Manchester.' 'Oh well, where were your parents from then?' In other words if you're black you'll never **belong** here and neither will your kids. My advice is, don't ever start by asking a black person questions like that unless you want to turn them off completely.*

Afro-Caribbean community worker

Make sure the questions you ask are based on concepts that are familiar to people in the community

If you ask a Mirpuri woman from a village background what her date of birth is she is not likely to know. The passport date is an official one but it's arbitrary. She could probably tell you roughly how old she was at Partition, but her birthday just isn't an important or relevant fact in her life. What's more important is the year she got married, when she had her first child, when her eldest son got married, when she became a grandmother and so on.

Asian community worker

Bear in mind three points when designing or asking questions

- **Is it simple?**

  If a single question is actually asking several things at once, it may be clearer to break it down into two or three more specific questions.

  e.g. Do you have any housing problems?

  This could cover a number of things: damp, noise, neighbours, lack of space, lack of running water. It might be appropriate to ask a series of more explicit questions.

- **Is it culture-specific?**

  A question based on one set of cultural values may be meaningless to someone from another culture.

  e.g. What kind of starchy foods do you eat?

  In Chinese languages there is no equivalent word to 'starchy' – the closest term would be 'rice-based' food, but this doesn't tell the questioner anything about other sources of carbohydrate in the diet.

- **Is it offensive?**

  A question that is quite acceptable to one person may be upsetting or rude to someone from a different culture.

  e.g. Did you have sex with your husband before you married?

  This question is asking about behaviour which is now considered the norm in some Western societies, but which completely contravenes the moral code of Islamic society. A Muslim woman might be shocked and angry to be asked something like this.

215

14.8 Difficulties you may encounter

Problems in asking questions

If the approach is not carefully thought out, research can produce false, inaccurate or misleading results for a number of reasons.

- People may not trust you.

  Members of the community may be justifiably suspicious or resentful of 'nosey' strangers. You may need to build up credibility by letting people judge you over a period of time, or through your actions, before they trust you enough to talk to you openly. People may mistrust you because of bad past experience with other people from your background, especially if you are a white person working with black communities.

- People may tell you what they think you want to hear.

  They may be reluctant to give you their own view, especially if they think it will meet with disapproval, ridicule or contempt.

- You may ask the wrong questions.

- You may be asking questions at the wrong time or place.

- People may have difficulty analysing what is second nature to them.

  Culture is transmitted largely at an unconscious level. People may not be able to talk like anthropologists about things they do without thinking.

- People's answers may be altered during translation.

- Your own age, sex, class, or skin colour may influence how people answer.

  Marked differences between interviewer and interviewee may affect the degree of confidence or embarrassment people feel in answering certain questions.

- People may mistake the ideal for the real.

  People may not be aware that they are telling you what they *think* they do, or what they think they *ought* to do, rather than what they actually do.

Problems of generalisations and stereotypes

Chapter 4 discussed some of the ways in which outsiders sometimes make false assumptions about minority communities and their culture. Well designed local research should aim to avoid some of these mistakes.

- Health workers sometimes draw half-baked conclusions based on too little information about what really goes on in a particular culture.

The conventional wisdom among professionals is that there are no problems among the Asian elderly because extended families look after their own so well. Of course, some families can and do, but this conventional wisdom actually means there are all sorts of difficulties that health workers are not picking up. I've come across families who were quite desperate but just didn't know that help was available.

Asian social worker

- Health workers may make generalisations from a non-typical group about the whole community.

A colleague of mine who worked as a district nurse in Brixton in the early 60s goes around telling everyone that West Indians don't use sheets and blankets, they just sleep in bedspreads or blankets. I never heard such nonsense. She may have come across some poor households in the early days when people had just arrived, but that was 30 years ago and even in those days it would have been absurd to generalise like that about the whole Afro-Caribbean population.

Afro-Caribbean community worker

- Health workers may overlook the range of variation and change within a community, even when their information is gathered from a random sample of people.

The problem is that outsiders tend to look for similarities between people in a particular community and they ignore the differences – in trying to make sense of a community they don't really understand, they want to find out what's 'typical'. Ask a French person what's typically British – they might say bowler hats, cricket, fair hair and blue eyes, fish and chips; but what's typical doesn't tell you much about age, sex and class differences in Britain, and about how much British society has changed in the last 50 years. What's 'typical' is likely to be a generalisation, a stereotype that bears no relation to any real individual within that social group.

White community worker

Local research should aim to build up a composite picture of the local community, not a series of generalisations and stereotypes.

14.9 *Effects of local research on the community*

- How will the research affect families and individuals within the community?

  Bear in mind that the existence of a research project or the presence of researchers could have a disruptive effect on the normal lives of people in the community. Try to make sure, for example, that the research does not intrude on or interfere with family relationships or community politics.

- Will the findings make any real difference to the health of the community?

  Local research of the type we are suggesting should not be research for its own sake; its immediate or long-term aim should be to promote positive change, either in the health of the community or in the quality of health care available to people in the community.

  It is, of course, possible that those responsible for doing the research are not the people responsible for implementing the recommendations; planners and decision-makers may not accept the proposals as a priority, or may find it difficult to take immediate action because of practical or financial constraints. But if the research is to gain the support and willing participation of community members, they need to see that it is at least attempting to achieve something that will be of practical benefit to the community.

Develop methods of research that can be used by local health workers and people from the community

One way that local research can be of immediate and practical value is if the research methods and techniques used are ones that can be learnt and used by local health workers and community members themselves in other areas of research they may want to look at later on. Providing local professionals and community representatives with the appropriate research skills and resources may in the long term be far more effective than using an outside team of 'professional' researchers who will eventually move on leaving nothing behind them.

Notes

1. Brownlee, Ann Templeton, *Community Culture and Care: A Cross-cultural Guide for Health Workers*, C. V. Mosy, 1978.
2. Townsend, Peter and Davidson, Nick, (eds), *Inequalities in Health: The Black Report*, Penguin 1982, Chapter 4: Inequality in the Availability and Use of the Health Services; Chapter 6: Towards an Explanation of Health Inequalities.
3. Box, Val, 'Rickets: What Should the Health Education Message Be?' in *Health Visitor*, vol. 56, April 1983, pp. 131–134.

15 Sources and resources

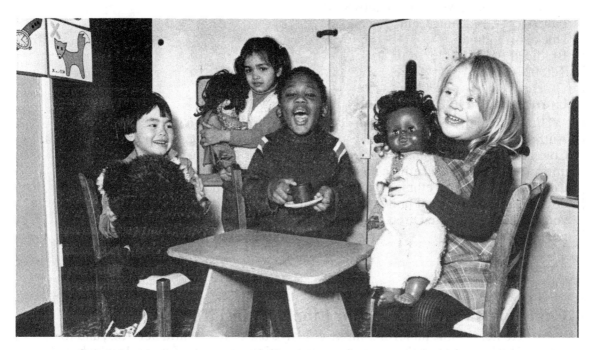

15.1 Agencies and organisations

15.2 Directories and other resource lists

15.3 Training resources for health workers and other professionals on working in a multiracial society

15.4 Film catalogues and other audiovisual resource lists

15.5 English as a Second Language: teaching materials

15.6 Addresses for directories, resource lists, film catalogues and teaching materials not available from bookshops

15.1 Agencies and organisations

Here are some agencies and organisations which you may find useful:

Centre for Ethnic Minority Health Studies

Aims to act as a resource, reference and research centre on ethnic minority health issues, and to organise training courses, seminars and conferences. Contact:
Maggie Pearson
Centre for Ethnic Minority Health Studies
Field House Teaching Centre
Duckworth Lane
Bradford BD9 6RJ
Tel: 0274-490324

Community Health Councils

The Community Health Council acts as a pressure group on the local Health Authority and can also initiate investigation of any complaints by patients. Your local Community Health Council secretary may be able to give you contacts and information about local ethnic minority health issues. Many Community Health Councils also have an ethnic minorities working party which is a useful forum for discussion. If you cannot find the address of your local Community Health Council you can get a complete Directory of Community Health Councils free from
CHC News
362 Euston Road
London NW1 3BL
Tel: 01-388 4943

Community Health Group for Ethnic Minorities

Aims to help ethnic minorities make effective use of the Health Services, and to inform Health Service policy makers of ethnic minority issues. Several locally based groups:
London: Philip Voon
CHGEM
2nd and 3rd Floor
13 Macclesfield Street
London W1V 7HL
Tel: 01-439 8765

Manchester: Milly Williams
Secretary
CHGEM Manchester
30 Warwick House
Central Avenue
Levenshulme
Manchester M19 2FF

Community Relations Councils

Community Relations Councils (CRCs) are locally based organisations set up to promote equality of opportunity for people of different racial groups. Your local Community Relations Council may have an officer who deals particularly in health matters who will be able to give you local contacts and information. The CRC will probably also have a Health and Social Services Committee or Panel, which meets regularly to discuss issues affecting the health and health care of ethnic minority groups.

If you are not sure whether there is a Community Relations Council in your area, you can get a free copy of the *List of Community Relations Councils* (a national register) from:
Information Officer
Commission for Racial Equality
10–12 Allington Street
London SW1E 5EH
Tel: 01-828 7022

English language classes

Many Local Education Authorities in urban areas run English as a Second Language (ESL) schemes for adults. Some ESL schemes have produced excellent material for English-language learners on a variety of health topics, including food and nutrition. Local ESL teachers may be willing to help in designing health education and other materials to help with communication with non-English-speakers, or to set up ESL classes in clinics, hospitals or other centres. Some education authorities also run home tutor schemes in which volunteer teachers work on a one-to-one basis with students.

You should be able to find out about these schemes by contacting the Education Department of your local Council.

If you have difficulty in finding out about language schemes in your area you may be able to get help or advice from a regional representative of NATESLA (National Association for Teachers of English as a Second Language to Adults). A list of regional representatives can be obtained from:
Marion Lazenby
Spring Grove Centre
Thornbury Road
Isleworth
Middlesex TW7 4HG
Tel: 01-568 3697 Ext 123

Health education units

Your local Health Education Unit can be contacted through the District Health Authority. Health Education Units can provide films, slides and leaflets on a wide range of health education topics. Some Health Education Officers will give talks and demonstrations on request.

Health Education Council

The Health Education Council is a national organisation set up to promote health education in Britain. One of its functions is to provide advice and resources for local Health Education Units. It also funds a number of projects concerned with ethnic minority health and produces health education material in a number of languages.

The HEC Resources Centre in London is open to anyone concerned with health education issues. For further information contact:
Resources Centre
Health Education Council
78 New Oxford Street
London WC1
Tel: 01-637 1881

Training in Health and Race

This project was established in September 1982. It is administered by the National Extension College and supported by the Health Education Council.

The overall aim of the Project is to work towards a health service more responsive to the needs of a multiracial society, through the provision of training and training materials for health workers. To achieve this aim the project is engaged in researching training needs, and finding effective ways of enabling trainers, tutors and other health educators to include multiracial health care in their training programmes. Contact:
The Project Coordinator
Training in Health and Race
18 Victoria Park Square
Bethnal Green
London E2 9PF
Tel: 01-980 6263

221

15.2 Directories and other resource lists

Titles marked with an asterisk are not available from bookshops or libraries. Addresses of issuing organisation are given at the end of this chapter.

Community Information (Asian Languages) Directory, Commission for Racial Equality and National Association of Citizens Advice Bureaux, 1980. Directory of leaflets on health, housing, social services, etc. available in Bengali, Gujarati, Hindi, Punjabi and Urdu. (Commission for Racial Equality)

*Directory of Information Material in Non-Asian Languages, London Voluntary Services Council, Migrant Services Unit, 1981. (Migrant Services Unit)

Health and Social Services for Ethnic Minorities in Britain: Bibliography, Dept. of Health and Social Security Library, updated 1982. (DHSS Library)

*Health Education Material for Ethnic Minorities, Health Education Council, 1982. List of books, pamphlets, notices, films, tape slide sets and kits for ethnic minorities and/or for health workers in multiracial areas. (Health Education Council)

*Henley, Alix and Taylor, Colette, *Register of Research Projects Related to the Health Care Needs of Ethnic Minorities,* King's Fund Centre, 1980. (The King's Fund Centre)

15.3 Training resources for health workers and other professionals on working in a multiracial society

Below is a selection of resources which can be used in training programmes on working in a multiracial society, and which we think are useful.

However, different training materials suit different groups of trainees. Some of these resources may need careful preparation or adaptation to make them appropriate to health workers. To be fully useful a training course cannot be completely prepackaged and churned out in the same form each time. It needs to be reworked not only for different kinds of trainees, but each time it is taught. If possible never use audio-visual or written materials that you have not seen or tried out yourself in advance.

Books and training packs

*Asian Foods and Diets: A Training Pack, Alix Henley, DHSS/King's Fund, 1982. Aims to enable health workers to discuss diets and dietary advice with Asian patients and clients in an informed and sensitive way. Contains trainers' information, slides, overhead projector transparencies, worksheets, trainees' booklets and language sheets. (National Extension College)

*Asian Names and Records: A Training Pack, Alix Henley and Colette Taylor, DHSS/King's Fund, 1981. Aims to enable health workers, records staff, receptionists, etc. to record and use Hindu, Sikh and Asian Muslim names correctly and prevent confusion in records. Contains trainers' information, overhead projector transparencies, worksheets, trainees' booklets and audio cassette. (National Extension College)

*Caring Communication, Joanna Grey, DHSS, 1982. Cross-cultural communication training manual, intended particularly for use with overseas nurses. Modules on communication skills include exercises on listening, asking questions, non-verbal signals, etc. Includes audio cassette exercises. (Local Industrial Training Unit or National Centre for Industrial Language Training)

*Cross-Cultural Training: Developing Skills and Awareness in Communication, Valerie Yates *et al.*, NCILT, 1982. A manual for trainers, designed to help people at work understand what cross-cultural communication consists of. First half of manual sets out aims and methods; second half is a materials bank with copies of worksheets and sample tape transcripts. (National Extension College)

*Helping Health Workers Learn, David Werner and Bill Bower, Hesperian Foundation, 1983. A collection of methods, aids and ideas for use by village instructors in Third World countries. Theoretical and practical emphasis on community-based approach to health, helping communities analyse and change their situation. Needs adapting, but key ideas very relevant to training of community health/outreach/link workers in Britain. (Hesperian Foundation)

London Against Racism, Greater London Council, 1984. Resource pack produced as part of GLC's London against Racism programme. Includes articles on racism, factsheets, and two pamphlets with questions and exercises: Roots of Racism and Patterns of Racism. (Ethnic Minorities Unit)

Providing Effective Health Care in a Multiracial Society: A checklist for looking at local issues, Training in Health and Race, 1984. Short pamphlet containing questions on different aspects of health care and examples of good practice. Useful reference text for nurse learners, medical students and other trainees. This project has several other training resources for health workers in preparation. (National Extension College)

Race Relations Teaching Pack, AFFOR, 1982. Designed for use in secondary school, contains teachers' instruction book, lesson plans, worksheets, audio cassette, reading list. Looks at immigration control, prejudice, racism. Needs adapting. (AFFOR)

Racism in the Workplace and Community, Open University, 1982. Open learning materials designed for people active in trade union and community organisations, to help them identify the origins and effects of racism in society. 22 topic units, notes for groupleaders, bibliography. (Community Education Office)

The Right to be Understood: a handbook on community interpreting, Jane Shackman, National Extension College, 1984. Handbook aimed at people who work in statutory and community agencies who either use, or recruit and train interpreters. Looks at role of interpreters, selection, recruitment and supervision, training of interpreters and training of staff who use them. Includes case studies, examples, detailed resources section, bibliography, useful addresses. (National Extension College)

White Awareness: handbook for anti-racism training, Judy Katz, University of Oklahoma Press, 1978. A group training programme for white people to explore and understand the conscious and unconscious nature of racism and its effects, and to develop action strategies to change behaviour. Basic programme adaptable to a range of situations; step-by-step training format includes instructions suggestions, recommended reading, sources of materials.

Audiovisual materials
Health

Mental Health, videocassette, colour, 30 mins, Skin Programme, London Weekend Television, 1981. The treatment of black people with psychiatric symptoms, dangers of misdiagnosis and mistreatment. (Concord Films Council)

Rickets are Back, videocassette/film, colour, 26 mins, World in Action, Granada, 1979. Looks at the new outbreak of rickets and osteomalacia and discusses possible preventative measures. (Concord Films Council)

Sea in the Blood: Thalassaemia, videocassette, colour, 70 mins, BBC, 1979. Discusses the nature and effects of thalassaemia, looks at real cases, discusses treatment and ante-natal diagnosis. (Concord Films Council)

Sickle Cell Anaemia, 20 slides, with audiocassette and booklet, 1979. Spenco Medical Corp, USA, ref. 76–224. (Spenco Medical (UK) Ltd)

Sickle Cell Disease: the Unkind Inheritance, 16 mm, colour, 45 mins, Film Drama, USA, 1977. Broad health-worker-oriented view of sickle cell disease. (BLAT Film Library)

The Great Health Robbery, videocassette/film, colour, 21 mins, Oxfam, 1981. Explores the effects of sales of drugs and baby milks in the Third World. (Concord Films Council)

Race/Racism/Race Relations

Cross talk, film, colour, 25 mins, BBC, 1979. Examines common communication difficulties between native English speakers and people who speak English as a second language: how to recognise and cope better with them. Prepared with a booklet *Crosstalk*, which amplifies the film and discusses how it can best be used in training staff. (Concord Films Council)

Institutional Racism, Tape/slide, 15 mins, London Borough of Lewisham and Turning Point, 1981. Broad introduction to racism in institutions – education, the law, etc. (Peter Anderson, London Borough of Lewisham)
*Also in videocassette from the Albany Video Project (Albany Video Project)

It Ain't Half Racist, Mum, film, colour, 30 mins, Campaign Against Racism in the Media, 1979. 'Open Door' programme showing the subtle and explicit racism of both popular comedy shows and serious current affairs programmes. (Concord Films Council)

Multiracial Videoscenes, Clarke, Jean, 30 mins. Videotape and Trainer's Manual, Leicester Polytechnic, 1982. Training material for professionals involved in helping/caring for/counselling clients from other cultures than their own. Manual explains approach, contains transcript, and suggestions for ways in which video can be used in training. Only sold to training agencies. (The Secretary, Student Counselling Service)

*Our People, film, Thames Television, 1979. Series of six films setting out the facts and history of immigration to Britain 30 mins each (Film Forum)
A booklet is available from Thames TV containing a summary of factual information about immigration and growth of racism, plus case studies, to accompany the film series. (Schools Publications Office, Thames TV)

*Recognising Racism, City of Birmingham Education Department, 1983. Filmstrip or tape/slide accompanied by a teacher's booklet, for use in Racism Awareness training. Looks at 'unintentional' racism in the education system.
Needs adapting for health service training. (Multicultural Support Service)

*The Enemy Within, Tape/slide, 30 mins, Catholic Commission for Racial Justice/British Council of Churches, 1981. Black people speak frankly of their experiences of racism. (Community and Race Relations Unit)

*The Eye of the Storm, film, colour, 25 mins, USA, 1973. Looks at an experiment to illustrate the effects of prejudice among schoolchildren. (Concord Films Council)

*Who Feels It Knows It, film, colour, 55 mins, National Film School, 1981. Life in the black communities of London through the eyes of a number of women. (Concord Films Council)

*Why Prejudice?, videocassette, colour, 20 mins, Scene Programme, BBC, 1980. Young people look at how racial prejudice is learnt and perpetuated. (Concord Films Council)

15.4 Film catalogues and other audiovisual resource lists

*Open University: Information sheets giving details about course material (films, books, TV programmes, etc.). Write specifying main areas of interest. (Open University)
Catalogue of Open University film and video material for sale (NOT hire).

*Information sheets giving times of Open University TV and radio programmes on general topics of interest. The following topic sheets are particularly relevant:
   Psychology, Family, Community, Public affairs and History, Communication/Educational Studies and General Courses.
Send stamped addressed envelope. (Information Officer, BBC, OU Production Centre)

*Concord Films: Extensive catalogue of films selected primarily to promote discussion for instruction and training. Covers documentaries, animated films and feature length productions concerned with contemporary issues, both at home and abroad. Sections on Race Relations, Medical Subjects, etc. (Concord Films Council)

*British Life Assurance Trust (BLAT) Extensive catalogue of films on medical and health education topics for professional and lay audiences. Includes films on health care systems in Third World countries such as Vietnam and Bangladesh. (BLAT Film Library)

15.5 English as a Second Language: teaching materials

Below are details of ESL teaching materials directly related to health and using the Health Service. These contain some visual material which health workers may find useful in communicating with clients who speak English as a Second Language.

*Swann, Sian, Mother and Baby Care, National Extension College, 1983. Contains tutor's handbook, photographs and other visual aids and four simple pictorial readers on crying, feeding, sleeping and safety. (National Extension College)

*Lewycka, M., Mares, P., and Whitaker, N., The HELP Maternity Language Course, Leeds City Council Printed Resources Unit, 1979. About 100 illustrated worksheets which cover most aspects of pregnancy, delivery, birth and the post-natal period. (Leeds City Council Printed Resources Unit)

*Nesbitt, Judith, Ante-Natal Language Teaching, Commission for Racial Equality, 1983. Comprehensive coverage of language needed for pregnancy, delivery, birth and the post-natal period, fewer illustrations. (Commission for Racial Equality)

15.6 Addresses for directories, resource lists, film catalogues and teaching materials not available from bookshops

AFFOR, 173 Lozelles Road, Birmingham, B19 1RN. Tel: 021-523 8076.

Albany Video Project, Douglas Way, London, SE8. Tel: 01-692 0231.

Information Officer, BBC OU Production Centre, Walton Hall, Milton Keynes, MK7 6BH.

BLAT Film Library, BMA House, Tavistock Square, London, WC1H 9JP. Tel: 01-387 4499.

Community Education Office, Centre for Continuing Education, The Open University, PO Box 188, Milton Keynes, MK3 6HW.

Commission for Racial Equality, 10–12 Allington Street, London, SW1. Tel: 01-828 7022.

Community and Race Relations Unit, British Council of Churches, 2 Eaton Gate, London, SW1. Tel: 01-730 9611.

Concord Films Council, 201 Felixstowe Road, Ipswich, Suffolk, IP3 9BJ. Tel: 0473-715754.

DHSS Library, Room A110, Alexander Fleming House, Elephant & Castle, London, SE1 6B7.

Ethnic Minorities Unit, Room 686, County Hall, London, SE1.

Film Forum, 56 Brewer Street, London, W1. Tel: 01-437-6487.

King's Fund Centre, 126 Albert Street, London, NW14 7NF.

Health Education Council, 78 New Oxford Street, London, WC1A 1AH.

Hesperian Foundation, PO Box 1692, Palo Alto, CA 94302, USA.

Leeds City Council Printed Resources Unit, 27 Harrogate Road, Leeds 7. Tel: 0532-623308.

Peter Anderson, PR Division, London Borough of Lewisham, Lewisham Town Hall, Rushey Green, Catford, London, SE6 4RU. Tel: 01-690 4343, Ext 373.

Migrant Services Unit, London Voluntary Service Council, 68 Chalton Street, London, NW1 1JR.

Multicultural Support Service, Bordesley Centre, Camp Hill, Stratford Road, Birmingham, B11 1AR. Tel: 021-772 7676.

National Centre for Industrial Language Training, Havelock Campus, Havelock Road, Southall, Middlesex.

National Extension College, 18 Brooklands Avenue, Cambridge, CB2 2HN. Tel: 0223-316644.

Open University, Education Enterprises Ltd, 12 Cofferidge Close, Stony Stratford, MK11 1BY.

Schools Publications Office, Thames TV, 149 Tottenham Court Road, London, W1P 9LL.

Spenco Medical (UK) Ltd., Tanyard Lane, Steyning, West Sussex, BN4 3RJ. Tel: 0903-815123.

The Secretary, Student Counselling Service, Leicester Polytechnic, PO Box 143, Leicester.

16 Reading list

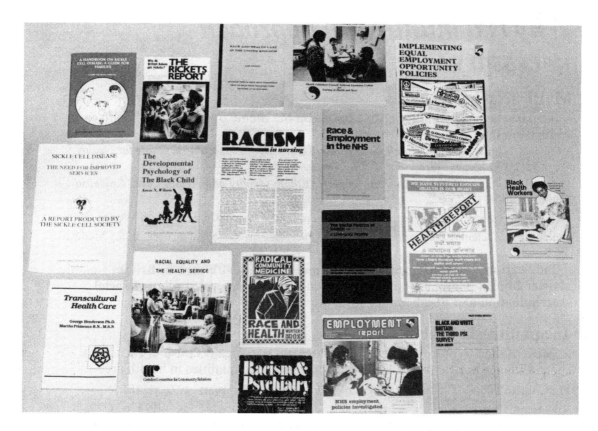

Introduction

This chapter gives suggestions for further reading. Each section sets out a reading list relating to one chapter, and is further subdivided into topics where appropriate. *Titles marked with an asterisk are not available from bookshops or libraries. Addresses of issuing organisation are given at the end of the chapter.

16.1 Why is a multiracial approach necessary?

Multiracial health care

To date the most comprehensive books on the theme of multiracial health care come from the USA.

Brownlee, Ann Templeton, *Community, Culture and Care: Cross-Cultural Guide for Health Workers*, C. V. Mosby, 1978.

Bullough, Bonnie and Bullough, Vern, *Poverty, Ethnic Identity and Health Care,* Appleton-Century-Crofts, 1972.

Henderson, George and Primeaux, Martha, *Transcultural Health Care*, Addison-Wesley, 1981.

Leininger, Madeleine, *Transcultural Nursing: Concepts, Theories and Practices*, Wiley Medical, 1978.

Publications dealing specifically with **multiracial health care in Britain** (mainly shorter books, pamphlets and articles), along with general studies of **racial discrimination and disadvantage** in Britain are listed in 16.2.

Inequalities in health

Most of the literature on this subject does not specifically consider racial inequalities in health. Three key works on general inequalities in health are:

Hart, Julian Tudor, 'The Inverse Care Law', *The Lancet*, 27 February, 1971, p. 412.

Townsend, Peter, 'Inequality and the Health Service', *The Lancet*, 15 June, 1974, p. 1179.

Townsend, Peter, and Davidson, Nick (eds.), *Inequalities in Health: The Black Report*, Penguin, 1982.

16.2 Racial inequality and health

Racial discrimination and disadvantage in Britain

Below is a selected list of research studies and other publications which have documented aspects of discrimination and disadvantage affecting Britain's black population.

Brown, Colin, *Black and White Britain: The Third PSI Survey,* Heinemann, 1984

Ethnic Minorities in Britain, Home Office Research Study, No. 68, HMSO, 1981.

*Open University, *Racism in the Workplace and the Community*, Open University Continuing Education Pack, 1983. (Open University)

Open University, *Ethnic Disadvantage in Britain*, (E345: Ethnic Minorities and the Community, Unit 4), Open University Press, 1982.

*Ouseley, Herman *et al.*, *The System*, Runnymede Trust and South London Equal Rights Consultancy, 1982. (Runnymede Trust)

Rampton, A. (ed.), *West Indian Children in our Schools: Interim report of the Committee of Inquiry into the education of children from ethnic minority communities*, HMSO, 1981.

Runnymede Trust and the Radical Statistics Race Group, *Britain's Black Population*, Heinemann, 1980.

Scarman, Leslie George, *The Brixton Disorders: Report of an Inquiry*, London HMSO, 1981, also available as *The Scarman Report*, Penguin, 1982.

*Simpson, Alan, *Stacking the Decks: A Study of Race, Inequality and Council Housing in Nottingham*, Nottingham and District Community Relations Council, 1981. (Nottingham and District Community Relations Council)

Smith, David J., *Racial Disadvantage in Britain: The PEP Report*, Penguin, 1977.

*Smith, David and Whalley, Anne, *Racial Minorities and Public Housing*, Vol. XLI, Broadsheet No. 556, PEP, September, 1975. (Policy Studies Institute)

*Smith, David J., *Unemployment and Racial Minorities*, PSI, No. 594, February 1981. (Policy Studies Institute)

*Young, Ken and Connelly, Naomi, *Policy and Practice in the Multi-Racial City*, Policy Studies Institute, 1981. (Policy Studies Institute)

Race and health in Britain

The following publications deal with aspects of racial inequality, health and health care needs.

Homans, H. and Satow, A., 'We too are strangers: Community nursing in a multiracial society', 'The nuclear family rules OK?', 'Fair service for all', 'Integration or isolation', 'Can you hear me?: Cultural variations in communication', series of five articles, *Journal of Community Nursing*, October 1982–February 1983.

**Asians and the Health Service*, Wandsworth Council for Community Relations, 1978. (Wandsworth Council for Community Relations).

**Black People and the Health Service*, Brent Community Health Council, 1981. (Brent Community Health Council)

**Ethnic Minorities and the Health Service*, Wandsworth and East Merton Health District, September 1979. (Wandsworth and East Merton Area Health Authority)

**Racial Equality and the Health Service*, Camden Committee for Community Relations, 1983. (Camden Committee for Community Relations)

*Torkington, N. P. K., *The Racial Politics of Health – A Liverpool Profile*, Merseyside Area Profile Group, 1983. (Merseyside Area Profile Group)

*Training in Health and Race, *Providing Effective Health Care in a Multiracial Society*, Health Education Council/National Extension College, 1984. (National Extension College)

16.3 Migration and health

The publications below deal with various aspects of migration and health. See also suggested reading in 16.1 and 16.2.

*Baker, R. (ed.), *The Psychosocial Problems of Refugees*, British Refugee Council, 1983. (British Refugee Council)

Berger, John and Mohr, Jean, *A Seventh Man: Migrant Workers in Europe*, Penguin, 1975.

Churches Committee on Migrant Workers, *Migrant Women Speak*, Search Press/World Council of Churches, 1978.

Humphrey, D. and Ward, M., *Passports and Politics*, Penguin, 1974.

*Levin, Michael, *What Welcome? Reception and Resettlement of Refugees in Britain*, Acton Society Trust, 1981. (Acton Society Trust)

**Migrant Workers and their Families*, Report of a series of seminars organised by the Earl's Court and Chelsea Migrant Workers Group/Kensington and Chelsea and Westminster Health Education Department, September, 1979. (Kensington and Chelsea and Westminster Health Education Department)

Moore, R. and Wallace, T., *Slamming the Door*, Martin Robertson, 1975.

Open University, *Migration and Settlement in Britain/Migrant Labour in Europe*, E345 Ethnic Minorities and Community Relations, Units 2 and 3, Open University, 1982.

*Tandon, Yash, *The New Position of East African Asians: Problems of a displaced minority*, Minority Rights Group, 1981. (Minority Rights Group)

16.4 Culture: a misleading explanation of health inequalities

Below is a selected list of publications which look specifically at culture and health care. A number of local Health Education Departments, Community Health Councils and Community Relations Councils have produced notes or pamphlets on the culture and health care needs of local communities, but these are not always easily accessible. We have chosen publications that are likely to be found in the libraries of nursing or medical schools, Health Education Departments, Community Relations Councils, etc. **Some are useful; others are less useful** because they present ethnic minority communities in a negative way, treating them as 'problems', or they fall into the trap of over-simplifying, generalising or stereotyping minority cultures in a way which does not help health workers to understand black people as **individuals. We ask readers to consider critically, doubt and question all of them!**

Brownlee, Ann Templeton, *Community, Culture and Care: a cross-cultural guide for health workers*, C. V. Mosby, 1978.

Dobson, S., 'Bringing Culture into Care', *Nursing Times*, 9.2.1983.

Harwood, Alan, (ed.), *Ethnicity and Medical Care*, Harvard University Press, 1981.

Henderson, G. and Primeaux, M., *Transcultural Health Care*, Addison-Wesley, 1981.

*Henley, Alix, *Asian Patients in Hospital and at Home*, King's Fund, 1979. (The King's Fund)

*Henley, Alix, *Caring for Hindus and their Families*, Health Education Council/DHSS/King's Fund, 1983. (National Extension College)

*Henley, Alix, *Caring for Muslims and their Families*, DHSS/King's Fund, 1982. (National Extension College)

*Henley, Alix, *Caring for Sikhs and their Families*, DHSS/King's Fund, 1983. (National Extension College)

de Lobo, E. H., *Children of Immigrants to Britain: their health and social problems*, Hodder and Stoughton, 1978.

*Mares, Penny, *The Vietnamese in Britain: a handbook for health workers*, Health Education Council/National Extension College, 1982. (National Extension College)

Sampson, Chris, *The Neglected Ethnic: Religious and Cultural Factors in the Care of Patients*, McGraw-Hill, 1982.

The publications below offer a detailed critique of 'culture' as an explanation of inequalities in health in the black population.

Black People and the Health Service, Brent Community Health Council, 1981. (Brent Community Health Council)

*Torkington, N. P. K., *The Racial Politics of Health,* Merseyside Area Profile Group, 1983. (Merseyside Area Profile Group)

16.5 *Communication*

Most of the publications below deal with aspects of communication in the context of health care, where practitioner and patient come from different cultural and/or linguistic backgrounds. We have also included some publications which consider general aspects of 'cross-cultural' communication, and some which deal with general principles of practitioner-patient communication.

Brownlee, Ann Templeton, *Community, Culture and Care: a cross cultural guide for health workers*. Chapter 3: Communication. Chapter 4: Language, St Louis, C. V. Mosby, 1978, 297 pp.

*Ewles, Linda and Shipster, Pieter, *One to One: a handbook for the health educator*, East Sussex Area Health Authority, 1980. (South East Thames Regional Health Authority)

*Fugelsang, Andreas, *About Understanding: ideas and observations on cross-cultural communication*, Dag Hammarskjöld Foundation, 1982. (Dag Hammarskjöld Foundation)

*Gumperz, J. J., Jupp, T. C., Roberts, C., *Crosstalk: A study of cross-cultural communication*, National Centre for Industrial Language Training, 1979. (National Centre for Industrial Language Training)

*Henley, Alix, *Asian Patients in Hospital and at Home,* King's Fund, 1979 Chapter 12: The Language Barrier. Chapter 14: Interpreters. (The King's Fund)

Homans, Hilary and Sato, W., Antoinette, 'Can you hear me? Cultural variations in communication' in *Journal of Community Nursing*, January, 1982, pp. 16–18.

*Mares, Penny, *The Vietnamese in Britain: a handbook for health workers,* Health Education Council/National Extension College, 1982, Chapter 16: Giving advice about nutrition. (National Extension College)

*Naish, Julia, *Report on 'Bengali Life and Language': a course for health visitors in Camden and Islington*, Camden Language Scheme, July, 1981. (Camden Language Scheme)

Savage, Felicity and Godwin, Peter, 'Controlling your language: making English clear' in *Transactions of the Royal Society of Tropical Medicine and Hygiene*, Vol. 75, No. 4, 1981, pp. 583–585.

Smith, V. M. and Bass, T. A., *Communication for the Health Care Team*, Lippincott Nursing Series, Harper Row, 1982.

Sutcliffe, D., *British Black English*, Basil Blackwell, 1982.

Talking with patients: a teaching approach, Nuffield Provincial Hospitals Trust, 1980. (Nuffield Provincial Hospitals Trust)

*Weinreich, Frances, *Report on 'Breaking the Language Barrier' Course for Health Visitors and Paediatric Nurses in Brent*, Neighbourhood English Classes, August, 1981. (Frances Weinreich)

*Werner, David and Bower, Bill, *Helping Health Workers Learn*, Hesperian Foundation, 1983. (Hesperian Foundation)

16.6 *Working with families and individuals*

Further general reading about family systems and family life in different cultures and communities.

Brownlee, Ann Templeton, *Community, Culture and Care*. C. V. Mosby, St. Louis, 1978, Chapter 5: The Family.

Cheetham, Juliet *et al.*, (ed.) *Social & Community Work in a Multi-Racial Society*, Harper & Row, 1981.

*Cheetham, Juliet, *Social Work Services for Ethnic Minorities in Britain and the USA*, 1981. (Juliet Cheetham)

Hiro, Dilip, *Black British, White British*, Penguin, 1973.

Khan, Verity Saifullah, (ed.), *Minority Families in Britain*, Macmillan, 1979.

Our Lives: Young People's Autobiographies, ILEA English Centre, 1979. (ILEA English Centre)

Rapoport, R. N. (ed.), *Families in Britain*, Routledge and Kegan Paul, 1982.

Watson, James L. (ed.), *Between Two Cultures*, Blackwell, 1977.

Specific ethnic minority communities in Britain

Barret, Leonard, E., *The Rastafarians*, Heinemann, 1977.

*Bonamy, David, *Immigrants from Bangladesh*, National Centre for Industrial Language Training, 1978. (National Centre for Industrial Language Training)

Blake, J., *Family Structure in Jamaica*, Free Press of Glencoe, Kingston, 1961.

Cashmore, E., *Rastaman*, Allen & Unwin, 1979.

Clarke, Edith, *My Mother who Fathered Me*, Allen & Unwin, 1966.

*Commission for Racial Equality, *Asian Links*, CRE, 1982. (Commission for Racial Equality)

Caribbean Links, CRE, 1982. (Interviews with Asian and Afro-Caribbeans in Britain about their links with the places they came from.) (Commission for Racial Equality)

*Cross, Colin, *What is Judaism?* Board of Deputies of British Jews. (Board of Deputies of British Jews)

Ellis, June, (ed.), *West African Families in Britain,* Routledge and Kegan Paul, 1978.

Foner, Nancy, *Jamaica Farewell*, Routledge & Kegan Paul, 1979.

*Henley, Alix, *Asian Patients in Hospital and at Home*, King's Fund, 1979. (The King's Fund)

Henriques, L. F., *Family & Colour in Jamaica*, McGibbon & Kee, 1960.

James, Alan, *Sikh Children in Britain*, Institute of Race Relations/Oxford University Press, 1974.

*Ladbury, Sarah, *Cypriots in Britain*, National Centre for Industrial Language Training, 1979. (National Centre for Industrial Language Training)

*Lynn, L. L., *The Chinese Community in Liverpool*, Merseyside Area Profile Group, 1982 (Merseyside Area Profile Group)

*Mares, Penny, *The Vietnamese in Britain: a handbook for health workers*, Health Education Council/National Extension College, 1982, Chapter 3: The Family. (National Extension College)

231

Pryce, Ken, *Endless Pressure*, Penguin, 1980.

Roberts, George W. and Sinclair, Sonja, A., *Women in Jamaica: Patterns of Reproduction and Family*, KTO Press, 1978.

Sharma, Ursula, *Rampal and his Family*, Collins, 1971.

Wilson, Amrit, *Finding a Voice*, Virago, 1978.

Black children in Britain

Coard, Bernard, 'What the British School System does to the Black Child' in *The School in the Multi-Cultural Society*, James, Alan *et al.* (eds.) Harper & Row, 1981.

*Commission for Racial Equality, *A Home from Home: black children in residential care*, CRE, 1977. (Commission for Racial Equality)

Caring for Under Fives in a Multi-racial Society, CRE, 1978. (Commission for Racial Equality)

Who minds? A Study of working mothers and child-minding in ethnic minority communities, CRE, 1975. (Commission for Racial Equality)

Gill, D. and Jackson, B., *Adoption and Race: Black Asian and Mixed Race Children in White Families*, Batsford Academic and Educational/British Agencies for Adoption and Fostering, 1983.

Milner, David, *Children and Race*, Penguin, 1975.

Stone, Maureen, *The Education of the Black Child in Britain: the myth of multiracial education*, Fontana, 1981.

Wilson, Amos, *The Developmental Psychology of the Black Child*, Africana Research Publications, 1980.

Further reading about family planning

Christopher, Elphys, *Sexuality & Birth Control in Social & Community Work*, Temple Smith, 1980.

Depo-Provera, The Campaign Against Depo-Provera, 1981. (CARD)

Mamdani, Mahmood, *The Myth of Population Control*, Monthly Review Press, 1972.

*Werner, D. and Bower, B., *Helping Health Workers Learn*, Hesperian Foundation, 1983, Chapter 23: The Politics of Family Planning. (Hesperian Foundation)

Further reading about the elderly

*Bhalla, A. and Blakemore, K., *Elders of the Ethnic Minority Groups*, AFFOR, 1981. (AFFOR)

*Glendenning, Frank, (ed.), *The Elders in Ethnic Minorities*, Beth Johnson Foundation, 1979. (Department of Adult Education, University of Keele)

*Haringey CRC, *The Ethnic Elderly,* Haringey CHC, 1979. (Haringey Community Health Council)

16.7 *Health beliefs and practices*

Bannerman, Robert *et al.* (eds.), *Traditional medicine and health care coverage: a reader for health administrators and practitioners*, World Health Organisation, 1983.

Bowens, Eleanor, E.,*The Anthropology of Health*, St. Louis, C. V. Mosby, 1978.

Brownlee, Ann Templeton, *Community, Culture and Care: a cross cultural guide for health workers*, C. V. Mosby, 1978, Part Three: The Health System of the Community.

Crozier, R. C., *Traditional Medicine in Modern China*, Harvard University Press, 1968.

Eagle, Robert, *A Guide to Alternative Medicine*, BBC, 1980.

Homans, H. and Satow, A., 'We too are Strangers: Community Nursing in a Multi-racial Society', in *Journal of Community Nursing*, November 1981, pp. 10–13.

Leslie, Charles, *Asian Medical Systems*, University of California Press, 1976.

Maclean, Una, *Magical Medicine: A Nigerian Case Study,* Penguin, 1977.

McMichael, Joan, K., (ed.), *Health in the Third World: Studies from Vietnam*, Spokesman Books, 1976.

*Mares, Penny, *The Vietnamese in Britain: a handbook for health workers*, Health Education Council/National Extension College, 1982, Chapter 5: Concepts of health and illness. (National Extension College)

Revolutionary Health Communittee of Hunan Province, *A Barefoot Doctor's Manual,* Routledge and Kegan Paul, 1977.

Storer, Jenny, '"Hot" and "cold" food beliefs in an Indian community and their significance', in *Journal of Human Nutrition*, 31, 1977, pp. 33–40.

*Werner, D. and Bower, B., *Helping Health Workers Learn*, Hesperian Foundation, 1983, Chapter 7: Helping people look at their customs and beliefs. (Hesperian Foundation)

Whang, J., 'Chinese Traditional Food Therapy' in *Journal of the American Dietetics Association*, Vol. 78, January 1981, pp. 55–57.

16.8 Foods and diets

Cameron, Margaret and Hofrander, Yngre, *Manual on Feeding Infants and Young Children*, Protein-Calorie Advisory Group, United Nations, 1976.

Carlson, E., Kipps, M. and Thompson, J., *An Evaluation of the Financial and Nutritional Viability of a Traditional Diet for Vietnamese Refugees*, Department of Hotel Catering and Tourism Management, University of Surrey, 1980.

Chang, K. C., *Food in Chinese Culture*, Yale University Press, 1977.

Chetley, Andy, *The Babykiller Scandal*, War on Want, 1979.

Dawar, Anne, 'Food for Thought in Work with Immigrants' *Nursing Mirror*, 18 October 1979.

*Department of Health and Social Security, *Catering for Minority Groups*, Catering and Dietetic Branch Manual, Vol. 6, 1982. (Catering and Dietetic Branch)

*Goel, K. M., *A Nutrition Survey of Immigrant Children in Glasgow*, Scottish Health Service Studies No. 40, Scottish Home and Health Department, 1979. (Scottish Home and Health Department)

Gopalan, C., Rama Sastri, B. V. and Balasubramian, S. C., *Nutritive Value of Indian Foods*, National Institute of Nutrition, Hyderabad, Indian, 1980.

*Henley, Alix, *Asian Foods & Diets: A training pack*, 1982. (National Extension College)

Hollingsworth, Dorothy, (ed.), *The Englishman's Food: A History of Five Centuries of English Diet*, Cape, 1958.

*Mares, Penny, *The Vietnamese in Britain: a handbook for health workers*, Health Education Council/National Extension College, 1982. (National Extension College)

*O'Brien, Maureen, *Hospital Food for Ethnic Minority Patients*, Haringey Community Health Council, 1981. (Haringey Community Health Council)

*Sheiham, Helena and Quick, Alison, *The Rickets Report*, Haringey Community Health Council, 1982. (Haringey Community Health Council)

*Suttcliffe, S. D., *Asian Families & Their Foods*, City of Bradford Metropolitan Council, 1978. (T. F. Davies Centre for Teachers)

Tan, Swee Poh and Wheeler, Erica F., 'Food Intakes and Growth of Young Chinese Children in London', *Community Medicine*, 1980.

16.9 Patterns of illness

Further general reading on patterns of illness;
Ethnic Differences in Common Diseases, Postgraduate Medical Journal, Dec. 1981, Vol. 57, No 674.

*McCarthy, Mark, *Epidemiology & Policies for Health Planning*, King's Fund, 1982. (The King's Fund)

Milunsky, Aubrey, *Know Your Genes*, Pelican, 1977.

Sickle cell disease
Anionwu, Elizabeth N., 'Sickle Cell Disease' *Health Visitor*, Vol. 55, July 1982, pp. 336–341.

Anionwu, Elizabeth N., 'Sickle Cell Menace in the Blood' in *Nursing Mirror*, 20 July 1978, pp. 16–19.

Anionwu, Elizabeth N. and Beattie, Alan, 'Learning to Cope with Sickle Cell Disease – a Parent's Experience' in *Nursing Times*, 8 July 1981, pp. 1214–1219.

Anionwu, Elizabeth N., Watford, Diana *et al.*, 'Sickle Cell Disease in a British Urban Community' in *British Medical Journal*, 24 Jan. 1981, Vol. 282, pp. 283–286.

Davis, L. R., Huehns, E. R. *et al.*, 'Survey of Sickle Cell Disease in England & Wales' in *British Medical Journal*, 5 Dec. 1981, Vol. 283, pp. 1519–1521.

Fleming, A. F. (ed.), *Sickle Cell Disease: A Handbook for the General Clinician*, Churchill Livingston, 1982.

Kenny, M. W., 'Sickle Cell-Disease' in *Nursing Times*, 4 Sept. 1980, pp. 1582–1584,

*Manchester Community Health Group for Ethnic Minorities, *Sickle Cell Disease in Manchester: A Discussion Document for All Interested Groups and Particularly for Health Professionals*, 1981. (CHGEM Manchester)

Murtaza, Lily, Stroud, C. E. *et al.*, 'Admissions to Hospital of Children with Sickle Cell Anaemia: a Study in South London' in *British Medical Journal*, 28 March 1981, Vol. 282, pp. 1048–1051.

*The Sickle Cell Society, *A Handbook on Sickle Cell Disease: a guide for families*, 1983. (Sickle Cell Society)

*The Sickle Cell Society, *Sickle Cell Disease – the Need for Improved Services*, 1981. (Sickle Cell Society)

Thalassaemia and other hereditary anaemias

Gorman, Angela, 'Thalassaemia' in *Nursing Times*, 31 July 1981, pp. 1348–50.

Modell, B., Benson, A. *et al.,* 'Incidence of Thalassaemia Trait among Cypriots in London', in *British Medical Journal,* 23 Sept. 1972, pp. 737–738.

Modell, B., Ward, R. H. T. *et al.,* 'Effect of Introducing Antenatal Diagnosis on Reproductive Behaviour of Families at Risk for Thalassaemia Major', in *British Medical Journal,* 7 June 1980, pp. 1347–1350.

Mouzouras, M., Ioannov, P. *et al.,* 'Thalassaemia as a Model of Recessive Genetic Disease in the Community', in *The Lancet,* 13 Sept. 1980, pp. 574–578.

World Health Organisation, *Report of a WHO Working Group on Community Control of Hereditary Anaemias*, 1981.

Hypertension and cerebrovascular disease

Beevers, D. G., Cruickshank, J. K., 'Age, sex, ethnic origin and hospital admission for heart attack and stroke', *Ethnic differences in Common Disease*, Postgraduate Medical Journal, Dec. 1981, Vol. 57, No. 674.

Langford, Herbert G., 'Is Blood Pressure different in Black People', *Ethnic differences in Common Disease,* Postgraduate Medical Journal, Dec. 1981, Vol. 57, No. 674.

Marmot, M. G., Adelstein, A. M. *et al.,* 'Cardiovascular mortality among immigrants to England and Wales', *Ethnic differences in Common Disease,* Postgraduate Medical Journal, Dec. 1981, Vol. 57, No 674.

Sever, P. S., 'Hypertension and the Environment' in *The Cardiovascular, Metabolic and Psychological Interface*, Proceedings of the Royal Society of Medicine, Series No. 14, 1979.

Sever, P. S., 'Racial differences in blood pressure: Genetic and environmental factors', *Ethnic differences in Common Disease*, Postgraduate Medical Journal, Dec. 1981, Vol. 57, No. 674.

Rickets and osteomalacia

Committee on Medical Aspects of Food Policy, *Rickets and Osteomalacia:* Report of the Working Party on the Fortification of Food with Vitamin D, DHSS/HMSO, London, 1980.

Dunnigan, Matthew, 'Measure of Success' in *Nursing Mirror*, 15 January, 1981, pp. 17–19.

Ford, J. A., McIntosh, W. B. *et al.*, 'Clinical and Subclinical Vitamin D Deficiency in Bradford Children' in *Archive of Diseases in Childhood,* 51, 1976, pp. 939–943.

Goel, K. M., Sweet, E. M. *et al.*, 'Florid and Subclinical Rickets among Immigrant Children in Glasgow', *The Lancet*, i, 1976, pp. 1141–1145.

Goel, Krishna, 'An Old Enemy Returns' in *Nursing Mirror*, 8 January, 1981, pp. 16–18.

Goel, K. M., Campbell, S. *et al.*, 'Reduced Prevalence of Rickets in Asian Children in Glasgow', *The Lancet*, ii, 1981, pp. 405–407.

*Manchester Community Health Group for Ethnic Minorities. *Rickets in Britain: A Discussion Document for All Interested Groups and Particularly for Health Professionals*. CHGEM (Manchester) Sept. 1980 (CHGEM Manchester)

*Manchester Community Health Group for Ethnic Minorities, *Rickets in Britain – A summary*. Oct. 1980. (CHGEM Manchester)

Preece, M. A., Ford, J. A. *et al.*, 'Vitamin D Deficiency among Asian Immigrants to Britain' *The Lancet*, i, 1973, pp. 907–910.

*Sheiham, Helena and Quick, Alison, *The Rickets Report*, Haringey Community Health Council, 1982. (Haringey Community Health Council)

**Stop Rickets Campaign: Resource packs for health service professionals and for the Asian community*. (Save the Children)

Mental health

**Aspects of Mental Health in a Multiracial Society*, Commission for Racial Equality, 1976. (Commission for Racial Equality)

*Burke, A. (ed.), *Racism and Mental Illness*, Transcultural Psychiatry Society, 1984. (Dr A. Burke)

Gaw, A. (ed.), *Cross-cultural Psychiatry*, papers from a conference held in 1979, John Wright – PSG, 1982.

Littlewood, Roland and Lipsedge, Maurice, *Aliens and Alienists: Ethnic minorities and psychiatry*, Penguin, 1982.

Rack, P., *Race, Culture and Mental Disorder*, Tavistock, 1982.

16.10 Responding to need

There are as yet no British publications that present a comprehensive overview of ethnic minority health needs and health service responses. Two useful American books discuss the provision of services to meet ethnic minority needs:

Brownlee, Ann Templeton, *Community Culture and Care: Cross-Cultural Guide for Health Workers*, C. V. Mosby, 1978, Part Three: The Health System of the Community.

Henderson, George and Primeaux, Martha, *Transcultural Health Care*, Addison-Wesley, 1981.

There are a number of short U.K. publications which provide a useful summary of research/issues/recommendations:

**Ethnic Minorities and the Health Service*, Wandsworth and East Merton Health District, 1979. (Wandsworth and East Merton Area Health Authority)

*Henley, Alix and Taylor, Colette, *Register of Research Projects related to Health Care Needs of Ethnic Minorities*, King's Fund, 1980. (The King's Fund)

**Racial Equality and the Health Service*, Camden Committee for Community Relations, 1983. (Camden Committee for Community Relations)

*Training in Health and Race, *Providing Effective Health Care in a Multiracial Society*, Health Education Council/National Extension College, 1984. (National Extension College)

The following articles describe specific needs/recommendations/health service responses.

**Asians and the Health Service*, Wandsworth Council for Community Relations, 1978. (Wandsworth Council for Community Relations)

Edwards, Susan, 'Giving an Asian Community a better health service', *Medical News*, 9.12.82

**North Kensington Moroccan Research Project Report*, Area Health Education Department, Kensington, Chelsea and Westminster Area Health Authority, 1979. (Kensington, Chelsea and Westminster Health Education Department)

**Sickle Cell Disease: The Need for Improved Services*, Sickle Cell Society, 1981. (The Sickle Cell Society)

**Study of Use of GP Facilities for Chinese Restaurant Workers in London*, Kensington, Chelsea, Westminster & N.E. District Community Health Council, 1976. (North East District Community Health Council)

**The Health of Traveller Mothers and Children in East Anglia*, Save The Children, 1983. (Save The Children)

Winkler, F. and Yung, J., 'Advising Asian Mothers' *Health and Social Services Journal*, 9 October 1981.

A detailed critique of ethnic minority needs and the health service response in Liverpool is contained in:

*Torkington, N. P. K., *The Racial Politics of Health – a Liverpool Profile*, Merseyside Area Profile Group, 1983. (Merseyside Area Profile Group)

Two studies have looked at the related area of social services provision, to determine how far current practices and procedures may result in unequal access or unequal treatment for ethnic minority families.

*Cheetham, Juliet, *Social Work Services for Ethnic Minorities in Britain and the U.S.A.*, Department of Social and Administrative Studies, 1981. (Juliet Cheetham)

*Young, Ken and Connolly, Naomi, *Policy and Practice in the Multi-racial City*, Policy Studies Institute, 1981. (Policy Studies Institute)

16.11 Ethnic minority staff in the National Health Service

Research on the position of ethnic minority health service workers:

*Baxter, Carol and Grant, Joan, *Nursing in Manchester: The Black Experience*, Community Health Group for Ethnic Minorities (Manchester), forthcoming. (CHGEM Manchester)

Enquiry into Training of Ethnic Minority Health Visitors, Camden Committee for Community Relations, 1982. (Camden Committee for Community Relations)

Ethnic Minority Hospital Staff, Commission for Racial Equality, 1983. (Commission for Racial Equality)

Doctors from Overseas: A Case for Consultation, Commission for Racial Equality/Overseas Doctors Association, 1976. (Commission for Racial Equality)

*Doyal, L. *et al.*, *Migrant Workers in the National Health Service*, Polytechnic of North London, 1982. (Geoff Hunt)

Hicks, C., 'Racism in Nursing', *Nursing Times*, 5 May, 1982 and 12 May, 1982.

*Smith, David J., *Overseas Doctors in the National Health Service*, Policy Studies Institute, 1980. (Policy Studies Institute)

*Thomas, M. and Williams, J. M., *Overseas Nurses in Britain: A PEP Survey for the United Kingdom Council for Overseas Student Affairs*, PEP, Broadsheet 359, 1972. (Policy Studies Institute)

*Walsh, Susan, *Overseas Nurses – Training for a Caring Profession?*, C.H.A.N.N.E.L., 1979. (RCN Personal Advisory Service)

Equal Opportunity

Free publications available from the Commission for Racial Equality:

Monitoring an Equal Opportunity Policy: A Guide for Employers.

Equal Opportunity in Employment: A Guide for Employers.

Why Keep Ethnic Records? Questions and Answers for Employers and Employees.

Racial Discrimination: A Guide to the Race Relations Act, 1976 (prepared by the Home Office).

Code of Practice for the Elimination of Racial Discrimination and the Promotion of Equality of Opportunity in Employment.

Other publications about Equal Opportunity

Equal Opportunities – Black and Minority Ethnic Workers: A Pack for Negotiators, National Union of Public Employees (London Division), 1981. (NUPE Divisional Office)

McNaught, A., 'Race Relations in the NHS', *Hospital and Health Services Review*, March 1982, pp. 86–88.

*Ouseley, Herman *et al.*, *The System*, Runnymede Trust and South London Equal Rights Consultancy, 1982. (Runnymede Trust)

Personnel: The Race Relations Act 1976, DHSS Health Circular HC(78)36, 1978. (DHSS Store)

Racial Equality and the Health Service, Camden Committee for Community Relations, 1983. (Camden Committee for Community Relations)

*Young, Ken and Connelly, Naomi. *Ethnic Record Keeping in Local Authorities: a discussion paper*, Policy Studies Institute, Interim Research Paper, September, 1981. (Policy Studies Institute)

*Young, Ken and Connelly, Naomi, *Policy and Practice in the Multi-Racial City*, Policy Studies Institute, No. 598, November, 1981. (Policy Studies Institute)

16.12 Health worker training and professional values

Little has so far been written on the question of developing a multiracial philosophy in U.K. health worker training. More has been done in North America, particularly in the field of nursing. The following publications consider training issues from several different viewpoints.

Burrows, Alison, 'Patient-centred nursing care in a multiracial society: the relevance of ethnographic perspectives in nursing curricula', *Journal of Advanced Nursing*, 8, 1983, pp. 477–485.

Ballard, Roger, 'Ethnic Minorities and the Social Services' in Saifullah Khan, V., (ed.), *Minority Families in Britain*, Macmillan, 1979.

Hall, Stuart, 'Teaching Race', *Multiracial Education*, Vol. 9, No. 1, Autumn 1980, pp. 3–13.

Katz, Judy, *White Awareness*, University of Oklahoma Press, 1980.

Leininger, Madeleine, *Transcultural Nursing: Concepts, Theories and Practices*, Wiley Medical, 1978, Part IV: Cultural Concepts in Nursing Curricula.

Miller, Audrey, 'Nurses' attitudes towards their patients', *Nursing Times*, 8.10.1979, pp. 1929–1933.

(ILT and NHS Awareness Training, National Centre for Industrial Language Training, Working Paper No. 34, 1982. (National Centre for Industrial Language Training)

*Ouseley, Herman *et al.*, *The System*, Runnymede Trust and South London Equal Rights Consultancy, 1982, Chapter 13: Training Programmes. (Runnymede Trust)

Peppard, Nadine, 'Towards Effective Race Relations Training', *New Community*, Vol. 8, 1980, pp. 99–106.

Satow, Antoinette, 'Racism Awareness Training: Training to Make a Difference', in Ohri, A. *et al.*, (eds), *Community Work and Racism*, Routledge and Kegan Paul, 1982.

Shaw, John, 'Training methods in race relations within organisations: an analysis and assessment', *New Community*, Vol. 9, No. 3, 1981, pp. 437–446.

*Werner, D. and Bower, B., *Helping Health Workers Learn*, Hesperian Foundation, 1983. (Hesperian Foundation)

16.13 Health education

Abbas, V., *A Theoretical Examination of the Factors involved in Health Education with Ethnic Minority Groups.* Dissertation submitted for the requirements of Diploma in Health Education, University of Leeds/Leeds Polytechnic 1981.

Box, Val, 'Rickets: What should the Health Education message be?' *Health Visitor*, Vol. 56, April, 1983, pp. 131–134.

Brownlee, Ann Templeton, *Community Culture and Care*, C. V. Mosby, 1978, Chapter 8: Education.

Health Education Material for Ethnic Minorities, Source list prepared by the Health Education Council, 1980. (Health Education Council)

Henderson, P. and Thomas, D. N., *Skills in Neighbourhood Work*, George Allen and Unwin, 1980.

*Jenkins, Janet, *Mass Media for Health Education*, International Extension College, 1982. (International Extension College)

Learmonth, Alyson, 'Asians' Literacy in their mother tongue and English', *Nursing Times*, 28 February, 1980.

Ross, S. E. and Rutter, A. C., *Healthiest Babies Possible: An Outreach Programme*, Vancouver Perinatal Health Project, City of Vancouver Health Department, 1980.

*Smith, Caroline, *Community-based Health Initiatives: a handbook for voluntary groups*, National Council for Voluntary Organisations, 1982, (includes Section on Women's Health Project, Hackney). (National Council for Voluntary Organisations)

Tauber, Ilse, J. *et al.*, 'Preliminary results of a Picture Recognition Study Amongst Bangladeshi Women' *Health Visitor*, Vol. 53, July 1980, pp. 251–263.

*Werner, David and Bower, Bill, *Helping Health Workers Learn*, Hesperian Foundation, 1983. (Hesperian Foundation)

16.14 Addresses for publications not available from bookshops

Acton Society Trust, 9 Poland Street, London, W1.

AFFOR, 173 Lozells Road, Lozells, Birmingham, B19 1RN.

Board of Deputies of British Jews, Woburn House, Upper Woburn Place, London, WC1H 0EP.

Brent Community Health Council, Rear Block, 16 High Street, London, NW10.

British Refugee Council, Bondway House, 3–9 Bondway, London SW8 1SJ. Tel: 01-582 6922.

Dr A. Burke, St George's Hospital, Blackshaw Road, London, SW17.

Camden Committee for Community Relations, 58 Hampstead Road, London, NW1 2PY. Tel: 01-387 1125.

CARD, c/o ICAS, 374 Grays Inn Road, London, WC1.

Camden Language Scheme, Haverstock School, Crogsland Road, London, NW1 8AS.

Catering and Dietetic Branch, Room 1062, DHSS, Hannibal House, Elephant and Castle, London, SE1 6BY.

Juliet Cheetham, Department of Social and Administrative Studies, Barnet House, Wellington Square, Oxford, OX1 2ER.

Commission for Racial Equality, 10–12 Allington Street, London, SW1E 5EH. Tel: 01-828 7022.

Community Health Group for Ethnic Minorities (CHGEM) Manchester, c/o Milly Williams, Secretary, 30 Warwick House, Central Avenue, Levenshulme, Manchester, M19 2FF.

Dag Hammarskjöld Foundation, Övre Slottsgatan 2, 752 20 Uppsala, Sweden.

DHSS Store, Scolefield Mill, Brunswick Street, Nelson, Lancs, BB9 0HU.

Haringey Community Health Council, Room 11, Tottenham Town Hall, High Road, London, N15 4RY.

Health Education Council, 78 New Oxford Street, London, WC1A 1AH.

Hesperian Foundation, PO Box 1692, Palo Alto, CA 94302, USA.

Geoff Hunt, Department of Sociology, Polytechnic of North London, 62–66 Highbury Grove, London, N5 2AD.

ILEA English Centre, Sutherland Street, London, SW1.

International Extension College, 18 Brooklands Avenue, Cambridge, CB2 2HN. Tel: 0223-353321.

Department of Adult Education, University of Keele, Keele, Staffs.

King's Fund, 126 Albert Street, London, NW1.

Kensington, Chelsea and Westminster Health Education Department, 304 Westbourne Grove, London, W11. Tel: 01-229 9001.

Learning Materials Service, Centre for Continuing Education, Open University, PO Box 188, Milton Keynes, MK3 6HW.

Merseyside Area Profile Group, Department of Sociology, University of Liverpool, Liverpool, L69 3BX.

Minority Rights Group, 36 Craven Street, London, WC2N 5NG.

National Centre for Industrial Language Training, Havelock Centre, Havelock Road, Southall, Middlesex, UB5 4NZ. Tel: 01-571 2241.

National Council for Voluntary Organisations, 26 Bedford Square, London, WC1 3HU. Tel: 01-636 4066.

National Extension College, 18 Brooklands Avenue, Cambridge, CB2 2HN. Tel: 0223-316644.

NUPE Divisional Office, 13/15 Stockwell Road, London, SW9 9AT.

North East District Community Health Council, 13 Ingestre Place, off Broadwick Street, London, W1. Tel: 01-437 5202.

Nottingham and District Community Relations Council, 37 Mansfield Road, Nottingham. Tel: 0602-586515.

Nuffield Provincial Hospitals Trust, 3 Prince Albert Road, London, NW1 7SP.

Policy Studies Institute, 1–2 Castle Lane, London, SW1E 6DR. Tel: 01-828 7055.

RCN Personal Advisory Service, Henrietta Place, London, W1.

Runnymede Trust, 37A Gray's Inn Road, London, WC1X 8PP.

Save The Children, Mary Datchelor House, 17 Grove Lane, Camberwell, London, SE5 8RD. Tel: 01-703 5400.

Scottish Home and Health Department, Room 207, Chief Scientists' Organisation, St Andrew's House, Edinburgh, EH1 3DE.

The Sickle Cell Society, c/o Brent Community Health Council, 16 High Street, Harlesden, London, NW10 4LX. Tel: 01-451 3293.

South East Thames Regional Health Authority, Thrift House, Collington Avenue, Bexhill-on-Sea, Sussex. Tel: 0424-222555.

T. F. Davies Centre for Teachers, Clifton Villas, Manningham, Bradford, BD8 7B7.

Wandsworth and East Merton Area Health Authority, Grosvenor Wing, St George's Hospital, Blackshaw Road, London, SW17 0QT. Tel: 01-672 1255.

Wandsworth Council for Community Relations, 57 Trinity Road, London, SW17. Tel: 01-767 3631.

Frances Weinreich, Neighbourhood English Classes, 49 Brookfield, 5 Highgate West Hill, London, N6 6AT.

An Appraisal by the Black Co-Author

I find this appraisal difficult to write because my contribution to the preparation of this book has been at a number of different levels – the main ones being as a consumer of the health service, a health worker within the service, a member of a minority community, and as co-author.

Alix Henley and Penny Mares were already significantly involved in the preparation of information and training materials on aspects of multiracial health care when I met them. I was at that time still at the stage of frustration - wondering what I ought to, should, and could do personally to improve my response to the situation of black people and the health service. In the months which followed, however, my involvement in the Community Health Group for Ethnic Minorities in Manchester helped me gain confidence and I viewed our getting together to produce *Health Care in Multiracial Britain* as the arrival of a machinery by which I could cope personally with an urge that had been developing within me since I started working in the National Health Service in 1970.

Having completed the major part of my contribution to this book in the UK I now find myself preparing this appraisal in a small town on the North Coast of Jamaica. However, rather than finding myself distanced from the kinds of problems confronting black people and the British health service, I find that after spending twelve years in the UK, I need (as a practice nurse/administrator) to spend a considerable amount of time trying to recapture 'the ways of my people' and making sure that the patients and I understand each other. This has reaffirmed a realisation of just how difficult it is to avoid sweeping generalisations and to write accurately about important and intricate aspects of people's lives. It has brought home the fact that the whole issue of which we are writing is about human interaction and people's struggle to live together.

Alix, Penny and I all realise that this is not without its faults. In discussions among ourselves we have come to terms with our limitations and recognised various weak areas. This analysis leads us to ask ourselves the following questions: since people's feelings are best described by themselves, should there not have been more black authorship involvement? Furthermore, should we not have sought the involvement of an Asian co-author?

This book would undoubtedly have been enriched by such quality of involvement. However, in 1981, when the book was in the preparation stage, there was a major obstacle to achieving this. It is best exemplified by Muhammid Ali's response on a

David Frost Show to the question about Ali's alleged interest in running for presidency of the United States of America. Ali replied as follows 'Just imagine that you have been a stoker on a ship all your career and suddenly you have been summoned forth to be Captain. I bet you the first thing which would spring to your mind is – My God, this boat is sinking!' This fully depicts the feeling of mistrust held by many black health workers when after years of being undervalued and sometimes exploited, they are suddenly consulted and expected to be 'experts'.

Also, the lack of pre-existing written information about certain less well-known groups of minority peoples was a major handicap to us in our work. Rastafarians are a case in point. This group probably exhibits more prescribed and proscribed health-related behaviour than any other single group in modern-day West Indian life in Britain. We have to admit that a greater degree of consultation and personal rapport with Rastafarians would have been ideal.

While many readers will realise the vast extent of community consultation and the degree of individual research which has gone into producing this book, there are others who will feel neither consulted nor represented. We hope that you will not only get in touch and educate us, but also that you may be encouraged to get involved and make your voice heard.

Working on this book has been a learning experience for us. We hope that you too may gain something from it.

Carol Baxter

Appendix 1
Consultation with the community

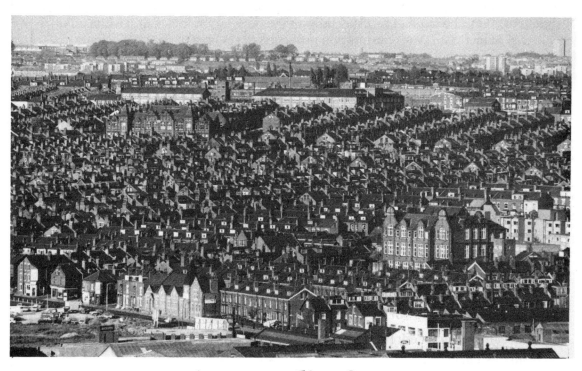

Appendix 2
Ethnic minority communities in Britain

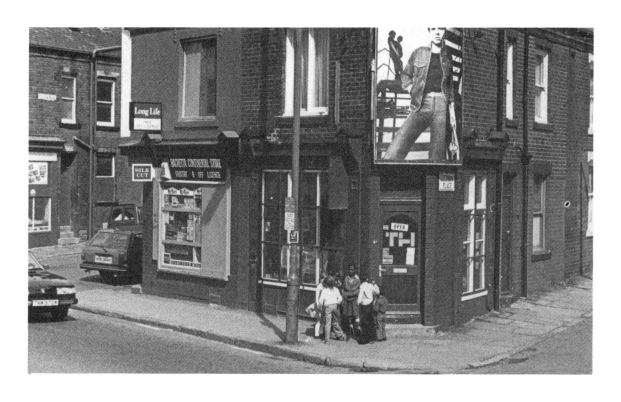

Appendix 1
Consultation with the community

At various points in this handbook we have argued the need for greater consultation with, and representation from, ethnic minority communities in order to improve and develop the quality of health care they receive. This is a principle which should of course be applied to all sections of the population, black and white alike. One way of increasing the consultation process is to set up a patient participation group, which a small but growing number of GPs and consultants are now doing. Some guidelines for setting up such a group, based on one GP's suggestions, are set out below.

Setting up a patient participation group

1. Partners and practice staff meet to decide on setting up a group and
   - agree objectives of group;
   - agree whom to invite to first meeting and
   - agree wording of invitation (if necessary arrange for translation into minority languages).

2. Check that neighbouring practitioners have no objections.

3. Collect names and addresses of secretaries of all organisations in the area, e.g.
   residents/tenants associations
   community associations
   community health projects
   Community Health Council
   local Council for Voluntary Services
   Inner City Forum
   church groups
   women's groups
   Citizen's Advice Bureau
   housing aid centres
   youth clubs

   Local organisations representing ethnic minority interests in the area might include:
   Sikh Gurdwara (Temple) Committee
   Afro-Caribbean Youth Centre
   Asian Women's Group
   Asian Youth Movement
   Indian Worker's Association
   Vietnamese Support Group
   Islamic Welfare Association
   Chinese Language School.

4. Invite each organisation to send a representative to the first meeting (preferably a patient of the practice). State the draft objectives of the proposed group, and suggest an agenda, e.g.
   - decide whether to set up a group;
   - revise objectives;
   - decide membership of group;
   - elect membership of group;
   - elect chairperson (preferably lay);
   - decide topics for discussion; and
   - decide how often to meet.

Bear in mind that in some cases ethnic minority representatives may need more encouragement and support than other participants before they feel confident that their contribution will be listened to, especially if the rest of the group is predominantly white.

Sample objectives

1. To help patients to have a say in the services provided at the health centre/surgery.

2. To encourage and discuss suggestions for improving services to patients.

3. To discuss general (not individual) complaints.

4. To inform professional staff how the services are running.

5. To discuss overall provision of health services in the district/area.

6. To produce a newsletter for patients in the practice (possibly with sections in community languages).

7. To discuss overall health education needs in the district/area.

8. To set up self-help and support groups, e.g. for mothers and toddlers, people giving up smoking, etc.

Source: adapted from Pritchard, P., *Manual of Primary Health Care: Its nature and organisation*, Oxford U.P., 1981, p. 120.

Appendix 2
Ethnic minority communities in Britain
Who do we mean by 'black' or 'ethnic minority' communities?

Many people, when they think of 'black' or 'ethnic minority' communities, tend to think only of the Afro-Caribbean and Asian population. These are probably the largest racial minorities in Britain, but the British population today includes many thousands of people from other ethnic minority communities.

This appendix gives very brief thumbnail sketches of the origins of many of those communities – small and large – in Britain. The information about language and areas of settlement given here is most relevant to the generation that migrated to Britain. It is likely to be less relevant to their children, grandchildren and great-grandchildren. Sources of further information about particular communities can be found in the general reading list in Chapter 16. The groups are arranged roughly in terms of the distance of country of origin from the UK. Some of the information and the layout of this appendix are taken from *Their Right to Health*, Health Education Council, 1982. Other reference sources are indicated in the text.

This is not intended to be a comprehensive list – if such a thing were possible. We are aware of large gaps. We have not, for example, included notes on people of Hungarian, Malaysian, Somali, Singaporean and Taiwanese origin, and notes about some communities are less detailed than others. This is not because these and other groups not included are unimportant, but because information about their migration and settlement in Britain has proved difficult to find.

People of Polish origin

The first major immigration from Poland to Britain was of Polish Jews fleeing persecution at the end of the nineteenth and the beginning of the twentieth century. They settled mainly in the East End of London, in Manchester and in Leeds. They spoke Polish and Yiddish.

The second major immigration occurred during and immediately after the Second World War, though there has been a trickle of people joining relatives ever since, and increased numbers recently since the military regime in Poland. During and after the Second World War most Poles settled in London, followed by Birmingham, Manchester, and Bradford, with smaller populations in Wolverhampton, Leeds, Nottingham, Sheffield, Coventry, Leicester and Slough. Most post-war settlers are Roman Catholics though there were also some Jews fleeing Nazi persecution immediately before and during the War.[1]

Other people of Central and Eastern European origin

Like the Polish Jews, Jewish refugees came to Britain at the end of the nineteenth and beginning of the twentieth century from Russia and Romania, where they were being persecuted. They settled mainly in the East End of London, where there was already a small European and Mediterranean Jewish community, Manchester and Leeds. Jewish refugees from Nazi persecution in Germany, Austria and the rest of Europe also came to settle in Britain during the 1930s and early 1940s, though as aliens under British law. Until 1939 many were refused permission to enter and were sent back to where they had come from.

During and immediately after the Second World War large numbers of other people from Central and Eastern Europe came to Britain as refugees or as European Voluntary Workers (a British government recruitment scheme). Apart from the Poles and Hungarians there were Ukrainians, Czechs, Romanians, Yugoslavs, Germans,

Latvians and Estonians. Many of this group are now elderly and may speak little English.

People of Italian origin

Most of the Italians who came to Britain have settled in London, Bedford and Hertfordshire, though there are smaller numbers in the Midlands, Glasgow and Cardiff. The peak of immigration took place in the 1950s and early 1960s when Italians were recruited by the hotel and catering industry, by foundries and the mining industry, to brick factories in Bedford and by the NHS to work as nurses and auxiliary staff. People came then on work permits and have since settled here. Since 1973, with EEC membership, permits have been unnecessary. Most, but not all, are from the south of Italy, are Roman Catholics, and speak a regional dialect, e.g. Sicilian, Neapolitan, as well as standard Italian. There were also some Italian prisoners of war who stayed in Britain after the Second World War.[2]

People of Portuguese origin

People came from mainland Portugal and the island of Madeira to Britain during the 1950s and early 1960s. Much of this migration was sparked off by direct recruitment by the NHS and the hotel and catering industry. The main areas of Portuguese settlement were London, the Channel Islands and south-east England. Most Portuguese people are Roman Catholic. There is a fairly high proportion of single women among the Portuguese in Britain, many of whom are now elderly and speak little English.[2]

People of Spanish origin

Most Spanish immigration to Britain took place in the 1950s and early 1960s and was of people, often directly recruited, coming to work mainly in hotels, catering and hospitals. The main areas of settlement were London and the south-east, Liverpool and Manchester. As in the Portuguese community, there is a fairly high proportion of single women who are now elderly and who speak little English.[2]

People of Moroccan origin

About two-thirds of the people of Moroccan origin in Britain live in north Kensington in London. Most of the men were recruited by agencies during the late 1960s to work in the hotel and catering industry and were joined by their families during the 1970s. Most people come from northern Morocco and speak Arabic and Spanish. Very few speak fluent English. Most Moroccans are Muslim.[3]

People of Greek Cypriot origin

Most Greek Cypriot migration to Britain took place in the 1950s and early 1960s. In 1974, during the war in Cyprus, several thousand Greek Cypriots sought asylum in Britain, but most of these later returned home. The main area of Greek Cypriot settlement in Britain is north-east London, though there are small communities in the Home Counties, Birmingham, Bristol, Manchester and Liverpool.

Cypriot men work mainly in the service industries, including catering and the retail trades, and as tailors and small factory owners and workers. Cypriot women work mainly in the clothing industry, often as home-workers. Greek Cypriots speak Greek as their mother tongue (Greek is written in the Greek alphabet). Most Greek Cypriots are Greek Orthodox Christians.[2,4,5]

People of Turkish origin

Most Turks came to Britain under work permit arrangements (organised by British employers) between 1950 and the mid-1970s. They work mainly in the clothing and catering industries. They speak Turkish, which has a strong Arabic influence, though it is written in the Roman alphabet like English and other European languages. Most Turks are Muslim.[2]

People of Turkish Cypriot origin

Most of the Turkish Cypriots in Britain migrated during the 1950s and early 1960s. The majority live in the Greater London area, with small settlements in the Home

Counties, Birmingham and Manchester. They work mainly in the clothing trade, as employers and employees. Turkish Cypriots speak Turkish as their first language. Turkish has a strong Arabic influence, though it is written in the Roman alphabet like English and other European languages. Most Turkish Cypriots are Muslim.[2,4,6]

People of Iranian origin

A number of people of Iranian origin now live in Britain as refugees or students. Most of the refugees are living in the London area. People from Iran speak Farsi as their mother tongue. This is written in the Arabic script. Most Iranians are Muslim, of the minority Shia sect.

People of Yemeni origin

There is a small, mostly male, Yemeni population in Britain, living mainly in Birmingham, Sheffield and Manchester, with smaller communities in Cardiff and Scunthorpe. The majority came to Britain from North and South Yemen during the 1940s, 1950s and early 1960s. There was some direct recruitment by British firms in Yemen and most Yemenis work in the heavy engineering industry. Very few men in Britain have brought their wives and families to join them. People from Yemen speak Arabic as their mother tongue. Educational facilities in Yemen have been relatively poor and some people may be unable to read or write. Most people from Yemen are Muslim.[7]

People of West African origin

Most of the West Africans who have come to Britain have been from Nigeria, although some came from Ghana and some from Sierra Leone. The majority of them came as students and returned home when they had completed their studies, though a few stayed on in Britain and a few returned here to work. Both these courses of action have been prevented by the 1971 Immigration Act. The language of education in Nigeria, Ghana and Sierra Leone is English, and West Africans in Britain speak English in addition to their mother tongue. Most West Africans are Muslim or Christian, the main Christian denominations being Anglican, Methodist, Baptist, Presbyterian, and Roman Catholic.[8]

People of Asian origin from East Africa

About a fifth of the people of Asian origin who have come to Britain travelled from East Africa. Their families had migrated to East Africa from northern India or Pakistan within the last 100 years. In East Africa they formed a largely commercial middle class living mainly in towns and cities.

East African Asians came to Britain from Kenya, Uganda, Tanzania, Malawi and Zambia, mostly in the 1960s. As British citizens with special UK and Colonies passports they had the guaranteed right to come to Britain at any time.

This guarantee was given to them in recognition of the fact that, as a minority in East Africa and as a group associated with British colonial rule, they were vulnerable to African nationalist feeling and might not always be treated favourably in East Africa. In 1968 the British government passed the Commonwealth Immigrants Act and broke their guarantee, forcing the British Asians in East Africa to join a queue for entry vouchers to come to Britain. This led to great hardship for many families.[9]

Most Asian people from East Africa came to Britain as whole families and often as forced migrants. Like other refugee groups they may include a higher proportion of elderly, ill or handicapped people than those groups that came to Britain to work during the labour shortages of the 1950s and early 1960s.

Ugandan Asians

In 1972 the Ugandan government expelled all Asian people from Uganda, whatever their nationality or type of passport. Just over half of the expelled Ugandan Asians came to Britain. Several thousand British passport holders were accepted, but only on a temporary basis, by India and are now in a queue to come to Britain.

The Ugandan Asian refugees were allowed to bring practically nothing with them and many were destitute on their arrival in Britain.

The first language of most Asian people from East Africa is either Gujarati or Punjabi; many people also speak English and Swahili. Older family members may speak little English. Most East African Asians in Britain are Hindu; there are some Muslims and a few Sikhs. There are also some Roman Catholics, generally or Goan origin, whose first language is usually English, and some members of other Christian denominations, mainly of south Indian origin. Many Asians of East African origin in Britain own shops and businesses, as they did in East Africa.

People of Kenyan origin

Apart from the Asians mentioned above, there are a few Kenyan Africans in Britain. Many of them came as students and some have stayed on and now work in professional fields. Since 1971 it has been virtually impossible for Commonwealth students to stay on in Britain or to return here to work.

People from Mauritius

Most people of Mauritian origin in Britain were recruited as nurses to work in the National Health Service. As Commonwealth citizens it was not necessary for them to obtain work permits to come to Britain until 1962. Since 1962 employers who wish to recruit Commonwealth workers have had to negotiate for them with the Department of Employment.

People of Pakistani origin

Most people from Pakistan in Britain came from one of three areas. The majority came from Mirpur in Azad (Free) Kashmir, north of Punjab; their first language is Mirpuri; a dialect of Punjabi. Some came from Punjab province; their first language is Punjabi. A few came from the North West Frontier Province and the north-western borders of Punjab Province; their first language is Pashto. Pashto and Punjabi are very different.

The language of education in Pakistan is Urdu, so anyone who went to school there reads and writes Urdu (which is written in Arabic script, from right to left). Not all areas of Pakistan are well provided with educational facilities. Most men from Pakistan speak and understand Urdu, generally as a second language, and most women understand it. A few people from Pakistan speak Urdu as their mother tongue. (Colloquial spoken Urdu and colloquial spoken Hindi are very similar. They are, however, written in different alphabets.) Most Pakistanis are Muslim.

Most people of Pakistani origin live in Yorkshire, Greater Manchester and Lancashire, and in the West Midlands, Glasgow and Cardiff, working mainly in the textile and engineering industries. Several British firms recruited workers in Pakistan immediately after the Second World War, particularly to work in the textile mills of West Yorkshire and Lancashire.

Most people from Pakistan, like many other Commonwealth groups (Pakistan has now left the Commonwealth), came to Britain during the late 1950s and early 1960s when Britain was suffering severe labour shortages. In general the men of the families came first and then applied for their wives and children to join them. Some Pakistani men are still waiting for entry clearance for their families to join them.[2]

People of Indian origin

Like people from Pakistan, most men from India came to Britain during the late 1950s and early 1960s, and their families were often not reunited for many years. People came to Britain from two main Indian states: Punjab in the north, and Gujarat on the west coast.

Most people in Britain of Indian **Punjabi** origin (the old province of Punjab was divided between India and Pakistan at Partition in 1947) are Sikh by religion, though there are a small number of Punjabi Hindus.

People from the Indian Punjab speak Punjabi as their first language and write Punjabi in the Gurmukhi alphabet, which is not used for any other language. There are large Punjabi Sikh communities in Leeds, West London, the West Midlands and Glasgow.

Most people in Britain of Gujarati origin are Hindus, like the majority of the Indian population. (The majority of people of **Gujarati** origin in Britain came here from East Africa, though some came directly from India.) People of Gujarati origin from India and from East Africa live mainly in North and South London, Leicester, Coventry and Greater Manchester. Gujarati is the official language of the state of Gujarat and is written in a form of the Devnagri alphabet. There are some Gujarati Muslims, particularly in West Yorkshire and Lancashire and in South West London.

The national language of India is Hindi. Hindi is studied as a subject in schools in northern India (as is French in Britain), and many northern Indian people with different first languages can communicate in Hindi. Though relatively few people of Indian origin in Britain speak Hindi as a first language, many speak it as a second language. Hindi is written in a form of the Devnagri alphabet.[2]

A few people in Britain originated in southern India, for example, in Tamilnad and Kerala. Southern Indian languages are of a different family from northern Indian languages and are unrelated to Hindi, Punjabi or Gujarati. People from northern and southern India may have no common language. The *lingua franca* in South India is English.

People of Bangladeshi origin

Most people from Bangladesh came to Britain in the late 1950s and early 1960s, though many Bangladeshi men are still waiting for entry clearance for their families to join them. Most came from the rural Sylhet District of Bangladesh and speak a Sylheti dialect which is very different from standard Bengali. There is no written form of Sylheti, so children at school learn to read and write Bengali, which is written in a form of the Devnagri alphabet. The main area of Bangladeshi settlement is the East End of London; there are also Bangladeshis working in manufacturing and catering throughout the country; most 'Indian' restaurants are staffed by Bangladeshis. Almost all Bangladeshis are Muslim.

People of Afro-Caribbean origin

Most people of West Indian origin came to Britain during the 1950s and early 1960s. Many of the early arrivals had been in the RAF or other armed services during the Second World War and had been stationed in Britain. Since skilled employment was difficult to get in the West Indies, many West Indians responded to British recruitment programmes and publicity about Britain's chronic shortage of workers.

The major direct recruitment was of workers for transport and the hotel industry: in the 1950s, the Barbadian Immigrants Liaison Service collaborated with the London Transport Executive and the British Hotels and Restaurants Association to recruit skilled labour in Barbados. London Transport set up recruitment and training centres for bus crews in Barbados, even taking London double-decker buses and English money out to Barbados to use in their training programmes. The National Health Service set up recruitment offices in the West Indies in the 1950s. Although most of the first immigrants were men, a high proportion of West Indian women also come to Britain on their own.

Over half the West Indians who came to Britain came from Jamaica. The others came mainly from Guyana, Trinidad and Tobago, and Barbados. Most people in the West Indies speak a local patois or Creole, the basis of which is usually English, and sometimes French very much influenced by West African languages. Most West Indians and their children and grandchildren in Britain speak a patois or Creole-influenced standard English, often as well as patois or Creole. There are West Indian or Afro-Caribbean communities in most of the industrial towns and cities of Britain.

Many West Indians are Christians: the largest group are Pentecostalists, including Jehovah's Witnesses and Seventh Day Adventists; some are Anglicans and Baptists; a few are Methodists and Roman Catholics. In Britain an increasing number of Afro-Caribbeans join Pentecostalist congregations, since they often feel unwelcome in white churches. An increasing number of young Afro-Caribbeans are Rastafarians.[10,11,12]

People of Colombian origin

Most of the Colombians in Britain were recruited through employment agencies during the 1970s to work in catering and other service industries, mainly in London. Since they are neither Commonwealth citizens nor from EEC countries, the terms of their employment in Britain are very restrictive and few of them are likely to be allowed to settle permanently. Their first language is Spanish and most are Roman Catholics.

People of Chilean origin

Most Chileans in Britain arrived after the overthrow of the Allende government in 1973. Chilean political prisoners were often 'adopted' – enabled to leave Chile and come to Britain – by local groups and so there are Chilean families living all over Britain. Those refugees who were political prisoners have suffered both physically and emotionally; this may have affected both their physical and mental health. Like other refugees, they may find it difficult to come to terms with their enforced departure from their own country. Their first language is Spanish and many Chileans are Roman Catholics.

There are also some refugees and residents in Britain from other Latin American countries. All speak Spanish as their first language except people from Brazil, who speak Portuguese.[13]

People of Vietnamese origin

Refugees began to leave Vietnam in 1975. Several thousand now live in Britain, many of whom have come via refugee camps in Hong Kong. The majority of Vietnamese in Britain come from North Vietnam but a few come from the South. Most are ethnic Chinese, who speak both Cantonese and Vietnamese (a few speak only Cantonese, a few speak Hakka or another Chinese language). The others are ethnic Vietnamese, who generally speak only Vietnamese. Most people read and write either Cantonese or Vietnamese; some are literate in both. Vietnam has no official religion, but most people are influenced by the three philosophical traditions of Buddhism, Taoism and Confucianism. Official policy has been to settle Vietnamese families wherever housing can be found; many live in rural areas far from other Vietnamese families or, for example, shops that sell familiar food. This can add to the stress of their resettlement in Britain.[14]

People of Hong Kong origin

The Hong Kong Chinese community in Britain is extremely widely scattered, working mainly in Chinese restaurants in almost every large and small town in Britain. There are sizeable communities in Central London, Liverpool, Cardiff, Manchester and Birmingham. Most people in Britain from Hong Kong and the New Territories speak Cantonese as their first language, though some people who originally emigrated to Hong Kong from mainland China speak other Chinese languages. Although all the different languages are written in one standard form, when they are spoken they are often not mutually comprehensible.

People of Filipino origin

Most people of Filipino origin in Britain came in the 1970s, and were recruited by employment agencies to work in the NHS, in the hotel and catering industries, and in private domestic services. Since they are not Commonwealth citizens or members of the EEC, Filipinos have to come on the work permit system which is severely restrictive. Most of those in Britain are women. After four years' 'approved' employment in Britain they may stay permanently. However, under current Immigration Rules they may never bring fiancés, husbands or children to join them. Most Filipinos are Roman Catholics. Their mother tongue is Tagalog.[15]

Notes

1. Patterson, Sheila, 'The Poles: An Exile Community in Britain', in Watson, James L. (ed.), *Between Two Cultures*, Blackwell, 1979.
2. *Their Right to Health: notes to accompany* Your Rights to Health *Booklets,* Health Education Council, 1982.
3. Fosdike, Hakima, 'Assessing the Needs of an Ethnic Community', *Midwife, Health Visitor and Community Nurse*, Sept. 1980.

4. Ladbury, Sarah, *Cypriots in Britain*, National Centre for Industrial Language Training, 1980.
   NCILT, Havelock Centre, Havelock Road, Southall, Middx. UB2 4NZ.
5. Constantinedes, Pamela, 'The Greek Cypriots: Factors in the Maintenance of Ethnic Identity', in Watson, James L. (ed.), *Between Two Cultures*, Blackwell, 1979.
6. Ladbury, Sarah, 'The Turkish Cypriots: Ethnic Relations in London and Cyprus', in Watson, James L. (ed.), *Between Two Cultures*, Blackwell, 1979.
7. Bush, Barbara, *Yemenis in Britain*, National Centre for Industrial Language Training, 1979.
   NCILT, Havelock Centre, Havelock Road, Southall, Middx. UB2 4NZ.
8. Ellis, June (ed.), *West African Families in Britain*, Routledge, 1978.
9. Tandon, Yash and Raphael, Arnold, *The New Position of East Africa's Asians: Problems of a Displaced Minority*, Minority Rights Group, 1978.
   Minority Rights Group, 36 Craven Street, London WC2N 5NG.
10. *Immigration: the fundamental facts and questions*, Catholic Commission for Racial Justice, 1978.
    Catholic Commission for Racial Justice, 1 Amwell Street, London EC1R 1UL.
11. Doyal, Lesley *et al.*, *Migrant Workers in the NHS*, Polytechnic of North London, 1980.
    Department of Sociology, Polytechnic of North London.
12. Smith, David J., *The Facts of Racial Disadvantage*, Political and Economic Planning, 1976.
    Policy Studies Institute, 1–2 Castle Lane, London SW19 6DR.
13. Mackillop, Jane, *Ethnic Minorities in Sheffield*, Sheffield District Education Committee, 1980.
    City of Sheffield Adult Education Department, PO Box 67, Leopold Street, Sheffield 1. Tel: 0742-77143.
14. Mares, Penny, *The Vietnamese in Britain*, Health Education Council, National Extension College, 1982.
    National Extension College, 18 Brooklands Avenue, Cambridge CB2 2HN.
15. *Filipino Migrants in Britain*, Catholic Commission for Racial Justice, 1980.
    Catholic Commission for Racial Justice, 1 Amwell Street, London EC1R 1UL.

Other titles available in NEC's health series

The Right to be understood: a handbook on community interpreting   Jane Shackman

This is a handbook aimed at people working in the statutory agencies eg: health, social services, education, housing, police and in the community eg: community relations, advice centres etc who either use interpreters to communicate with their non-English speaking clients, or recruit and train interpreters.

The handbook is designed as a practical resource and covers issues like:

★ the role of the interpreter
★ why trained interpreters should be used
★ selection, recruitment, support and supervision of interpreters
★ styles of interpreting and where interpreters should be used
★ setting up a community interpreting service
★ conditions of employment of interpreters (sample job descriptions, pay etc)
★ training of interpreters and training of users.

The Right to be Understood is written in an accessible style using case studies and examples and photographs. It includes a detailed resources section with a bibliography and list of organisations.

It has been produced with support from The Wates Foundation and the Local Government Training Board.

0 86082 469 1   162pp   A4

The Vietnamese in Britain: a handbook for health workers
Penny Mares

This is a handbook designed as a resource for health workers, trainers, other professionals and volunteers who are working with the Vietnamese and/or who are interested in the broader issues of working effectively in a multiracial society.

The handbook is divided into four main sections which cover:

1. **Background:** *From Vietnam to Britain; Life in Vietnam; Family life* and *Finding out about your client.*
2. **Health:** *Concepts of health and illness: Using the health services; Mothers and babies; Death and mourning* and *Emotional health.*
3. **Diet:** *Vietnamese food in Britain; Eating patterns; Buying, storing and preparing food; Food groups; Beliefs about food; Food in hospital; and Giving advice about nutrition.*
4. **Resources:** *Sources of information, advice and support; Appendices and bibliography.*

0 86082 318 0   180pp   A4

Caring for Muslims and their families: religious aspects of care
Alix Henley

Caring for Muslims and their families is the first of three short books in the 'Asians in Britain' series which look at the religious practices and customs of each of the three main religious groups in Britain. The books are aimed particularly at health workers but will also be of interest to social and community workers, teachers, other professionals and the interested general reader.

Caring for Muslims and their families begins by summarising briefly the basic beliefs and values of Islam and goes on to outline the most important practices and customs followed by Asian Muslims in Britain. The final chapter is aimed specifically at tutors and trainers who wish to use the book as a basis for training.

0 86082 321 0   86pp   A5

Caring for Sikhs and their families: religious aspects of care
Alix Henley

Caring for Sikhs and their families concentrates on those features of Sikh religious practice that are likely to be important for health workers and other professionals in hospitals and in the community, setting them in the context of the religious beliefs and values from which they spring. The final chapter is written for trainers who may wish to use the book as a basis for training.

0 86082 351 2   75pp   A5

and
Caring for Hindus and their families: religious aspects of care   Alix
Henley

Caring for Hindus and their families should provide health workers with a basis of
knowledge from which to discuss with practising Hindus their needs and wishes in an
informed and sensitive way.

0 86082 387 3   83pp   A5

Publications from Training in Health and Race

Black Health Workers: Report on a one-day seminar for black professional health workers

This report focuses on racial inequality in employment practices in the NHS, showing
clearly the nature of the discrimination faced by black health service workers. This
ranges access to basic training courses, the racist attitude of some white staff and
patients, and unequal employment, promotion and post-basic training opportunities.
Detailed recommendations for change are also included in this report.

0 86082 573 6   32pp   A5

Black Women and the Maternity Services

Black Women and the Maternity Services looks at the perceptions and experiences of
the maternity services of thirty young Afro-Caribbean women, from the antenatal
period, the stay in hospital, to delivery and sources of support they received from the
maternity services on their return home. Detailed recommendations to make the
maternity services more sensitive, appropriate and supportive to young black women,
are included.

This book is essential reading for health service workers, especially those involved in
the maternity services, for social workers, teachers, youth club and community
workers, and other professionals responsible for the provision of services and facilities
to black pregnant women and mothers.

0 86082 609 0   48pp   A4

Providing Effective Health Care in a Multiracial Society: A Checklist for Looking at Local Issues

This publication was produced because of THR's concern about the lack of
coordinated effort within the National Health Service to meet the health needs of
black and ethnic minorities in Britain. Aspects of health care covered are:
Communication; Records; Health Education; Hospital Care; Maternity Provision,
Foods and Diets; Family Planning; the Elderly; Psychiatric Services; Child Health;
Screening and Counselling; Staff Training and Employment. Questions, information
and recommendations for good practice on these aspects of health care form the main
part of this publication. It is hoped that it will provide some practical suggestions on
how to improve service provision and promote direct consultation between health
authorities and black and ethnic minority communities.

0 86082 442 X   24pp A4

To find out more about these and other NEC publications write or phone for our
catalogue.
Publications Dept.
National Extension College
18 Brooklands Avenue
Cambridge CB2 2HN
(0223) 316644